THE AGING PROCESS

A Health Perspective

The AGING PROCESS
A Health Perspective

Molly S. Wantz
Ball State University

John E. Gay
Louisiana State University

Winthrop Publishers, Inc.
Cambridge, Massachusetts

Library of Congress Cataloging in Publication Data

Wantz, Molly.
The aging process.

Bibliography: p.
Includes index.
1. Aging. 2. Geriatrics. 3. Gerontology.
I. Gay, John E., joint author. II. Title
QP86.W28 612′.67 80-22157
ISBN 0-87626-008-3

Cover and interior design by MaryEllen Podgorski

17 Dunster Street, Cambridge, Massachusetts 02138

10 9 8 7 6 5 4 3 2 1

This book is dedicated to all of us who aspire to be healthy, contributing centenarians.

Contents

Foreword

A printer by the name of Benjamin Franklin decided to make Cicero's celebrated essay on aging available to his contemporaries. In his foreword to the new edition, Franklin noted: "I have, Gentle Reader, as thou seest, printed this Piece of Cicero's in a large and fair Character, that those who begin to think on the Subject of OLD-AGE (which seldom happens till their Sight is somewhat impair'd by its Approaches) may not, in Reading, by the Pain small Letters give the Eyes, feel the Pleasure of the Mind in the least allayed."

Franklin did much else to increase the pleasures and reduce the miseries of old age. He not only invented the bifocal but through his own life created a memorable image of an ingenious, effective, worldly, and wise old man. Indeed, until very recent times Franklin had relatively little competition as a model of Grand Old Age in American culture. His "colleagues" were mostly such as "Uncle Sam," who, although drawn from an actual person, is essentially a fictional mascot, and Santa Claus, a mythological figure based loosely on the life of a saint who, at last report, has officially been certified as a never-was.

Were Franklin writing the foreword to this book he might not think it necessary to bring out the LARGE TYPE. More Gentle Readers today think about aging before they have sprouted their own silver threads or acquired bifocals. He might also be delighted by the fact that he did not have to rely entirely upon essays from antiquity, no matter how sagacious. Instead, he would be able to offer his readers a wealth of empirical knowledge gained by the now vigorous fields of gerontology and geriatrics. We will probably never outgrow the wisdom of our elders such as Cicero and Franklin. However, it is to our advantage to consult the emerging sources of knowledge as well.

If each of us is personally to become a model of Grand Old Age (move aside there, Ben, Santa, and Uncle), then it would certainly be helpful to bring a healthy body along with us. Molly Wantz and John Gay have done their part by pouring many of the riches of current knowledge into this book. You will find here not only specific information on many health-related topics but also a sound and straightforward framework that increases the utility of the information. The authors make it clear that "aging" is not a sudden transfiguration but part of the continuity of life. Youthful readers may gain increased appreciation of where they have been as well as where they are going, while elderly readers may find it easier to make sense out of changes they have been noticing.

Through its attention to social and behavioral as well as physical dimensions of health, this book serves as a useful introduction to a broad range of age-related phenomena. We have here, then, not only an up-to-date treatise on aging and health but also a sound foundation for further explorations in gerontology and geriatrics.

Robert Kastenbaum

Preface

The path of history is strewn with relics of methods that were supposed to increase one's life span. From the early searches of Ponce de Léon for the fountain of youth to the current-day proponents of novocaine, human beings have traditionally been interested in prolonging life.

This book has two goals: The first goal is to provide information and concepts on the physical and psychosocial experiences of those who have already approached the upper end of life's continuum. The second goal is to provide information and concepts on the physical and psychosocial changes that young adults have already experienced and will continue to experience throughout their remaining years. In other words, this book provides information *for and about* aging.

Young adults are at a time in life when the pattern of aging has been established in both mind and body. They want to know why they grow old, what they can expect with their parents and grandparents, what is going to happen to their own bodies, and what measures, if any, they can employ to inhibit the process.

This book is divided into five parts. Part 1 begins with a basic concept of aging and explores the historical search for longevity by looking at a vast array of theoretical possibilities. Part 2 explores the psychosocial aspects of aging in respect to the many factors that affect an individual's level of mental health and aging. Parts 3 and 4 examine those physical changes which seem to be "normal" parts of physiological aging and then they examine those physical changes that are directly related to chronic and degenerative diseases. Part 5 examines nutritional and exercise practices, two significant factors in the total aging process.

We believe that aging is a continuous lifelong experience which begins at birth and ends at death. It is a complex interaction of the physical, mental, social, spiritual, and intellectual dimensions of each human being. Throughout most of the chapters the reader will see examples of the physical and psychosocial aspects of aging at various developmental stages of life and see how the dynamic interaction of these aspects of aging affect people as they live.

Acknowledgments We wish to thank the following people for their assistance in the preparation of this book: Kacey Gay, Virginia Ingram, Jane Lesh, and photographer John Porter.

MOLLY S. WANTZ
JOHN E. GAY

PART ONE

Concepts and Theories

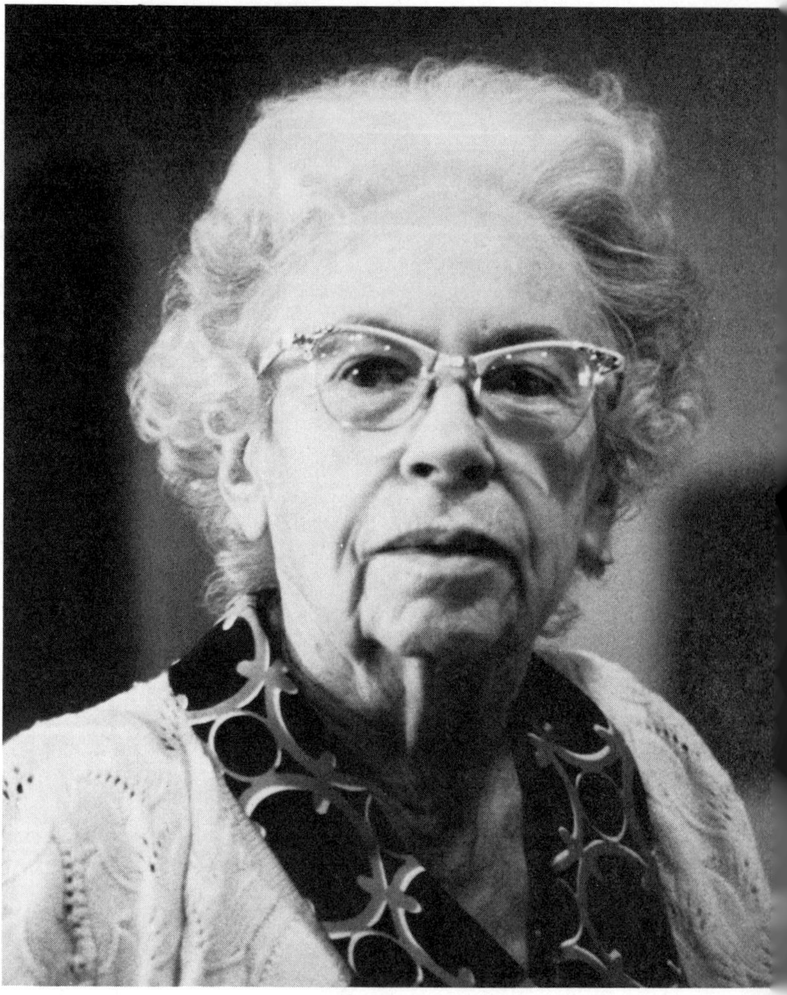

■ Chapter 1

Introduction

Major Concepts

1. The aging process is a continuous and dynamic lifelong interaction of multiple factors.
2. The aging process is influenced by intrinsic and extrinsic factors.
3. Multiple variables influence the lifestyle of the older adult.

The Aging Process

From the moment of conception until death each individual experiences the aging process. This process is similar to that of all other people and yet it contains differences that make it a unique experience. When a child is born it is immediately affected by its physical and psychosocial environment. It is warmed by clothing, housed, fed, and taken care of, loved, or neglected. The child soon develops skills for interacting and surviving in its environment. As the child ages and moves into childhood, adolescence, and young, middle, and older adulthood, it learns to perceive and relate to all kinds of situations. Each situation becomes a learning experience for future decisions.

The aging process is characterized and influenced by each of the following components: physical, mental and social dimensions, perceptions, relativity, and dimensional reciprocity.

The Dimensions of Aging Each person ages biologically, psychologically, and sociologically. Biological aging generally denotes a person's relative position in terms of his or her life span. It involves the physiological changes that occur during the aging process. Sometimes it is difficult to determine whether physiological change is the result of intrinsic factors of aging, such as genetic predisposition to diabetes or the greying of hair, or whether the physical change results from extrinsic factors of aging, such as stress, disease, or poor nutrition. The most common and reliable method of measuring biological aging is in terms of chronological age.

Psychological aging denotes an individual's ability or capacity to adapt to both familiar and unfamiliar situations. This part of the aging process is most often measured by observing the behavior of an individual as he or she adapts to these situations. Comparisons are made of the individual's behavior with what has been established as a typical or normal behavior for an age group. For example, we expect young children to be self-centered, desire immediate attention to their problems, and eventually have a desire to succeed. Typically, we can expect the adolescent to display sudden changes in mood and to be self-critical. Young adults are often sensitive to the economic and social status of the family and many times are sensitive to their own inadequacies. In later years feelings include happiness, friendliness, satisfaction, and occasionally discouragement and guilt. All of these feelings and many others are generally considered to be normal for each age group. Psychological aging, then, is related to some degree to chronological age.

Sociological aging denotes the performance of prescribed social roles at given ages. This type of aging is measured by developing a composite list of an individual's performance of specific social roles at specific ages. A comparison can then be made with established social developmental patterns. For instance, children begin developing social skills by learning to cooperate, working in a group, and belonging to a gang. Adolescents are influenced by the peer group, they are socially insecure, and most become interested in the opposite sex. In early adulthood a family pattern and career are established and social and political groups are identified. As age continues, careers reach a peak, parents become grandparents, men and women become widowed, and age usually requires retirement from a lifelong career. These are examples of specific social roles which are generally performed at specific ages. Sociological aging is closely related to chronological aging and to a lesser degree to psychological aging.

Individual Perception of Aging People perceive aging within their own frames of reference based upon their experiences with other people and upon their race, economic status, and occupation. Each generation perceives the next generation to be old, but the degree to which the perception is positive or negative depends upon the older people with whom one interacts. For example, if the interactions take place exclusively with older people who are ill and in poor health, it is quite likely that the perception that develops will be that old means being sick. If, however, there is interaction among all types of people, more alternatives are presented from which a different perception can be developed.

Relativity of Aging Aging is also related to specific events or circumstances that occur in life. People's motives and perceptions greatly influence their response to aging. For example, a boy whose father dies is sometimes told, "Now that your father is gone, you'll have to be the man of the house." He may assume this role because he wants to help his mother and because someone expects him to do so. In one respect, the boy is aging because of his response to an event in his life. Another example can be seen in the girl who is physically mature at an early age.

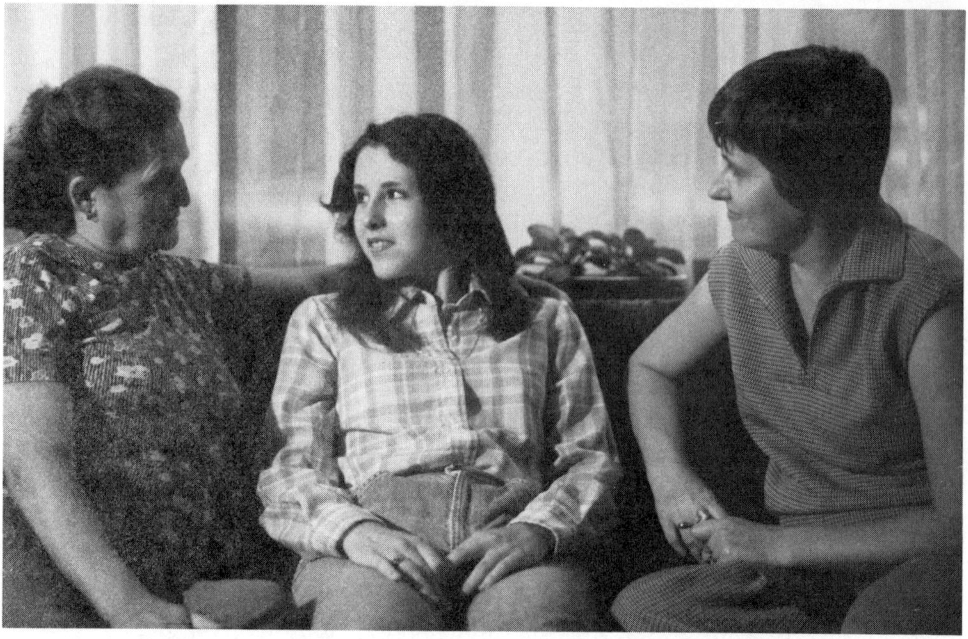

Figure 1.1 Your ideas about aging, whether positive or negative, arise from your own experiences with older people.

She may be expected to assume a more mature behavior long before she is psychologically ready. A third example might be the adult who becomes widowed, withdraws from circles of friends once shared with a spouse, and drastically reduces all social interactions.

One of the best examples which illustrates how a specific situation influenced people's perception and motivation, and thus influenced physical, mental, and social aging, is the Great Depression. During this time the country experienced reduced industrial production, reduced or cessation of growth in construction, widespread unemployment, and decline in the growth of the labor force. Starvation, illness, anxiety, depression, fear, desolation, and death were common. Young people who grew up during these times carried into adulthood feelings of apprehension and cautiousness and a need to be frugal. These in turn affected the degrees of aging. Today's economic conditions bring back the same sense of insecurity that was felt during those depression years.

As young people think about their future they voice concern over what lies ahead for them as they approach older ages. Inflation affects all segments of the population, but it hits the older person much harder. Social security insurance, originally designed to supplement one's income, provides only a small portion of income. Private pension plans are not able to keep up with inflation. Furthermore, not all people retired from the labor force are covered by such plans. Reduced income and spiraling costs create anxiety, frustration, and feelings of insecurity.

The emotional ties and security of living in one's home are threatened by increased energy and home maintenance costs. This affects the emotional well-being. Rapidly increasing gas prices and the limited availability of gas have a tremendous impact. Many older people cannot afford to operate cars or use public transportation. This has an effect on their social and psychological well-being because the lack of transportation makes them socially isolated. Food prices have increased because the costs of energy used for food production and transportation have risen. Thus, many older people eat less. This affects not only their physical but also their emotional well-being.

Perhaps because of rising inflation, increased unemployment, and more social welfare programs, the older generations of the future will be totally dependent upon society and the government. Or, as the number of older people increases, we may see more knowledgeable individuals who are more vocal, politically active, and powerful and who will have more control over their own destinies.

Each of the above examples represents a physical, mental, or social event that can occur in life. Each can stimulate some degree of aging. In each of these situations only one behavioral response was presented, but there are many viable alternatives from which a person can choose to adapt to the situation. The manner in which an individual perceives the situation and the motives which provide the drive will determine the extent of aging that might take place.

Dimensional Reciprocity The physical, mental, and social dimensions of aging are sometimes in opposition to each other, but more often they are related and overlap. In everyday living it is difficult to separate these dimensions. An example can be seen in the following hypothetical situation:

> Gina is 66 years old and has been retired for a year. She has always been an active woman and her health has been relatively good. After her retirement she was unable to find a way to use her extra time. She spent many of her days brooding because her friends were

> able to continue to work. As the days passed, her anxiety and stress mounted. Her health began to fail and a visit to the doctor revealed that her blood pressure was dangerously high.

So far we can see that each dimension has had a negative influence on the other.

> Gina took the prescribed medication for her elevated blood pressure. She assessed her situation and decided to do something with her free time. She became an active member of the Retired Seniors Volunteer Program and met many new people. Her social interactions improved and as a result of this she felt better about what she was doing with her life. She reduced her anxiety and stress and her blood pressure returned to normal. She now feels good both physically and mentally.

This situation illustrates the reciprocity that takes place between the dimensions of health and aging. The dimensional reciprocity and its effects on a person can be either positive or negative.

■ Intrinsic Components of Aging

Intrinsic or internal components of aging are based upon biological and physiological factors and influence one's potential longevity. Intrinsic factors include such things as longevity patterns, sex, race, intelligence, personality, and genetic diseases. An individual has little or no control over the internal components of aging.

Longevity is determined at the moment of conception. The genetic blueprint received from one's parents determines potential height, hair and eye color, sex, size of nose, and other characteristics. This same genetic blueprint may possibly have in its design the length of an individual's life span.

Theoretically, an individual could live to be 1000 years or more. No scientific data can prove or disprove this theory. Claims have been made of individuals who have passed their 150th birthdays, but not one of these claims has been authenticated. The oldest recorded and authenticated age is reported to be 114.

This would indicate that if an individual's genetic blueprint contained a long life span, the person could reach a minimum age of 114 and very possibly longer.

Since it is impossible for one to visibly examine his or her genetic blueprint, he or she must rely on studies of inherited life span by examining such things as genealogical records, life insurance records, and family histories of the general population. In general, it can be said that children of long-lived parents will live longer than children of short-lived parents.

Sex and Race Sex and race are important factors correlated to longevity. Women have a longer projected life expectancy than men. Life expectancy for a female born in 1976 is 76.7 years, compared to 69.0 years for a male born the same year (6). It is not clear whether women live longer because of biological factors or whether they live longer because of a combination of biological and psychosocial factors. From menarche to menopause the endocrine metabolism of females provides a degree of protection against cardiovascular problems. Men do not have the benefit of this protection. Once menopause is completed the death rate between male and female narrows. Other factors that may account for extended female longevity are differences in physical activity levels, stress from occupation, weight control, and tobacco use. It has been speculated that as women become more "liberated" and assume behaviors and practices previously seen in males, the life expectancy gap may approach the same level for both sexes.

Life expectancy for the white population is 73.5 years and for all other races it is 68.5 years. Death rates for races other than white are higher for both male and female between ages 45 and 74, but after age 75 the death rate for whites exceeds that of all other races (8) (Table 1.1).

Intelligence Although intelligence is greatly influenced by psychosocial factors and disease processes, it seems to be a reliable indicator of possible life span. Among college graduates, honor students have a greater life expectancy than other graduates (5, 8, 9). High-level executives appear to have a longer life expectancy than lower-level employees (4). In nursing homes and other institutions, aged individuals who have higher intelligence levels seem to fare better than those who have

Table 1.1 Death Rates by Age, Sex, and Race for 1976 (Rate per 100,000 population)

Age	White Male	White Female	All Other Male	All Other Female
45–54	7.7	4.1	14.0	7.7
55–64	19.2	9.4	28.1	15.9
65–74	42.8	21.1	48.5	30.1
75–84	96.0	59.8	86.5	62.2
85+	187.7	148.2	115.2	91.8

Source: Monthly Vital Statistics Report: Advance Report, Final Mortality Statistics, 1976. D. H. E. W. Publication No. (PHS) 78-1120, Vol. 26, No. 12, Supplement (2), March 30, 1978, p. 1.

lower intelligence levels (3). People who have higher intelligence levels have probably developed effective decision-making skills and are better able to make choices which positively influence their health and consequently their longevity. As individuals who have higher intelligence reach later years, they have a tendency to become more financially secure. In their retirement years they are better able to self-select a lifestyle that allows them to continue activities that enhance rather than atrophy physical, mental, and social well-being. This in turn enhances their life span.

Personality The development of personality is a complex and continuous interaction between heredity and environment. The results of Friedman and Roseman's study (2) indicate that personality may also be an intrinsic factor that influences life expectancy. Friedman and Roseman have identified the type A and B personalities. The type A personality (Figure 1.2) describes the individual who is competitive, never seems to have enough time, never relaxes, and is constantly on the go. This type of individual appears to be more prone to heart attack than the type B person who "goes along" with life events. Personality influences the adoption of abusive behaviors, such as overeating and tobacco and alcohol abuse. All of these have been well-documented as having a negative influence on health and ultimately on life span.

Figure 1.2 Do you think you are a type A or a type B personality?

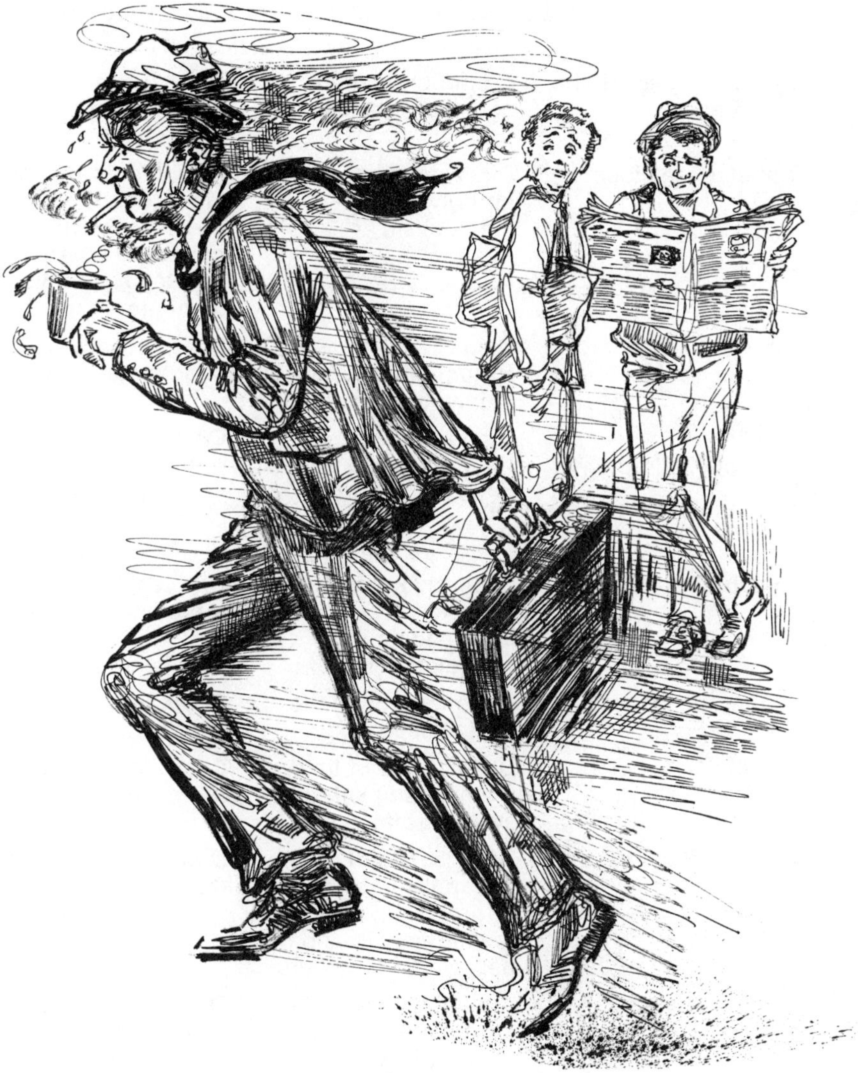

Genetic Diseases Diseases of a genetic origin can also influence longevity. The development of genetic diseases can terminate life a few days after birth or allow a person to live to middle age. Table 1.2 outlines specific genetic diseases and their

Table 1.2 Diseases of a Genetic Origin That Influence Life Span

Disease	Description	Prognosis
Cystic fibrosis of the pancreas	Disturbance of all secretory glands	Death usually in early childhood from lung problems
Diabetes mellitus	Disturbance of carbohydrate metabolism	Insulin controls the disease, but often it predisposes the patient to other problems such as circulatory deficiency
Fabry's disease	Disturbance of lipid metabolism; results in kidney malfunction	Death usually by middle age
Familial hypercholesterolemia	Blood plasma alterations; abnormal deposits of lipids	Contributes to premature atherosclerosis and coronary heart disease
Hemophilia	Excessive bleeding caused by deficiency in a specific coagulation factor	Can result in death if patient is injured
Huntington's chorea	Degeneration of the brain tissue	Death usually in middle life
Infantile Gaucher's disease	Disturbance of lipid metabolism; all body systems affected	Death usually during first year of life
Niemann-Pick disease	Disturbance of lipid metabolism; results in retarded physical and mental growth and neurologic disorders	Death usually by age three
Sickle-cell anemia	A hemolytic anemia attributed to physical alterations of hemoglobin molecules; reduced hemoglobin and red blood cell fragility	Death usually in childhood or adolescence
Tay-Sachs disease	Disturbance of lipid metabolism; affects nervous system	Death usually by age three

effect on longevity. The quality and quantity of life, as they relate to genetic diseases, are most effectively dealt with through genetic counseling by competent specialists.

In one's genetic blueprint, it is believed, the ultimate plan has been established for the functional changes that will take place as the body ages. In general, children of parents who retain good vision, hearing, heart action, and other functions can expect the same as they age. Of course, this would be unlikely if the individual deals ineffectively with stressful situations, is obese, consumes tobacco or alcohol in excessive amounts, or follows other negative psychosocial or physiological practices.

■ Extrinsic Components of Aging

Environmental or extrinsic components include such things as employment and economic level, education, health practices and related diseases, and societal attitude. Most of us have some degree of control over these factors and they all influence, in varying degrees, the total aging process.

Employment and Income The way one lives is determined largely by income and employment. The type of food that one eats and the type of health care one receives are dependent upon the amount of money that is available.

In 1976, 93% of the males and 91% of the females age 16 and over were employed. Race was also a factor in employment rates. White males and females were employed at a higher rate than were black males and females. In the labor force 41% of the males and 64% of the females constituted white-collar workers. White-collar male workers earned $13,455 (average income) in 1976 and white-collar female workers earned $8,099. Blue-collar male workers earned $12,469 (average income) and female blue-collar workers earned $6,808. The greatest percentage of males, 26%, was employed between the ages of 25 and 34. This also was seen for females ages 25 to 34, with 24% of them being in the work force. As age increases, there are fewer men and women employed (13, pp. 289, 389, 406, 411).

Inadequate diet, poor living conditions, and job-related and financial stress have an effect on the overall level of health. This in turn may predispose an individual to diseases which shorten the potential life span.

Education Generally, the higher the educational level, the more opportunities for higher paying jobs and higher standards of living. In addition, the person who has had a good education has had the opportunity to learn more about health and health care and will have developed skills for seeking additional information and health care services.

In 1976 more than 60% of the white population 25 years or older had completed four years of high school or more, compared to less than 45% of the black population. As age increases, the level of educational attainment decreases. For example, in 1976, 83% of the men and women of both black and white races had completed four years of high school or more. Between the ages of 35 and 64 the percentage was 64, and for those 65 years and over the percentage was only 37 (13, pp. 124, 137).

Health Practices Poor diet, lack of exercise, and tobacco and alcohol consumption have a negative effect on health.

In this country for all age groups except the elderly, overnutrition seems to be more of a problem than undernutrition does. Many, if not all, commercially prepared foods are supplemented with additional nutrients. Between 1970 and 1976 statistics showed that there was an increase in the intake of protein, fat, iron, magnesium, thiamine, riboflavin, niacin, vitamin B_6, and ascorbic acid (13, p. 118). Caloric intake averaged approximately 600 calories over the recommended daily dietary allowance. Excessive calories and saturated fats contribute to the development of obesity, arteriosclerosis, diabetes, and other health problems that affect one's potential life span.

Inactivity seems to enhance lower levels of health. The sedentary person experiences physical atrophy, obesity, and heart disease, especially when combined with other factors such as overeating, smoking, stress, alcohol abuse, and others. In this country almost 50% of the population over the age of 20 exercise on a weekly basis. A slightly higher percentage of women, 48.7%, exercise weekly compared to 48.6% of the men. As age increases in both males and females, the regularity of exercise decreases. There is also a greater difference in exercise patterns between males and females after age 65. The most frequently practiced form of exercise for both sexes is walking (13, p. 112).

Many experts feel that in order to maintain or reduce weight, to keep joints flexible, and to strengthen the cardiovascular system, an individual should participate in a complete exercise program which includes activities for strength, flexibility, and endurance and involves a 30-minute (minimum) workout 3 days a week. Although scientific evidence has not been able to prove that regular exercise delays the aging process, exercise will help reduce many health problems which can shorten the potential life span.

Alcohol and Tobacco Excessive use of drugs has varying effects on the individual who uses them. In this country the most frequently used drug is alcohol. According to a survey conducted in 1976 by the National Institute on Drug Abuse, 32% of youths between the ages of 12 and 17 were current users of alcohol compared to 59% of the adults. The second most frequently used drug was tobacco; 23% of youths between the ages of 12 and 17 were current users compared to 41% of the adults (7).

Although the number of alcoholics or problem drinkers does decline with age, it is estimated that there still are millions of alcoholics over the age of 60. There are several reasons why many older alcoholics are not easily identified.

1. Many older people live alone and have minimal social contact with other people. Drinking becomes a pastime.
2. Family members are reluctant to confront the older alcoholic about the disease.
3. Medical personnel often associate the clinical symptoms of alcoholism with other degenerative diseases. They are also reluctant to confront the older alcoholic.
4. Older alcoholics are more likely to deny their problem with alcohol than are younger alcoholics.

Several factors contribute to the development or continuation of alcohol problems in the older population. One of the most significant factors is loneliness. Living alone and having little social contact with family or friends enhance alcohol abuse. Bereavement over the loss of a spouse or friend is another source of stress. Some use alcohol to alleviate the stress. A loss of a sense of self-worth associated with retirement stimulates or increases drinking practices. The use of alcohol becomes a way to fill time and inactivity. In addition, retirement communities in which social drinking is regularly practiced also enhance problem drinking.

Alcohol is a drug that has lethal potential. Each year the

number of people who become addicted to alcohol increases. Alcoholism can result in fatal automobile accidents, loss of job and subsequently reduced income and health problems such as cirrhosis of the liver, premature arteriosclerosis, and heart disease.

The number of tobacco users seems to be relatively high considering all of the evidence which indicates that cigarette smoking contributes to serious health problems. The incidence of lung cancer, bronchitis, emphysema, and heart disease is much

Figure 1.3 Increased incidence of cigarette smoking by young females may result in shortened projected life spans among women.

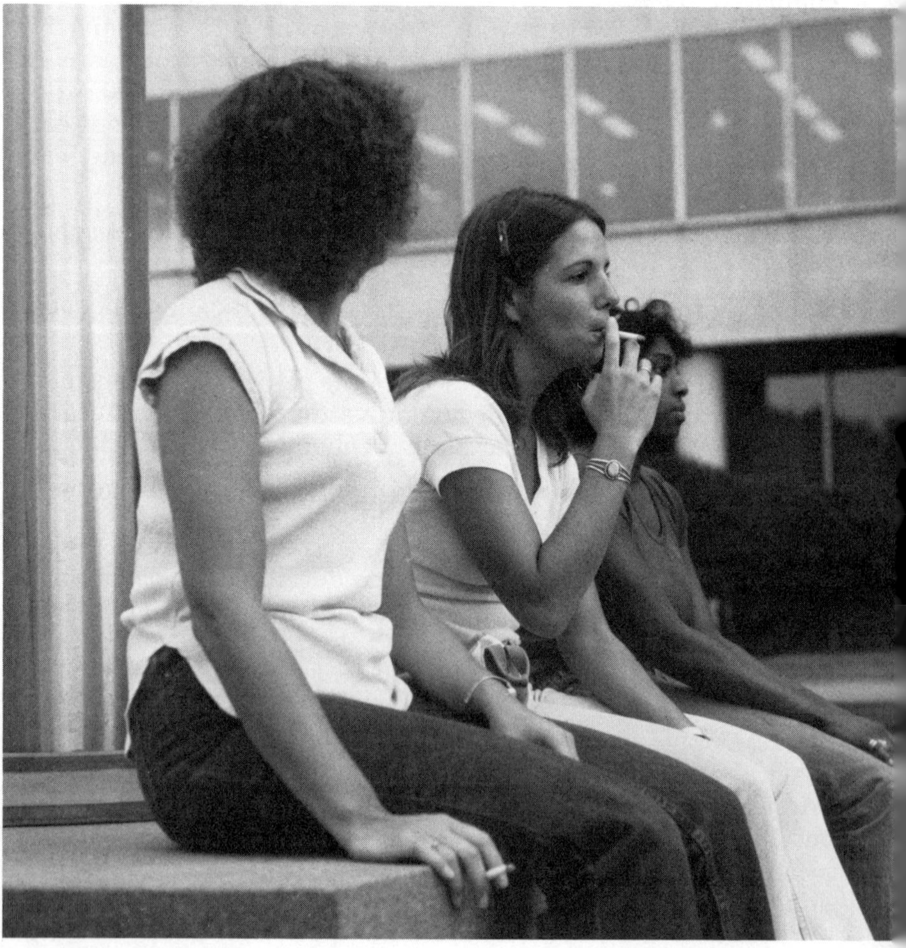

higher for smokers than for nonsmokers. Illnesses and days lost from work are also higher for smokers.

The choice to use and abuse cigarettes and alcohol is strictly an individual decision. No one is forced to use either substance. The cessation or reduction in the use of both would increase the likelihood of achieving one's potential life span.

Societal Attitudes A person's behavior is generally related to the expectations of society. In other words, an individual usually behaves the way he or she feels that others expect him or her to behave. A variation from society's expectation labels us. Many times we expect young children to behave in a more mature manner before they are ready. When they behave according to how they feel, we hear parents say, "Act your age. Don't be a baby." Adolescents are often pushed into adult behavior long before they are ready. Older adults are expected to be unproductive, inflexible, senile, and asexual. These are examples of societal attitudes that continue to perpetuate negative stereotypes of the elderly.

Alex Comfort, renowned gerontologist, claims that 25% of what we experience as aging is of a physical nature and 75% is sociogenic, a combination of sociological and psychological factors. According to Comfort, "It is the role which our folklore, prejudices, and misconceptions about age impose on the old" (1). Hundreds upon hundreds of jokes about aging have appeared in a vast array of literature. Most jokes concentrate on physical ability or appearance, age concealment, old maids, or mental abilities, and all reflect aging in a negative manner. Most jokes are more negative toward women than toward men.

Susan Sontag claims that ". . . aging enhances a man but progressively destroys a woman" (12). Society seems to accept a male with greying hair, middle-age spread, wrinkled face, and sexual interests but does not accept these changes or behaviors in females.

Children, as a part of society, also view aging negatively. In a study at the University of Maryland 180 children between the ages of 3 and 11 were asked how they felt about growing old, what they knew of older people, and how they interacted with older people. For the most part, the children had negative feelings about the physical and behavioral characteristics of age, describing aging as sad, sick, and ugly. They expressed warm affection for older adults by describing them as good, friendly, rich, or wonderful (11). In other words, the children liked older people but did not like the idea of getting old.

Society's attitude is an extrinsic component of the aging process. If older adults succumb to the expectation of society, they will be "old." An older adult who varies from societal's expectation is often considered abnormal, bizarre, or worse yet, mentally incompetent.

As the predictions for population change occur, we will begin to see a change in society's expectation of the older adult. For example, the median age will pass 30 by 1981, be 35 by the year 2000, and approach 40 by the year 2030. One out of six Americans in 2030 will be over age 65 (14). With the increase in median age will come changes in attitudes, politics, industry, clothing, advertisements, housing, and consumer goods.

■ Demographics

Population As of April, 1976, the estimated population of the United States was 214,649,000. There were more females than males. The 65 and over age group comprised 10.7% of the total population. Figure 1.4 shows the percentage of men and women ages 65 to 80+. Figure 1.5 shows the ratio of males to females for white, black, and Spanish races.

Figure 1.4 Women (12.3% of total female population) and men (8.9% of total male population) 65 years or older, 1976.

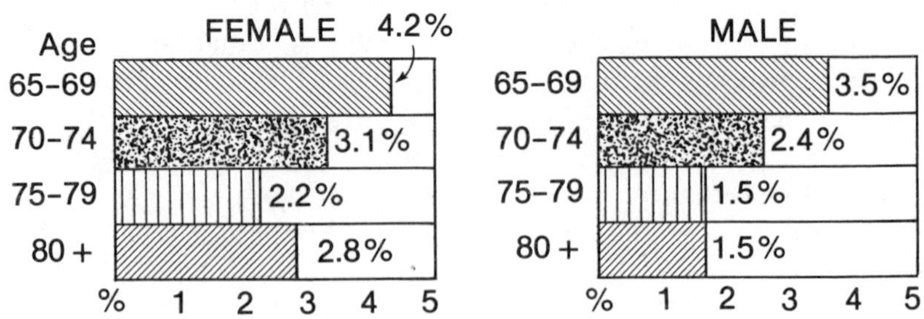

Source: The U.S. Factbook, 1978, p. 29.

Figure 1.5 Ratio of males to females by age group and race, 1976.

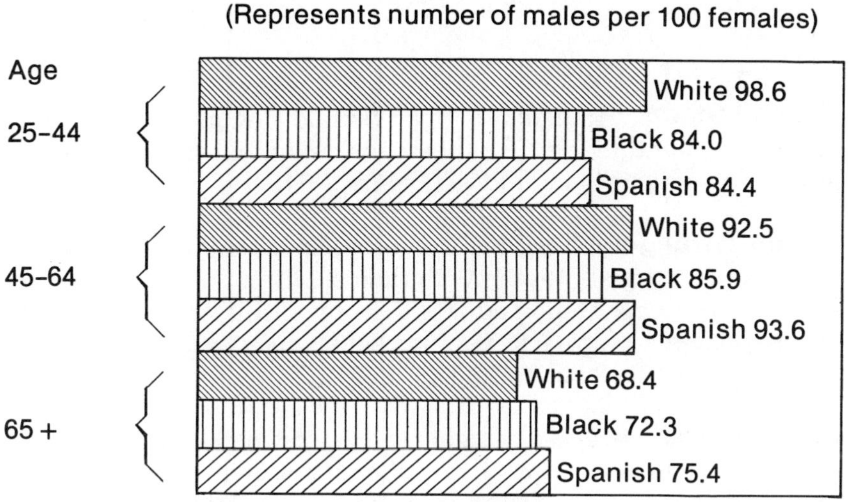

Source: *The U.S. Factbook,* 1978, p. 25

Figure 1.6 Marital status of men and women 65 years old and over, 1976.

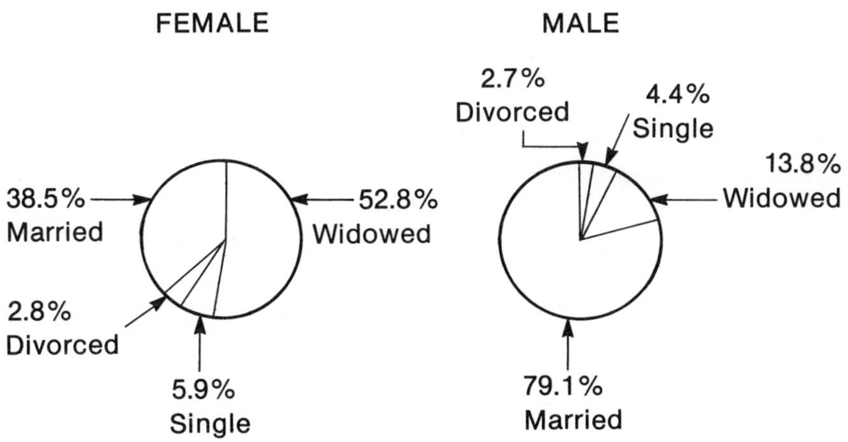

Source: *The U.S. Factbook,* 1978, p. 29

Marital Status In general, it can be said that most older men are married and living with their spouses and most older women are widowed and living alone (Figure 1.6).

Living Arrangements Since most men are married, over three-fourths are also living with their spouses. Two-fifths of older women are living alone and less than two-fifths are living with their spouses. Contrary to popular belief, a very small percentage live in an institutional setting (Figure 1.7).

Labor Force Because of age, the greatest percentage of older men and women are not in the labor force. A little less than one-fifth of the males and an even smaller portion of females are employed (Figure 1.8).

Figure 1.7 Living arrangements of men and women 65 years old or older, 1976.

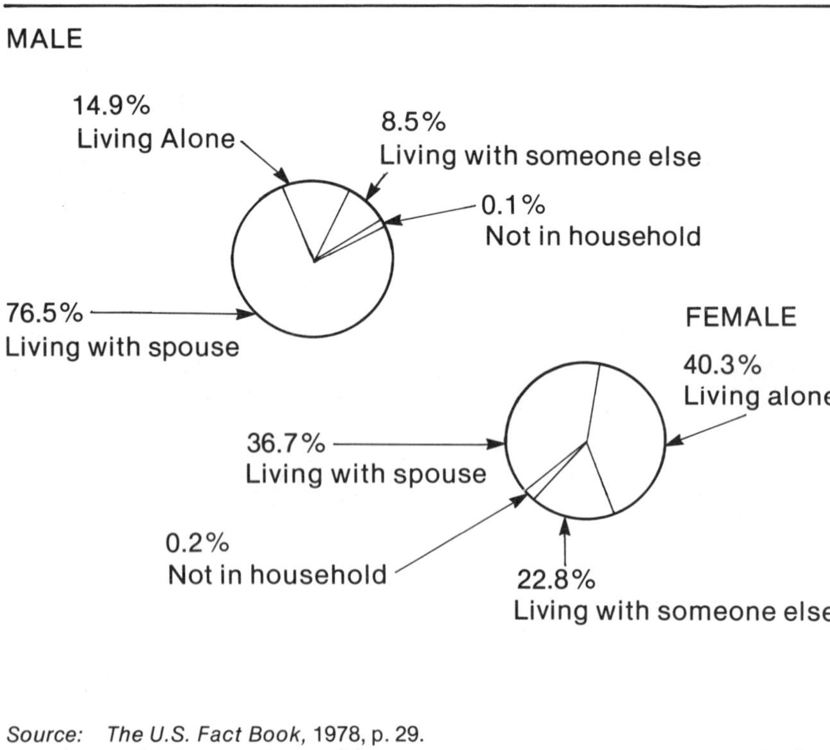

Source: The U.S. Fact Book, 1978, p. 29.

Figure 1.8 Percentage of men and women 65 years old or over in the labor force, 1965 and 1976.

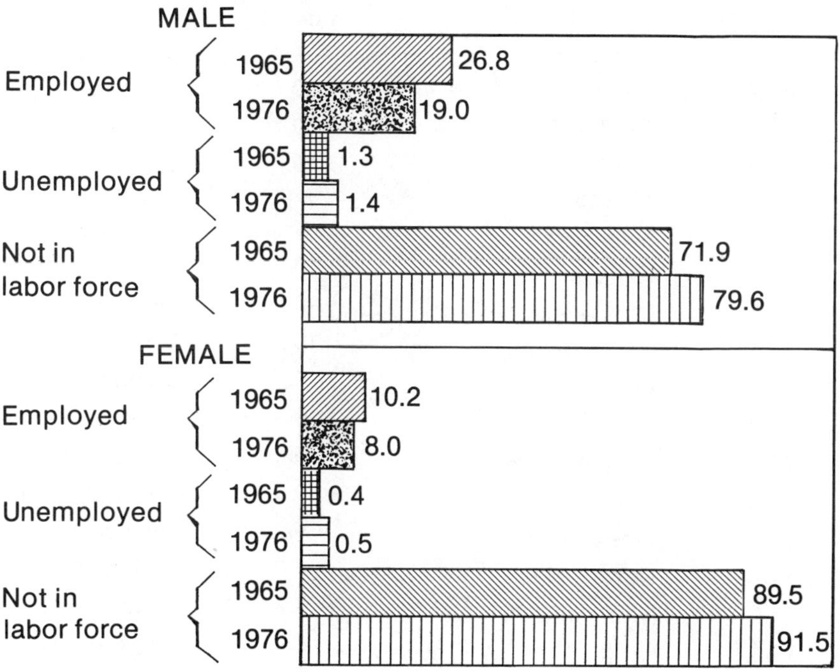

Source: The U.S. Factbook, 1978, p. 29.

Geographical Location In one state, Florida, 16.4% of its population was 65 years or older in 1976. Arkansas was ranked second with 13.1% and seven states had from 12.3% to 12.8% over age 65. The remainder of the states ranged between 2.4% and 11.8% (Table 1.3).

■ Summary

Aging is a continuous and dynamic lifelong process. The components of the aging process are physical, mental and social dimensions, individual perceptions, relativity, and dimensional

Table 1.3 Percentage of Population by State for Ages 65 and Over, 1976

Percentage	State	Percentage	State
16.4	Florida	10.4	Arizona
13.1	Arkansas	10.4	Illinois
12.8	Iowa	10.4	Washington
12.7	Missouri	10.3	District of Columbia
12.6	Nebraska	10.2	Ohio
12.5	Kansas	10.2	Indiana
12.5	Rhode Island	10.2	Montana
12.5	South Dakota	9.9	California
12.3	Oklahoma	9.7	Idaho
12.0	Maine	9.6	Texas
11.8	Pennsylvania	9.4	North Carolina
11.8	West Virginia	9.2	Louisiana
11.7	Massachusetts	9.2	Michigan
11.7	North Dakota	8.9	Georgia
11.4	New York	8.8	Delaware
11.4	Oregon	8.7	Wyoming
11.3	Wisconsin	8.4	Colorado
11.2	Minnesota	8.4	Maryland
11.1	New Hampshire	8.4	South Carolina
11.1	Vermont	8.0	New Mexico
11.0	Mississippi	7.7	Nevada
10.9	Kentucky	7.7	Utah
10.7	New Jersey	6.8	Hawaii
10.7	Tennessee	2.4	Alaska
10.6	Alabama		
10.6	Connecticut		

Source: Ben Wattenberg, *The U.S. Factbook* (New York: Grosset & Dunlap, 1978), p. 28.

reciprocity. The degree to which an individual experiences the aging process depends upon intrinsic and extrinsic components. Intrinsic components include such things as longevity patterns, sex, race, intelligence, personality, and genetic diseases. Extrinsic components include such things as employment, income, education, negative health practices, related diseases, and society's attitudes. Over 10% percent of the population in the United States are men and women over the age of 65. In general, older men are married and living with their spouses and older women tend to be widowed and living alone. Few people over the age of 65 are in the work force.

References

1. Comfort, Alexander. "Age Prejudice in America." In *Focus: Aging*, pp. 84–88. Guilford, Conn.: Dushkin Publishing Group, 1978.
2. Friedman, M., and Roseman, R. "Association of Specific Overt Behavioral Pattern with Blood and Cardiovascular Findings." *Journal of the American Medical Association* 169 (1959):1286.
3. Goldfarb, A. "Predictors of Mortality in the Institutionalized Aged." In *Predictions of Life Span*, edited by E. Palmore and F. Jeffers, p. 132. Lexington, Ky.: Heath Lexington Books, 1971.
4. Hinkle, L., Whitney, L., Lehman, C., Dunn, J., Benjamin, B., King, R., Plakun, A., and Flehinger, B. "Occupation, Education and Coronary Heart Disease." *Science* 161 (1968): 238.
5. Jarvick, L. F., and Falek, A. "Intellectual Stability and Survival in the Aged." *Journal of Gerontology* 18 (1963):173.
6. Monthly Vital Statistics Report, Provisional Statistics. *Annual Summary for the U.S., 1976*. DHEW Publication No. (PHS) 78–1120, Vol. 25, No. 13, December, 1977.
7. National Institute on Drug Abuse, *Nonmedical Use of Psychoactive Substances*. Washington, D.C., 1976.
8. Palmore, E., and Jeffers, E., eds. *Predictions of Life Span*. Lexington, Ky.: Heath Lexington Books, 1971.

9. Quint, J., and Cody, B. "Preeminence and Mortality: Longevity of Prominent Men. *American Journal of Public Health* 60 (1970):56.

10. Roseman, R., and Friedman, M. "Behavior Patterns, Blood Lipids, and Coronary Heart Disease." *Journal of the American Medical Association* 184 (1963):934.

11. Serock, K., Seefeldt, C., Jantz, C., and Galper, A. "As Children See Old Folks." In *Focus: Aging*, pp. 101–103. Guildford, Conn.: Dushkin Publishing Group, 1978.

12. Songtag, Susan "The Double Standard of Aging." In *Focus: Aging*, pp. 93–100. Guilford, Conn.: Dushkin Publishing Group, 1978.

13. Wattenberg, B. *The U.S. Factbook.* New York: Grosset & Dunlap, 1978.

14. ———. "The Greying of America." In *Focus: Aging*, pp. 2–11. Guilford, Conn.: Dushkin Publishing Group, 1978.

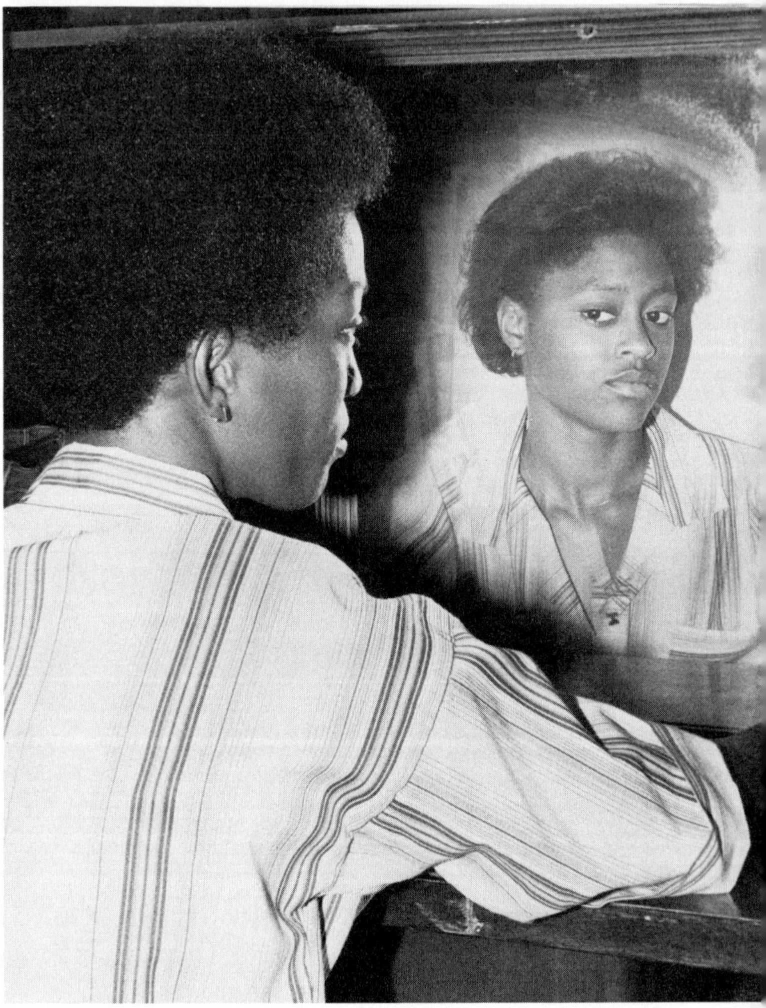

■ Chapter 2

Aging: An Historical Search— Reality and Theory

Major Concepts

1. There is no magic remedy to prevent or retard the aging process.
2. Various theories have been advanced to provide the individual a variety of answers on the aging process.
3. Research on theories of aging has brought about the interests of other professionals as well as lay individuals.

Aging has been thought to be the ongoing process throughout life that brings birth to it's inevitable reality. The idea that birth is the predetermined focus eventually leading to death tends to obscure the complexity of an individual's aging process and their effects on each individual (1). This complicated aging process occurs at all physiological levels but it can be strengthened or diminished by various psychological and social pressures. Aging can be the combination of a variety of events that either inhibit or enhance the individual's life span.

There have been various theories of aging, and countless other theories are introduced every year by health scientists. But the aging process cannot be assumed to be a single entity. Recent aging theories have been put forth by scientists in the fields of biology, sociology, and psychology, but there is little agreement among them on a particular age group or on the aging process.

Understanding the aging process can at times be difficult. The difficulties in an individual's perceiving the aging complex from within are often hindered by the onset of senescence. *Senescence* is defined as the increasing "vulnerability" of a specific organism as it progresses through its expected life span. The classic concept of physiological aging has come from researchers in gerontology and medical microbiology and has been passed on to the public via the media. Health-related fields may ease the aging perception by adopting a broad focus of aging in order to reach a better understanding of interrelated sciences and the basic foundations of aging in today's society, as well as its interplay with perception (11).

■ Life Expectancy and Life Span

In order to define the aging process, it is essential to explore how past cultures have defined the aging process and the individual. These historical definitions may help us examine some portion of the aged population and examine the concept of life span versus life expectancy (8). Life expectancy can best be defined as the average number of years lived by individuals born during a designated period of time. Life span can best be defined as the *maximum* length of life potential attainable in the individual's culture. Scientifically, the human life span can be somewhere between 120 and 150 years if it is unaffected by disease processes. To the amazement of most health scientists, this span has yet to be accurately recorded. The initial difficulty in examining historical definitions of the aging process is that there is an almost total absence of accurate and reliable data on past generations. There are hardly any written records and the information available on life spans in the nineteenth century is mostly conjectural.

■ Problematic History of Aging

How long early man lived was determined by how well he or she was able to avoid disasters and survive natural inhibitors and epidemics. Analyses of the remains of several ancient civilizations indicate that the normal length of life was approximately 18 years. Those who survived beyond age 26 were undoubtedly considered the elders. A major drawback in utilizing historical information is that it lacks physiological accountability. Specific physical changes and their influences on the aging process in earlier societies were seldom documented. Various societies whose growth was unrestricted and in which hazards were reduced succumbed to early deaths (10). High mortality rates were attributed to wars, overpopulation, and famine. Early societies had not only high mortality rates but also high birth rates. With guaranteed food supplies, alterations in food production, more protective housing, and increased medical care came an increase in longevity. It became necessary to consider family size in evaluating the aging process.

Life expectancy at birth was greater than it was at adolescence. If one managed to survive the childhood diseases, one could look forward to reaching the teen years. For example, historical accounts describe the destruction brought about by plagues and wars, both of which have had major influences on longevity. Figure 2.1 illustrates the life expectancy at birth at various points in man's history. As illustrated in Figure 2.1, by the early 1300s life expectancy at birth ranged from 33 to 36 years (14). This information must be viewed with skepticism because some historical documents once considered representative have generally recorded the information only on the upper classes. Not until recently was it known that the high infant mortality was not recorded. Records usually assumed to be reliable included only those individuals who survived early childhood. Archives, registers, and legal documents dealing with inheritance have

Figure 2.1 Life expectancy at birth at various points in man's history. By the middle of the twentieth century, life expectancies were 73.0 for females and 66.5 for males.

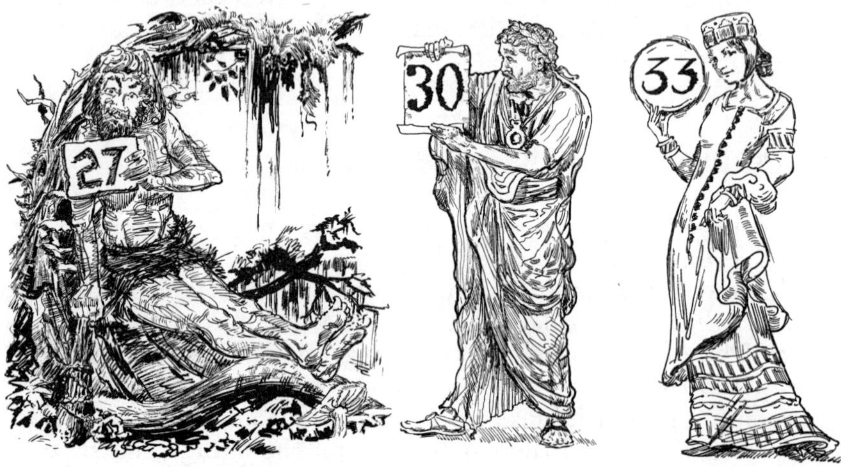

provided valuable information on the health status of individuals during the aging process. Recent articles in periodicals have tended to discuss social aging instead of physiological aging. As previously indicated, social status often precluded individuals from the fulfillment of the average life span. Members of the upper class often lived far beyond the average life span of those of the lower classes. Unlike the rest of society, members of the upper class could flee if disease or war threatened. They also had the available resources to escape malnutrition, the effects of severe weather, and the chronic problems of insufficient shelter (3).

■ Environmental and Social Factors

There are several physical correlates to environmental and social factors as they relate to the aging process. Other than genetically determined differences, the physical environment does "affect" one's metabolism and thus it directly affects one's longevity. Such related effects include exterior temperature as related to total body temperature, eating habits, and calorie expenditure (13).

Early twentieth-century experiments indicated that it

Figure 2.2 Your physical environment and your longevity are directly related.

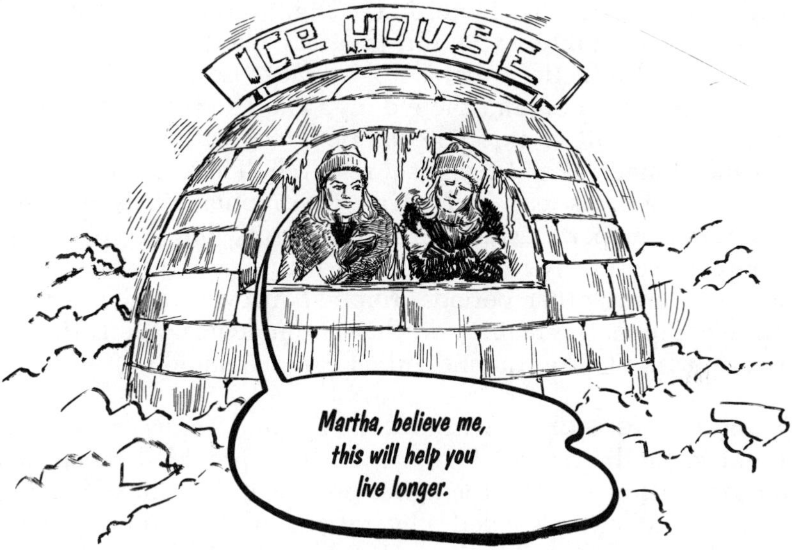
ICE HOUSE
Martha, believe me, this will help you live longer.

might be possible to increase longevity by dropping the body temperature. This method of reducing the body temperature has been suggested by many sciences, but it is not subscribed to by any body of scientists. Pharmacologists and physicians have debated the use of *cryogenics* and *chemotherapy* to bring about a reduction in body temperature and promote longevity. These methods involve a massive drop in temperature in order to reduce basal metabolic functioning (17).

Longevity and Social Factors History has shown the complexity of the interplay between longevity and social factors ranging from legal statutes to education and religion. In all likelihood, the purposes behind many of the religious practices were to help the masses rationalize the high rates of child mortality and to console them. It is evident that after the middle 1700s people could expect greater longevity for the mortality rate among individuals between the ages of 45 and 70 had declined by 50% (9).

The proportion of individuals ending life prior to the age of 50 due to disease has steadily decreased, but the postnatal death rate has not changed significantly. Infant and child mortality rates have traditionally been extremely high because medical techniques to deal with infectious diseases have not been available. The primary factor in the slight reduction (worldwide) in postnatal fatalities was the progress made against infant diseases and infectious diseases that cause degenerative effects among the newborn and the elderly. The elderly have continued to die as a result of chronic conditions not within the reach of advanced medical and technical research. These diseases include cancer, heart disease, and organ dysfunction. This disease syndrome, in part, explains the propensity for the older age groups to suffer lower longevity during various periods in time but not during other periods. Implicit in every society's age stratification is the realization that chronological age is the basic determinant of what the individual can and should do.

Aging in Literature Attitudes toward and norms of aging are found in the literature of today. Aristotle provided Renaissance authors with a view of the aging process in his time. William Shakespeare has provided illustrations of the conventional attitudes of aging in his time. His characters tend to emphasize the deterioration of physical ability during the aging process. These are evident in his descriptions in *King Lear, As You Like It,* and *Macbeth.* It was thought at this time that aging meant the loss of teeth, hearing acuity, and virility, the greying and loss of hair, increased presence of wrinkles, distasteful odors, loss of eye and nose control, and slight loss of sight. As if this physical trauma were not enough to demoralize aging individuals, individuals past the age of 40 were supposed to have dulled mental powers. These negative characteristics of old age (past the age of 40) have transcended the virtues of positive aging.

Scientific Analysis and Life Expectancy Scientific investigation has emphasized the importance of record-keeping and has taken a closer look at mortality figures. Vital statistics have disclosed that during the past decade ten or more years of life expectancy were to be expected over previous life expectancies. Many health scientists think that the mean age expectancy of 43 was realistic in developing countries and that a mean age of 55 was realistic in industrialized countries (12). At the turn of the century the age of 50 was equivalent to the age of 70 today. After World War II there was another significant change in life

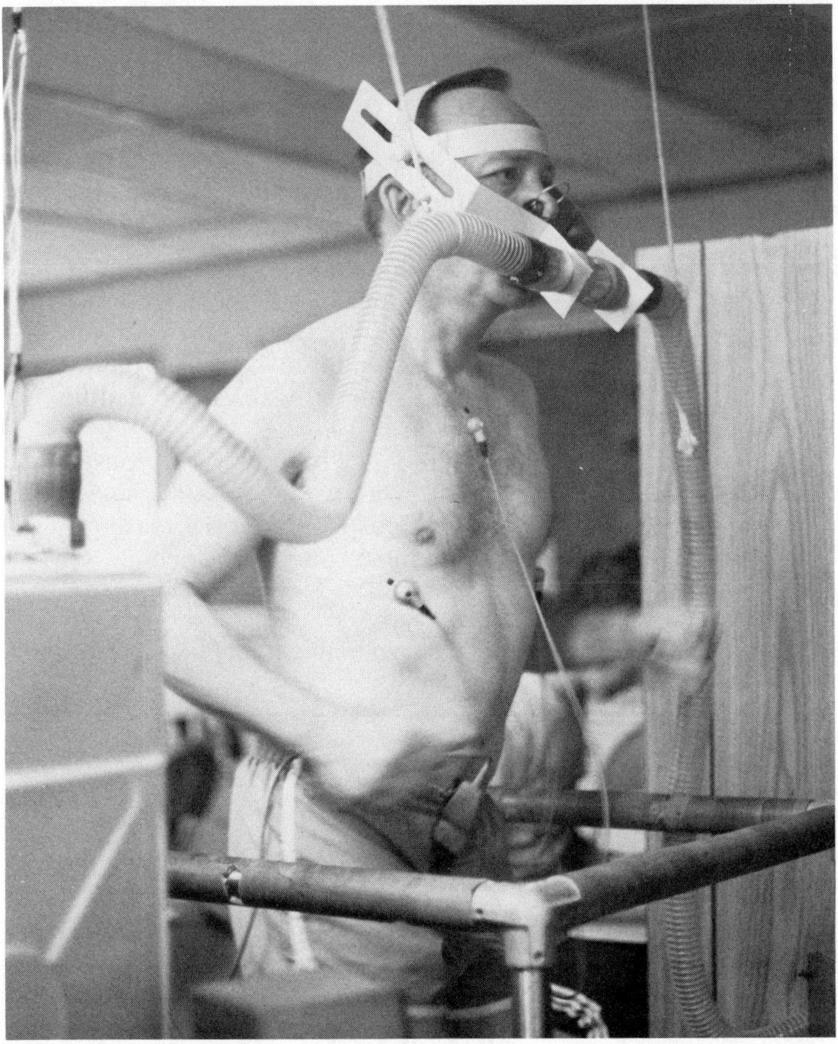

Figure 2.3 Scientific testing is important in the analysis of reasons for greater longevity.

expectancy. Life expectancy was increased to 60. An indication of this was the proportion of people over 50 in the labor force. For example, 3% of the labor force was over 50 in 1915 but by 1978 19% of the labor force was over 50 (12).

Life expectancy rates have been calculated by private organizations and government agencies that need measures of the various factors affecting a population's life span. Rates are based on intercorrelations of scientific perspectives and social issues in aging. Geneticists are able to evaluate not only basic biology at the molecular level but also cellular deterioration with age. The computation of factors in conjunction with vital statistics preestablishes one's life expectancy.

Economics and Longevity In our culture there is discrimination against age. It is especially evident in politics, government, and the business world and in some professions, for example, medicine and law. Examples are minimum ages for political office and maximum working ages for educators and public servants.

There has been a significant change in society's response to all stages of the aging process. Today young adults are at the center of our youth-oriented society and old people are increasingly discriminated against. For the most part, old people are

Figure 2.4 There is no generally accepted theory to explain the aging process.

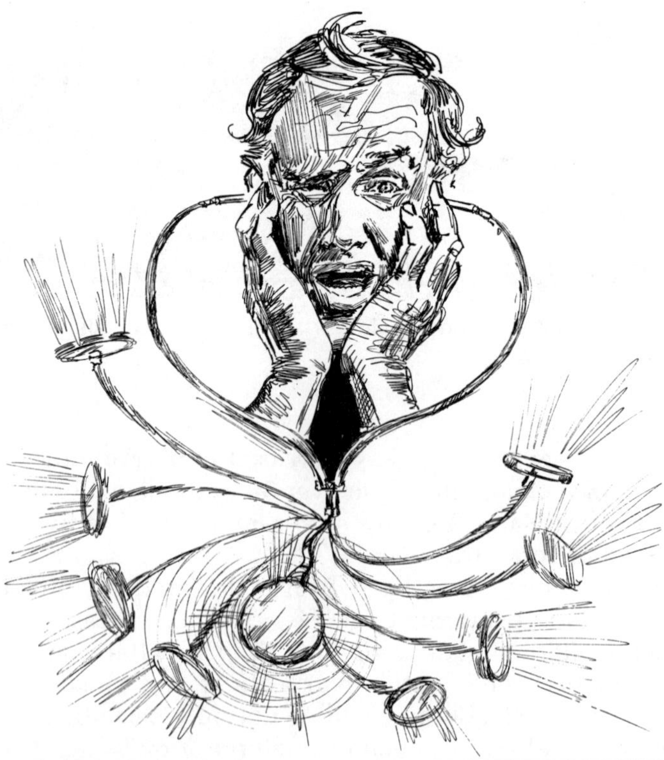

unwanted and are left to their own devices to get satisfaction from life. They are restricted to the company of people their own age and status in the social system. The social problems of aging, in part, result from the fact that the preparation for young adulthood (work and child rearing) is a basic part of our society but the psychological preparation for later life is left to each individual to handle his or her own way.

■ Aging: Theories Past and Present

Many biological and physiological theories on aging have been discussed. These theories may be grouped into two categories: (1) the cellular theory and (2) the genetic theory. These theories are universally accepted because they are not drastically changed by external influences and because they involve all members of the species.

Cellular Theory The question of whether cellular aging is due to intrinsic or extrinsic factors should be examined before the cellular theory is discussed. Could it be that the cellular theory

Figure 2.5 Typical cross section of an artery clogged with fatty deposits.

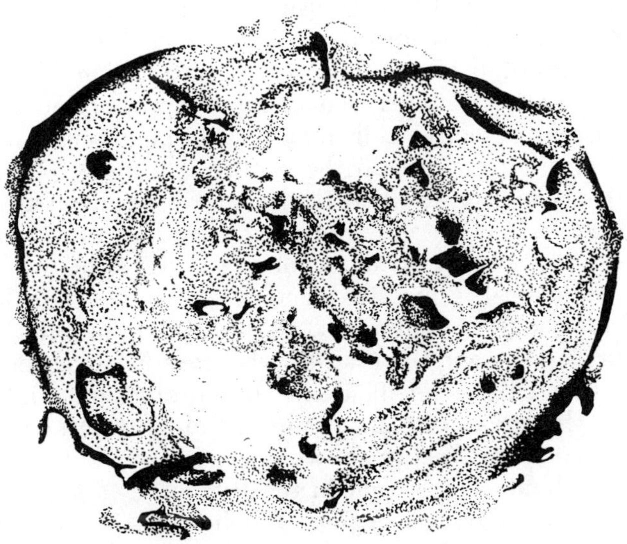

Figure 2.6 Typical human cells.

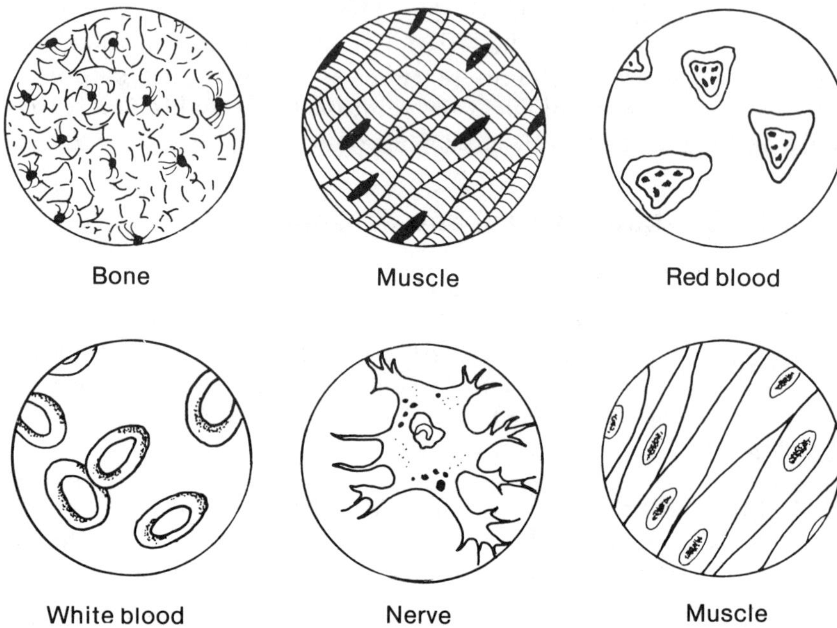

of aging may be related to organismic aging (longevity)? There are a number of explanations for cellular aging. The most popular and widely accepted one is the *error accumulation hypothesis* (18). This hypothesis states that cellular reproduction is not perfect and that defective cells may be produced within the body as a result of abnormalities in the synthesis process (18). As mentioned in Chapter 1, allied health professionals assume that these cells are defective and that their functions are impaired. This process supposedly occurs at one or more cellular levels. An example would be the massive accumulation of intercellular changes (intercellular mutations). The cellular mutation subtheory is far less acceptable than the theories discussed below. It has been shown that the incidence of chromosome defects perpetuates the age of cellular tissue. Although there have been few experiments, this theory shows promise and could be the center of biochemical research in the future.

Protein and Cellular Aging. Biochemists William Raush and T. K. Hansen have experimentally attempted to support the hypothesis that accumulation of insufficient proteins is responsible for cellular aging. The total mechanisms that produce abnormal proteins are a matter of speculation, but the observation of their existence has provided a basis for the concept of age-related loss of the physical and psychological functional capacity. The hypothesis is based on the premise that this accumulation will in time affect everyone and that it is a normal aspect of the aging process.

Toxin Theories. Other attempts to explain the aging process have suggested that preestablished aging patterns are caused by the dilution of essential enzymes and the accumulation of harmful metabolic waste and by-products. The dilution theory is little likely to be substantiated under close

Figure 2.7 Metabolic waste product theory: aging through accumulation of harmful wastes and by-products.

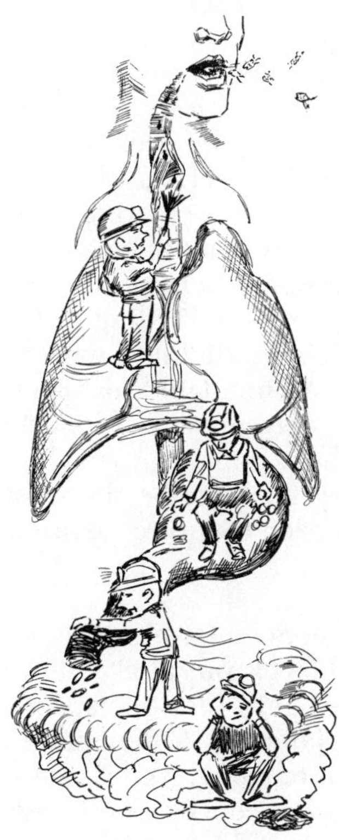

investigation because cellular dilution studies have failed to produce conclusive evidence on toxin poisoning in the body. Indeed, few, if any, studies have been able to explain the toxin theory. It seems that the toxin theory cannot totally apply to specific aging and it does not apply to those cells classified as nondividing cells, such as neurons and muscle tissue (7).

Preestablished biological aging patterns give credence to the theory that there is a biochemical "time clock" in the body which monitors cell divisions and the time spans for these divisions and thus controls and initiates the aging process. A prime example of this theory is the variety of cardiovascular diseases afflicting other healthy individuals. This theory is popular among health professionals because the results of populations monitored, i.e., cardiovascular patients, are consistent. To date, no significant study has been conducted on large enough numbers to provide undisputed evidence. Since the aging process varies in different populations, there seems to be some indication that the hypothesized time clock could be controlled by genetic factors. Evidence on predetermined longevity must be viewed, in the purest sense, as hypothetical because there is little empirical evidence to support the theory.

The most acceptable of the toxin theories indicates that compounds broken down in the cells simply cannot be removed. As a result, there is a buildup of harmful protein *toxins* that act as a toxic poison to the system, creating accelerated aging in many critical body organs. This theory provides a satisfactory explanation for the observed changes in the nondividing cells, but it does not totally explain dividing cells. It is mathematically unexplainable because an individual would only produce double the normal amount of accumulated toxins in a normal life span. Could this be the sole determinant of longevity? There is little empirical evidence that toxins accrue with chronological age, but the cellular theory seems to be the most plausible and it provides a viable approach to future research in aging theories (1).

Genetic Theory Genetic determination of the life span operates at not only individual levels but also within the various species. Genetic makeup determines that one species will live longer than another species. James C. Korenchevsky indicates that there is a genetic upper limit to aging. And, as stated in Chapter 1, one's longevity is *determined* at conception. Longevity may be altered under various environmental conditions and absence of disease

(15). Environmental variations may to some extent determine variations in longevity, but they do not override genetic factors. In other words, an organ may be genetically programmed to atrophy due to a certain experience of a given environmental condition (10). An example of this would be in the increase in malfunctions of the respiratory system among coal miners.

Parental Influences. Subfactors, including maternal and paternal influences, parental age at birth, genetic mutations, birth order, and marital status, have been shown to hinder or promote longevity. Although there seems to be a definite relationship between parent and offspring longevity, there seems to be no difference whether it was the male or female who lived longer (1). The discrepancies in findings of various health professionals give little credit to this aspect of genetic influence. These studies have been described as trying to understand longevity in terms of time alone, putting aside associated factors of longevity and leaving unexplained the variances in the genetic theory. The absence of findings can be dealt with as a social theory, even if the male genetic influence is known. It is difficult to determine whether parental influences are, for the most part, genetic or social.

Parental age at birth has long been considered a factor in determining the longevity of offspring. It is assumed that there is no change in genetic influence with increasing age of the offspring (1). Generally speaking, the importance of parental age as a longevity predictor shows increased validity when contrasting maternal to paternal age. Telerchy Yerushalry (15) has found that the younger the mother, the larger the number of abnormal pregnancies. Social and physiological explanations indicate a higher incidence of abnormal births among younger females, but this is innate in social research reporting systems. As the age of the mother progresses between the twenty-fifth and thirty-fifth years, so does the longevity of the successively born offspring. Therefore, the birth order may be yet another determinant of longevity.

It has been hypothesized that if maternal age were to be controlled, the mother's reproductive abilities might be diminished with additional births. Sociologists say that the first born are more culturally esteemed and have a cultural advantage. Biologists say that the first born may be severely disadvantaged due to initial birth traumas (15). These thoughts, *while worth noting*, are only a minor factor in theorizing longevity.

Biological Determinants and Genetics. Biologists and allied health professionals generally agree that nongenetic and genetic factors combine to alter the protein enzyme reproduction, thus causing cell irregularities. Hypothetically, this alteration affects the offspring through postnatal accumulation. In essence, this is a mutation. It therefore seems logical that the rate of mutations would account for the age at death and the totality of the aging process (7).

Marriage. Research has indicated that marriage increases longevity. This longevity seems to be attributed to the fact that society frowns on individuals in poor health marrying. Statistics indicate that once an individual is married the environment is favorable to longer life (5). This is credited to positive mental health and emotional support, planned and adequate nutrition, as well as personal health care in time of illness.

Charles Timiras states that longevity can be directly related to marital environments. However, this factor will be much less important in the years to come as lifestyle changes and cohabitation is accepted. A significant factor in Timiras' theory may be that medical and economic changes facilitate marriages that would have never taken place in years past. Sociologists say that in the future marriage will be less crucial as a factor in longevity.

Heredity Factors as a Genetic Base. For centuries researchers have thought that outbreeding (intermarriage) is directly related to longer life spans. Anthropologists say that intermixed breeding is prone to producing longer-lived offspring, that is, longer-lived in terms of their parents' longevity. It has been hypothesized that if social mores were to be eliminated, interbreeding would produce individuals prone to longer lives. These social mores include marrying outside religion, ethnic backgrounds, and social classes. These social factors in various societies determine marriage patterns, resulting in social control of genetic patterns. Geographic and social mobility encourages and discourages outbreeding (17). This social phenomenon influences longevity through the available genetic pool; in other words, it limits the potential "mate pool." If one were to assume that both genetic and social factors existed, it would be possible that the differences in longevity would be reduced. However, this social factor of longevity cannot be significant in determining genetic pools, and therefore it is a moot point.

Race Factors. To determine whether or not race is a genetic component, it is necessary to compare white versus nonwhite mortality with an equal socioeconomic status or compare racial mortality differentials versus social status. One problem to be examined in the future is the unreliability of determining race from color of skin (10). Race factors have undermined all studies in this area of research and have thus tainted these studies. There is a tendency among sociologists and allied health professionals to interpret trends in racial mortality as a sign of sociological differences. This is best illustrated with the increase in black male deaths due to heart disease. Is society or genetic inbreeding responsible?

Sex Factors. As indicated in Chapter 1, research indicates that there is a genetic female superiority in life span at all age levels. Females have a lower death rate at virtually all ages beginning with stillbirths (10). This is not only in the United States but also in all industrialized countries. The basis for this is a genetic factor. This biological factor involves the XX and XY chromosomal differences. The XX chromosome combination is generally stronger. Statistics compiled by the Center for Disease Control in Atlanta, Georgia, indicate relatively fewer chronic disease cases among women.

Sex is passed on through the X and Y chromosomes. All normal females have two X chromosomes and all normal males have an X and a Y chromosome. A female may only pass on an X chromosome, but a male may pass on either an X or a Y chromosome, for each sperm contains one or the other. Thus, the male determines the sex of the offspring. The X chromosomes carry other genetic material as well, and it is now thought that the Y chromosomes may also carry material that affects the aging process.

The chromosomal influence operates under the affect of genetically based secondary sex characteristics. Social factors that tend to reduce the male life span are secondary considerations, but they do produce evidence that environmental factors play sexual and social roles in longevity (10). Recently, male deaths have increased due to accidents, cancer, and heart disease. This may also be associated with stereotyped male behavior and lifestyles. Preferential treatment for the young female may explain potential female genetic superiority. Often the female is given greater care during early developmental years. But a change may be forthcoming. This is indicated by changing socioeconomic factors, white longevity superiority declining via interbreeding, and higher female mortality due to occupational trends.

Hypothetical Theories

Autoimmune Theory The autoimmune theory is a hypothetical derivation of cellular mutation theories which explains a person's resistance to aging being directly related to disease immunity. The theory attempts to associate diseases with individual aging processes. There seems to be some validity to the theory because the majority of deaths are due to diseases associated with the aging process. It is thought that the interaction in the protein process results in certain chemical compounds called *autoantibodies* that may cause cellular damage (19). Such damage is often reflected in the disease process and eventual death. The greatest number of age-related deaths, including cancer, cardiovascular disease, and diabetes, have been thought to have this autoimmunity (15). Whether or not factors other than mutations are involved in this process is highly controversial. Ironically, social settings that produce exposure to mutant agents may enhance the reduction of longevity.

Nutrition Theory Minimal food consumption has been shown to decrease obesity and therefore a decrease in disease-related deaths. It has been hypothesized that minimal eating has a definite effect on extending one's life span. Life insurance companies report that obesity is directly related to higher mortality from the major degenerative diseases. Obesity has been directly related to environmental psychological conditions. Thus, ethnic eating habits as well as individual habits influence longevity in terms of caloric intake and nutrition. Additionally, one must consider the factor of energy expenditure being related to longevity (9). However, this factor cannot alone be responsible for reduced longevity; it may be only a contributing factor. Occupational groups may account to some degree for this energy expenditure. Additional eating factors may include social class and living conditions.

The various theories of aging and development can provide a useful basis for understanding the foundation from which a logical progression may be made in comprehending human longevity. Some theories indicate that a person's lifestyle during the first half of life dictates the difference in later life. The theories suggested to the point indicate that there is possibly a change of life crisis when society places restrictions on productivity in later years. Theories help professionals and lay people to understand the broad outlines of lifecycles and ask questions. Theories tend not only to be general in nature but also unrealistic (9). Theories do not give much indication of how cultural differences and social classes interact with overall growth and development, and how they therefore affect longevity.

For some individuals, aging may mean physical survival and providing one's offspring with the opportunity to survive. For others, aging may mean facing illness, poverty, social isolation, and few psychological goals. Research on the effects of physiological well-being and social class, ethnic heritage, and sexual differences is now being conducted at universities, private research institutes, and gerontology centers.

Theories are based on empirical research. Therefore, theories and research must proceed in similar directions. This may lead to developing research in growth and development. It seems incredible to hypothesize that one may gain significant information about aging by studying a parent and offspring rather than conducting a longitudinal study over a period of 25 years. The Andrus Gerontology Center at the University of Southern California is the forerunner in this research.

Wear and Tear Theory Probably the most reliable theory of aging is that the human organism wears out (7). Theoretically, it is very similar to that of any mechanical device. Aging is believed to be the result of the gradual deterioration of organs necessary for life. However, Howard Curtis indicates that there is no conclusive evidence that physical stress alone is responsible for decreasing one's life span (10). The effects of severe chemical stress have been shown to shorten one's life. An example would be the excess use of alcohol, narcotics, tobacco, etc. Once these excesses are removed, the individual may return to predetermined longevity. The total rate of metabolism appears to be a factor in the aging process. The wear and tear theory hypothesizes that lowering the metabolic rate could postpone some of the physiological consequences of aging. This may be done through environmental methods or chemical methods! However, the interrelation of various body systems is probably more implicated in the aging process than is significant failure of a particular organ. Although medical research has indicated that transplants may extend longevity, health professionals are inclined to believe that it is not likely that transplants will significantly affect longevity.

Waste Product Theory. Another widely accepted theory is that of metabolic waste accumulation. This theory differs from the protein toxin theory in that a variety of waste products accumulate. Researchers have suggested that organisms age because cellular poisons or waste products hamper their functioning. It has been hypothesized that waste products accumulate with age and are a symptom of aging rather than a cause of aging. This was evidenced while studying *collagen,* a fibrous protein substance that is formed slowly in some tissues and eliminated only at a slow rate. Some researchers believe that these fibers are not eliminated and that in time they may tend to shrink and constrict the growth of various body tissues. Timiras found that these strands of protein change with age. This may be due to changes in the linkages between the interwoven strands of the protein. The accumulation of collagen and its change with age are physiologically related to loss of oil in skin cells and slowness in the healing process in later life. *Lipofuscins,* another waste product, is thought to build up in some nerve cells with age and give rise to irregular pigmentation. This is also thought to be a symptom of aging rather than a cause of aging (18).

A more recent hypothesis indicates that a possible shift in calcium deposits often occurs late in an individual's life cycle. This calcification is viewed most regularly in elderly individuals and suggests a defect in calcium metabolism (18). However, it may not be the dominant factor in the aging process. Recent research has suggested that this process is yet another factor in the breakdown of one of the many interrelated factors of metabolic waste and cellular aging.

Subsequent theories that rate mention are: (1) The radiation theory: Ionizing radiation is thought to cause an acceleration of the aging process via interaction with cellular processes. (2) The cybernetic theory: The central nervous system deteriorates to a point that it fails to control various organisms' cellular function, thus resulting in eventual debilitation. (3) The virus theory: Individual viruses and their effects are thought to influence rates of aging. (4) The stress theory: It is thought that normal stress causes a wearing down of bodily functions. Stress affects all organs in the body and with additional years of stress may cause death. (5) The evolution theory: Humans are evolving toward a more successful adjustment to the habitat. Humans are not totally adapted to the present environment and therefore must continue to adapt physiologically. It may be the body trying to search for death when attempts to adapt are foiled.

It may be assumed from the above that there is a tremendous amount of research to be done on the specific cause of the aging

Figure 2.8 Collagen fiber growth may, over time, tend to shrink and constrict the growth of various body cells.

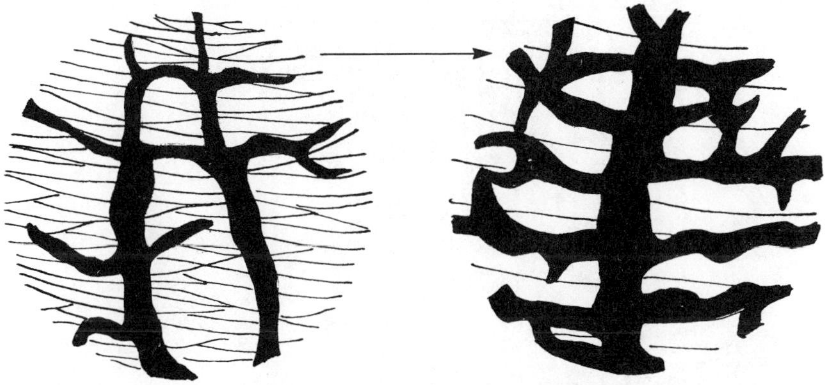

process. Can it be that the fountain of youth lies in the cellular process of aging? Although a strong argument may be made for many other theories, could this be the most promising? Eternal longevity does not lie in the prevention of disease; it lies in the mechanisms that regulate human life.

There seem to be some overriding social issues involved with the extents of human life expectancy. If people live longer, there will be more people inhabiting the earth. Thus overpopulation will be a certainty. Under current social mores, this would mean increased numbers utilizing limited care facilities and retirement facilities and "grey unemployment." Who will support this older population? Probably the most critical question asked by allied health professionals and sociologists is, "Will extended life also add vitality to one's later years?" Attempts to lengthen life will, without doubt, increase the "later disease affliction rate." There will have to be both economic and social advances for the older population if full benefit for later life is to be expected. Undoubtedly, there are innumerable questions to be answered in this area.

■ Summary

There have been a number of theories, hypotheses, and conclusions about the aging process. Cultures have defined aging as it directly related to their social values. Probably the most

Figure 2.9 Environmental stress may play a significant role in aging.

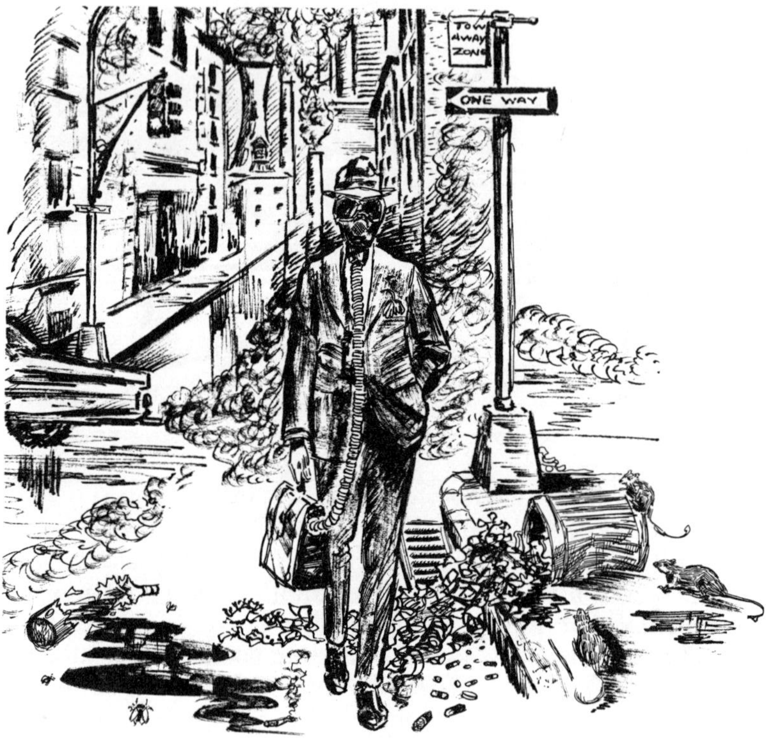

significant theories have been the cellular, genetic, and autoimmune theories. No significant evidence has been found that correlates all theories in the human's total environment. One's forefathers probably provide the most important input into one's longevity. Longevity and life indicators pose a variety of interesting questions about an individual's life.

References

1. Bakerman, Seymour. *Aging Life Process.* Springfield, Ill.: Charles C. Thomas, 1969.
2. Benet, Sula. "Why They Live to Be 100 or Even Older in Abkhasia." *New York Times Magazine,* 26 December, 1971.
3. Birren, James E. "Behavioral Theories of Aging," *Aging:*

Some Social and Biological Aspects, Pub. No. 65. Washington, D.C.: American Association for the Advancement of Science, 1960.

4. ———. *The Psychology of Aging.* Englewood Cliffs, N.J.: Prentice-Hall, 1964.
5. Blood, R. O. *The Family.* New York: The Free Press, 1972.
6. Botwinick, Jack. *Cognitive Processes in Maturity and Old Age.* New York: Springes, 1967.
7. Clark, A. M. *Genetic Factors Associated with Aging.* New York: Academic Press, 1964.
8. Comfort, Alex. *Aging: The Biology of Senescence.* New York: Holt, Rinehart & Winston, 1964.
9. ———. "The Prospects of Longevity." Paper presented at the meeting of the Gerontological Society, San Juan, Puerto Rico, December, 1972.
10. Curtis, Howard J. *Biological Mechanisms of Aging.* Springfield, Ill.: Charles C Thomas, 1966.
11. Hayflick, Leonard, "Aging Under Glass." *Experimental Gerontology* 5 (1970): 291–303.
12. Lehman, Harvey. *Age and Achievement.* Princeton, N.J.: Princeton University Press, 1953.
13. Reed, Homer. "Changes in Psychological Test Performance Associated with the Normal Aging Process." *Journal of Gerontology* 18 (1963): 271–274.
14. Richardson, B. E. *Old Age Among the Ancient Greeks.* Baltimore: Johns Hopkins Press, 1933.
15. Rockstein, Morris. "The Biological Aspects of Aging." *The Gerontologist* 8 (1968):124–25.
16. Selye, Hans. "Stress and Aging." *Journal of the American Geriatrics Society* 18 (1970): 669–80.
17. Shock, Nathan. *Perspectives in Experimental Gerontology.* Springfield, Ill.: Charles C Thomas, 1966.
18. Timiras, P. S. *Developmental Physiology and Aging.* New York: Macmillan, 1972.
19. Walford, Roy L. *The Immunologic Theory of Aging.* Baltimore: Williams & Wilkins, 1969.

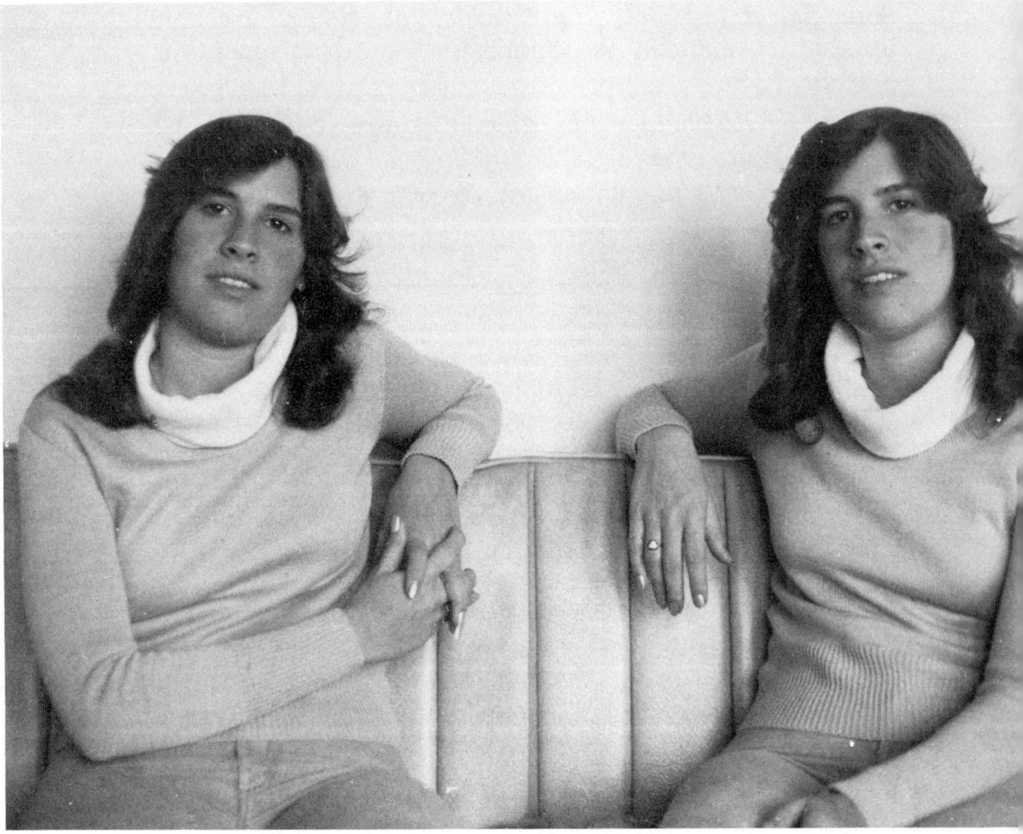

■ **Chapter 3**

Longer Life: Theoretical Possibilities

Major Concepts

1. Extremely diverse patterns of aging exist in the world.
2. Senility is considered by some professionals as a myth and by others as a progression in the aging process.
3. There are a number of hypothetical means by which life may be extended.

To Be Or Not To Be

So many of my friends are gone,
It's as if I were once part of a forest
And now I'm a lone tree
That has withstood a lot of storms
And may or may not
Withstand the next one.
But it's not up to me.
I find that comforting, God.
I'd hate the job of deciding whether
To be or not to be
At this stage of the game.
I have my up times and my down
And what I decided would depend on
How I felt at the moment
And I certainly don't have all the facts.
How do I know if I'm through here
Or if there's more for me to do?
When I was younger I was big on "running my own life."
(Tried to run quite a few other people's lives, too—Forgive me for that.)
Now I'm quite content to let You make the major decisions.
Funny thing. I know whenever You call me,
I won't be ready to go,
But that's life. Or should I say Death?

Anonymous

Diversity of Aging

In society there are widely divergent patterns of aging which scientists see through the eyes of statistics. They use a device called a life table (Figure 3.1), which is a survival schedule for a defined population. Life tables have long been used to probe for patterns and causes of aging in many societies.

In animals, death is the last in a rapid sequence of reproductive and developmental processes. It has been noted that for efficient completion of the life cycle, animals must complete life processes in a short time span (9). In animals one can see that definite life termination processes are present and are under the control of genetic mechanisms. It is thought that environmental factors have less of an effect on people than on animals. Clear-cut instances of programmed aging are exhibited in the deterioration of renewable parts of the organism. The failing of organs results from programmed aging processes, as are the death of the red blood cells at a characteristic age and the individual's "renewing" processes.

An individual functioning under favorable environmental and nutritional conditions has a relatively high death rate in prenatal, neonatal, and infantile periods. These death rates decline rapidly, reaching a minimum at an age which corresponds roughly with puberty. With young adulthood, these death rates rise slowly. From age 30 an individual's mortality rate rises, by

Figure 3.1 Example of a life expectancy table.

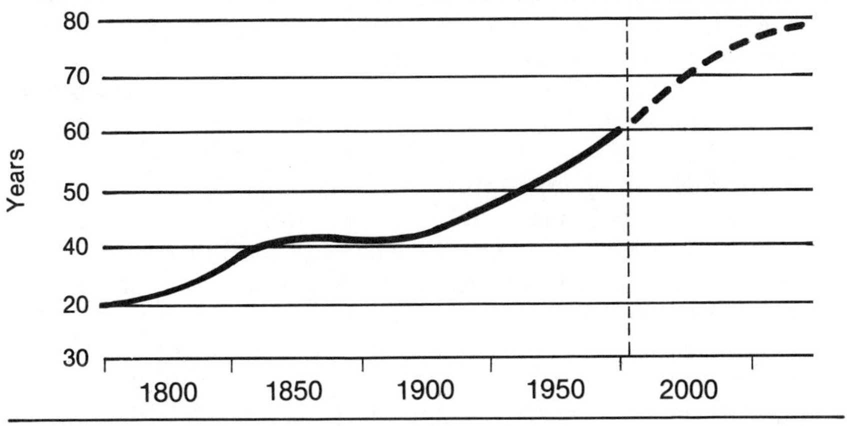

Figure 3.2 Changes begin early in life.

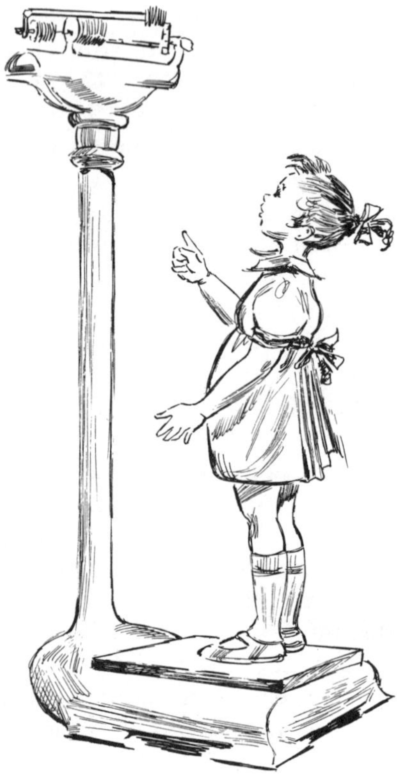

a law of geometric increase, more rapidly with increasing age. For instance, diseases and degenerative effects compound with additional years and additional *onsets*.

Factors that influence aging in a population are varied and diverse. The survival of an individual must be viewed in relation to his or her *total* environment. There are complex personality patterns that interact with the environment which may result in a struggle for existence (18). This is often best illustrated through life tables in which for each age mortality rates are contrasted with environmental factors. Exterior temperature of the environment is often reflected in longevity. Since the sequence of *senescent* changes also progresses more rapidly, longevity seems to decrease as temperature increases. This temperature is important in supporting the concept that aging is

Figure 3.3 Some researchers feel that aging is programmed.

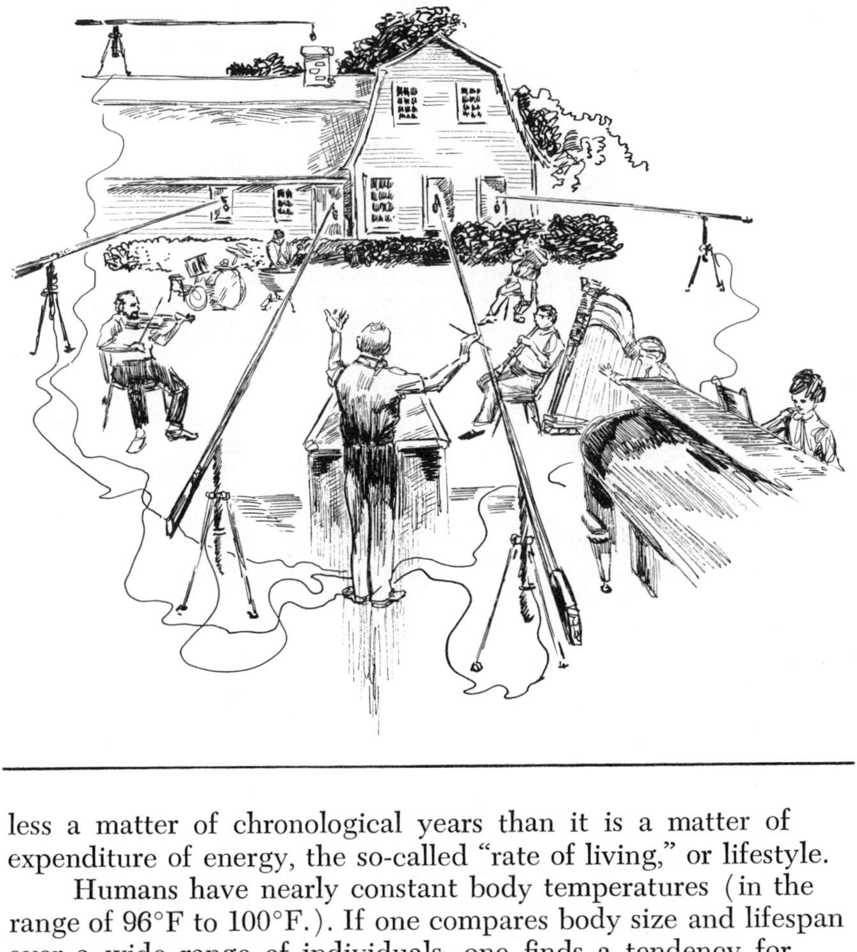

less a matter of chronological years than it is a matter of expenditure of energy, the so-called "rate of living," or lifestyle.

Humans have nearly constant body temperatures (in the range of 96°F to 100°F.). If one compares body size and lifespan over a wide range of individuals, one finds a tendency for larger individuals to have a higher mortality rate early in life and to be proportionately longer-lived than smaller individuals in later life (21). There seems to be no scientific basis for such deviations and reversal.

Improved disease prevention and cures over the past century have reduced mortality rates in early years significantly. However, mortality rates of later years have not been reduced significantly. Hence, the death rate rises more steeply. Despite the improvements in survival at early ages, the maximum age to which individuals live has not increased appreciably, even

Table 3.1 Death Rates by Sex, Age, and Cause, 1976 (rates per 100,000 population)

	All Ages		15–24		25–44		45–64		65+	
	Male	Female	Male	Female	Male	Female	Male	Female	Male	Female
(1.)	Heart disease (383.5)	Heart disease (293.4)	Accident (94.1)	Accident (25.3)	Accident (65.7)	Cancer (32.5)	Heart disease (554.9)	Cancer (264.0)	Heart disease (2906.9)	Heart disease (2039.3)
(2.)	Cancer (196.6)	Cancer (156.0)	Suicide (18.5)	Cancer (5.1)	Heart disease (40.3)	Accident (16.7)	Cancer (338.7)	Heart disease (184.4)	Cancer (1324.0)	Cancer (741.0)
(3.)	CVA (77.1)	CVA (98.1)	Cancer (8.0)	Suicide (4.8)	Cancer (27.5)	Heart disease (12.6)	Accident (65.0)	CVA (50.2)	CVA (694.7)	CVA (694.5)
(4.)	Accident (67.3)	Accident (27.7)	Heart disease (3.4)	Heart disease (1.9)	Suicide (23.3)	CVA (6.8)	CVA (63.1)	Cirrhosis (26.0)	Pneumonia, Flu (259.6)	Pneumonia, Flu (177.6)
(5.)	Pneumonia, Flu (36.1)	Pneumonia, Flu (26.6)	Pneumonia, Flu (1.6)	Pneumonia, Flu (1.4)	Cirrhosis (12.4)	Cirrhosis (6.1)	Cirrhosis (56.9)	Accident (23.7)	Accident (133.8)	Arterio-sclerosis (125.8)

Source: Statistical Abstract of the United States, 1978, p. 76.

though the expectation of life from birth has doubled over the past century.

Changes in the Individual Death rates in a population increase proportionately with increasing chronological age. The incidence of many diseases, such as cardiovascular disease and cancer, increases with age. Since the diseases generally take decades to develop, characteristically they appear in individuals in later life. The individual changes with time in a manner that it is believed may increase susceptibility to certain diseases.

Aging: A Disease or Result Age has been characterized as those alterations found in individuals who leave no diagnosable disease. Possibly, these changes attributed to aging are to be thought of in time as the early signs or states of specific disease processes (23). One can also think of aging as the forerunner of a variety of diseases. For this reason, diseases may be referred to as a *sign* of aging.

In describing age-related changes that take place with time, there is an inclination to include persons who have degenerative diseases. To characterize aging, repeated observations must be made of a person as that person moves through life. This method of observation is essential if variances are to be avoided when groups are compared using such variables as race, age, income, health status, and education. In longitudinal (long-term) studies individuals are compared to themselves at a previous age. Research adjustments have not been made for the variables listed above. Therefore, most information dealing with aging is based on cross-cultural studies (short-term), which are subject to cultural, economic, environmental, and other biases.

Researchers must also provide a reliable and meaningful picture of aging and a unifying conceptual framework. Data collected in other aging studies must be cumulative instead of expanding descriptive data. It is necessary, therefore, to go beyond the data and trace the links between the various facets of aging. To date, individuals working in the field have been rather slow to use an integrative approach. Research findings have not been comparable and the impact of the data falls short of its total worth. The future dictates integrative perspectives capable of lending order to conflicting findings and providing straightforward avenues to explain why men and women age and a more concentrated effort on various isolated aspects of aging.

Figure 3.4 Do you really need to rest?

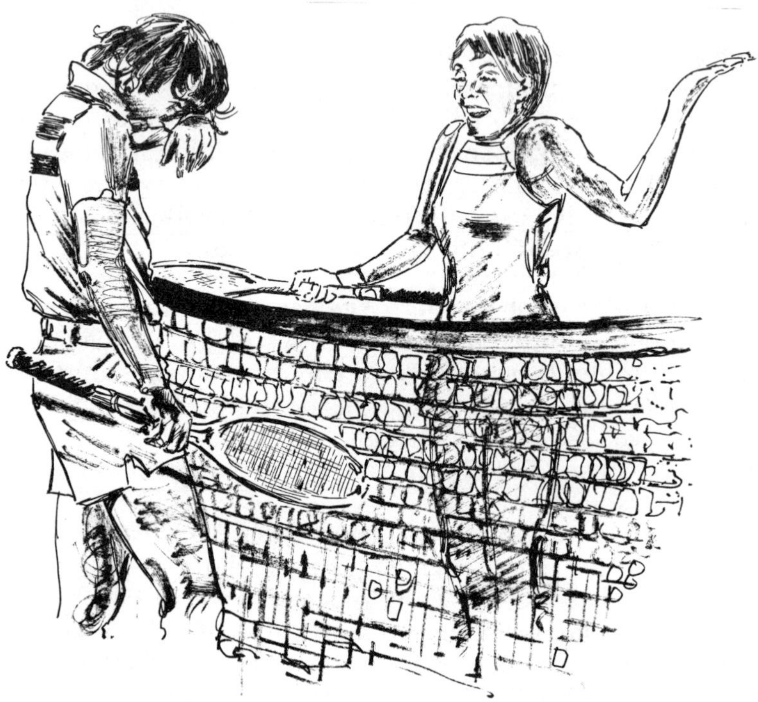

Aging and Conditions of Rest In most instances, patterns of age differences appear in various physiological characteristics. Some individuals are well "maintained" even in advanced age (18). Other individuals peak physiologically in middle life and then decrease in later life. However, the most common pattern is a gradual decline in adulthood, with rapid declines in the sixth and seventh decades.

Blood Flow. Under strenuous conditions, the normal biochemical characteristics of the blood are maintained into advanced ages. There is no systematic change in the blood with age under these conditions. This is not surprising since the life of each cell of the body depends upon the stability of the internal environment. The various physiological mechanisms that regulate blood composition are capable of maintaining stable values even in advanced age if no extra demands are placed on the system (12). Some physiological characteristics continue to increase after reaching maximum body size and sexual maturity and are followed by decrements in late middle age and old age. These include normal cell division as well as variations in body size.

Organs. The most common pattern of age differences in physiological characteristics is a gradual reduction in performance of many organ systems. Some of the physiological functions which decline with age when measured under resting conditions include: speed of conduction of the nerve impulse, cardiac output, renal blood flow and filtration rate, basal metabolism, vital capacity, and excretion of sex hormones. Age changes may arise from intrinsic and extrinsic causes. The common denominator for these factors is that they decrease the ability of the organism to perform functions that may be necessary for staying alive. Most show a gradual decrease that begins in the forties and continues throughout life.

As mentioned earlier, intrinsic factors occur inevitably, regardless of the environment. They may be considered a natural property of the organism and result from one or more of the processes and structures characteristic of living systems, in much the same sense as the eventual wearing out of an automobile engine is an intrinsic part of its nature and the result of continued "normal" operation. Extrinsic factors are environmental influences. They may be modifiable to some extent and they may have an immediate interest to practitioners.

Extrinsic factors may be of different magnitude in different environments. They include such factors as radiation, temperature, physical injury, diet, and such agents as harmful bacteria and viruses. Psychological and sociological events, influenced by the individual's own emotional makeup, may modify aging (5).

The Search for Youth Since the beginning of time people have searched for a magic potion to thwart old age. Potential prospects have ranged from the tiger testicle remedies (drunk to produce youth) to rejuvenation via contact with sexually active teen-agers, to modern mythology utilizing the drug procaine to promote youth.

Many individuals have tried in vain to follow the lead of Ponce de León in a search for the magic formula or cure for the aging process. Such a cure is hypothetical at this time. However, health professionals continue to search for a deterrent within the innermost mechanisms of the human body. This deterrent may have its beginning with intracellular actions (22). Further examination by professionals has given indications that causes may be due to biological decay and minimal levels of operation at which organs in the body are capable of supporting total life (this was discussed in Chapter 2). It is interesting to ponder how many individuals would desire to prolong life if it meant they would have to live with various infirmities for a prolonged period of time. This thought might be enough to cause aging health professionals to give up the search.

Possibilities for Longevity Various possibilities exist for retarding, but probably not for abolishing, the effects of time and environment or the aging process. The effects of disruptive environmental factors already have been reduced by public health measures (24). These include information on diets, promotion of safety practices, and other measures. Better diet and hygiene as well as prevention and treatment of new and degenerative diseases will, no doubt, further increase the mean age of death. Nonetheless, senescence and death are inescapable consequences of human biology.

Possible means of postponing or counteracting these effects may exist in the experimental reduction of body temperature to a value allowing efficient function (e.g., 33°C to 34°C), the discovery of special chemical substances to promote the growth or division of cells that normally limit the function of old organisms, the development of agents to reduce the rate of formation of cross linkages in proteins, and the development of *in vitro* (outside the body) and *in vivo* (inside the body) techniques for the replacement of wornout organs or their parts. Presently such means are strictly hypothetical (24).

Senility—A Myth? Psychological age usually refers to one's capacity for emotional adaptation to one's environment. This would include such things as sensory functions and memory. Such age can be reflected as *social age* (13). This is not sociological age which refers to one's function in a total society. What this does refer to is one's role in the family, at work, in the community, as well one's interests and activities in the home. There is no single process in aging that produces the sociological and psychological infirmity called senility. This progressive loss of energies and ability to recall seems to be on a psychological time

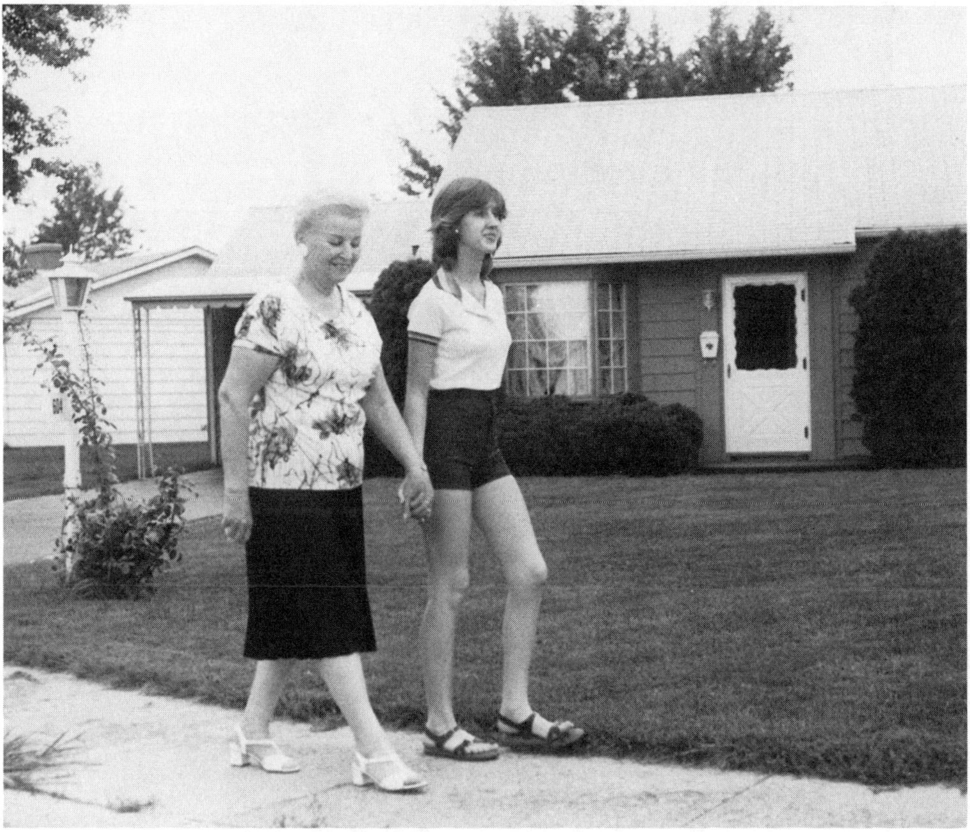

Figure 3.5 Aging is an inescapable consequence of human biology—for everyone.

clock. Sooner or later, no matter how well one looks after the body, the loss will eventually take place. Most individuals try to ignore these facts until they are forced to face them.

Psychological aging has been referred to as senility by many individuals. Senility is an archaic, general term that was used to refer to mental infirmities thought to be the result of aging. Scientists in biology, health, and chemistry now know that the symptoms related to aging and thought to be senility are specific degenerative diseases that are often treatable or arrestable. Sociologists and psychologists agree that the aging process covers a wide realm that encompasses the sensory and psychomotor processes. Such functions in turn affect perceptions and memory. Thus, various factors are thought to directly affect the onset of senility.

The importance of these changes lies in the impact they have on the social functioning of the individual. Such a change

Figure 3.6 "Old" is what one perceives.

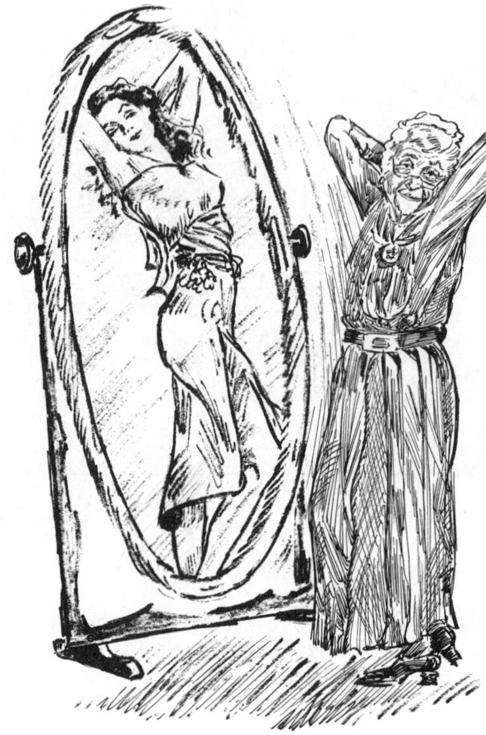

is not programmed into the individual. In other words, it does not have to occur genetically. For example, a 70-year-old does not have to be senile because his father was senile.

One's sensory processes are often the means through which the mind experiences the world. In order to adapt and interact with one's environment, one must be able to investigate one's surroundings. This sensory process of investigation is far from complex. Sensory organs (the eyes, ears, nose, mouth, and skin) pick up information about the environment and transmit that information to the brain. Psychologists prior to the 1960s thought that the onset of mental infirmity or senility destroyed one's sensory perception; such thinking no longer is realistic. For example, vision is adaptable. The lens of the eye must change shape in order to be able to focus on both near and distant objects. As physical age increases, the ability of the eye to change shape and focus on near objects decreases. This loss of one's visual acuity does not indicate mental infirmity, only the loss of one sensory organ's efficiency.

Another example is hearing acuity. Hearing involves many reactions. The essential one is detecting the pitch and intensity of sound. As individuals age, their reactions to pitch and intensity change. But there is no evidence that the ability to distinguish sound intervals changes with age. The intensity threshold does not change with age, but certain frequencies cannot be heard. This may mean that the loss of hearing indicates a degree of senility. If individuals cannot hear various sounds or see their environment, they cannot react to their environment. Some social scientists consider these factors in determining senility.

Presbycusis is the gradual loss of acute hearing. The perception of high-frequency sounds is usually affected first. Loud noises may later alter middle- and low-frequency ranges as well. Males tend to show hearing loss earlier than females do. If the speculation that more males than females have been exposed to high-level occupational noise is correct, sex differences in auditory loss could be due to environmental exposure rather than to inherent differences. It is hypothesized that high-volume noise occupations may increase female hearing loss in the 1990s because more women will be working in high-volume noise occupations.

Intelligence Psychologists say that intelligence is both an individual's potential and an applied ability. However, it is difficult to measure applied ability. Measured intelligence is actually mental ability in terms of responsiveness. Through intelligence, learning, and memory, individuals may create a mirage of mental images, but the images may diminish with age. Thinking, problem solving, and creating may be more drastically affected by advancing age. Psychologists have indicated that if various functions such as vision and hearing decline with age, they could serve as barriers to the development of concept information (3). It is thought that stimulus reaction time decreases as age increases. That is, when not given enough time, some individuals tend to be confused by tasks that require reaction to and synthesis of stimulus. Some sociologists believe that this is an expected social factor rather than individuals' aging processes.

However, most gerontology tests are prepared by individuals from various disciplines. As a result, measurable data are sometimes inconclusive, at best, and may not truly measure intelligence. The tests are similar to those taken by racial groups and may not truly measure intelligence.

■ Myths or Theoretical Possibilities?

Cryogenics As mentioned in Chapter 2, decreasing the body temperature by 2°C to 3°C could increase one's life span by up to twenty years (10). This could be done by controlling the environment in which one lives. The basis for this hypothesis seems to be built on the premise that cellular deterioration may be retarded.

Hibernation It has been hypothesized that in future space travel hibernation may be a way of providing the longevity needed to exist in outer space. Scientists have hypothesized that humans who hibernate may live eight to ten times longer than if they do not hibernate. Does it seem possible that one's physiology may attain a chronological age of 800 years? The process is based on suspended animation, which, ideally, is the reduction of bodily functions to minimal standards while supporting life. Life support systems may be used as adjunct body systems to further eliminate elapsed body time. In essence, body time is limited genetically. If body time can be slowed, then chronological time may become greater than elapsed body time.

Hormone Replacement Hormone replacement has been thought to retard total skin aging, impaired memory (and therefore senility), and declining vigor. It has become popular today among individuals seeking youth in latter years, but its practical use as an aging deterrent is still experimental (12). Do one's hormone-producing glands "wear out?" And if they do, will synthetic hormones replace those no longer produced? If this possibility were scientifically approachable, then it might have

Figure 3.7 "Honest, Ralph, this *really* works!"

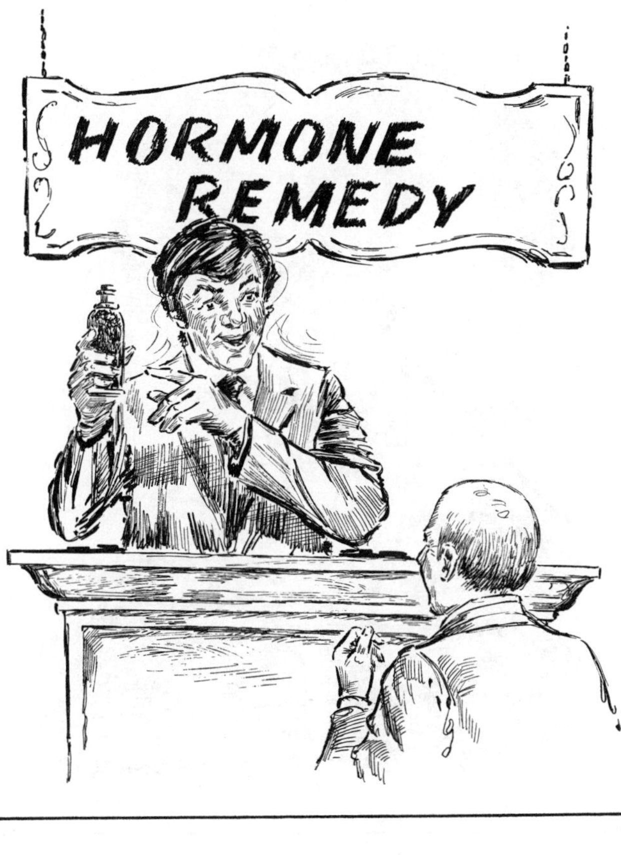

more promise than other theories. Can androgenic hormone replacements be the answer to maintaining one's masculinity?

Optimal Health Maintenance As mentioned in Chapter 1, the maintenance of physical and mental health to the highest level through diet, exercise, control of stress, and medical care is most often defined by health professionals as optimal health maintenance (20). Mental well-being may be obtained through meditation, philosophy, religion, love, and self-usefulness. Maximum physiological conditions may not always be the sign of optimal well-being. The total person must be considered. Cardiovascular and respiratory fitness must be examined in a

Figure 3.8

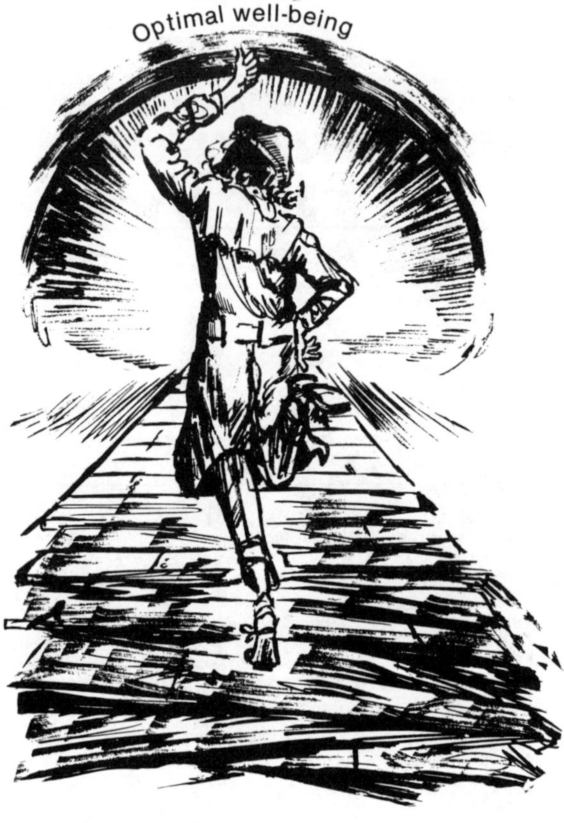

total fitness assessment without concentrating on an individual's physical appearance. All too often physical appearance is diagnosed as physical well-being. However, one's diet may be the basis for many physical problems and this will be discussed in Chapter 9.

High Oxygen Environment A high oxygen environment is said to compensate for reduced oxygen transport with age. As the individual ages, cardiovascular output decreases; therefore, one's oxygen supply to the various organs is diminished. The diminished oxygen environment is thought to be insufficient for vital cell reproduction. Once cell reproduction is inhibited, the aging process may accelerate. Conversely, it is hypothesized

Figure 3.9 Cloning may be a future means of reproducing oneself and thus extending one's longevity.

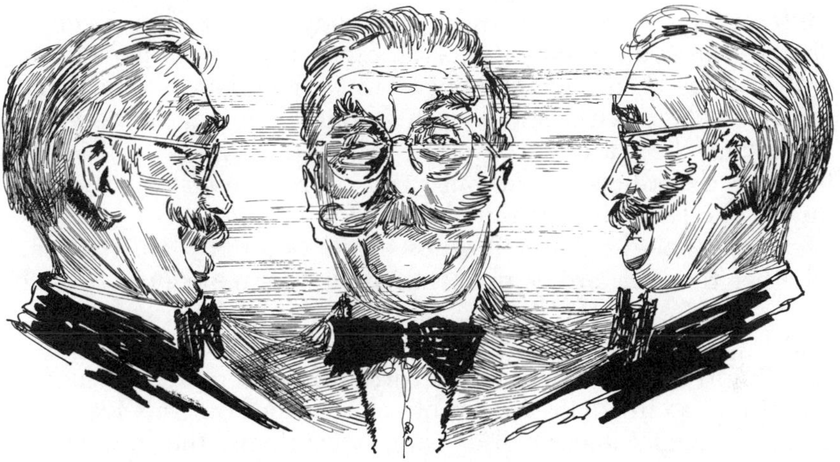

that supplying a high oxygen environment may inhibit this process.

Replication of Organs Replication of existing organisms through genetic manipulation such as cloning may be possible in the future, but can one consider this increasing or replacing one's longevity? *Cloning* has been acclaimed as a means by which to reproduce oneself asexually. Test tube research has indicated that this could be the "fad" of the future. Cloning experiments may replicate individuals vital to national affairs or persons needed for national defense. If such a process were developed and medically sanctioned, it would be theoretically possible to have a stand-in for the president of the United States. Absurd, yes, but possible.

Biorhythms and Disease It is thought that biorhythms are a matter of coincidence. Scores of internal cycles operate within the human body, each cycle peaking and dipping regularly during the course of the day. Both rhythmic cycles and the disturbance of these regular patterns may be important in medicine. The mere fact that a rhythmic cycle exists indicates any number of diagnostic and therapeutic practices. For example, it suggests that certain times of the day may be better than others for administering medication to patients.

Specific examples are cell mitosis and cancer. *Circadian rhythms* (often referred to as the body clock) have been observed in cell division (mitosis), especially in cells associated with surface tissue, which is constantly sloughing old cells and replacing them with new ones. The skin, ears, hair, and eyes are among these areas. The prime example is skin cells. Scientists feel that they show a peak rate of division during sleep, usually during the late hours of the night (8).

It is thought that cell mitosis follows a circadian pattern, whether the cells are components of skin tissue of organs, such as the liver, or of the nucleic acids. Some physicians suggest that in the case of cancer cells, in which the rate of mitosis is significantly greater than in the surrounding normal cells, one might find a circadian rhythm of cell division. But this is not the case. Although cancer cell division is rhythmic, the frequency of the rhythm varies widely. However, this does not seem to be the case with breast cancer; these cells divide according to daily rhythms (11).

A person who has a genetic predisposition to develop abnormal timing is like a poorly constructed watch that is likely to lose or gain time. The watch works for a while and then suddenly starts to break down, often for no reason at all. If this theory is correct, people who discover that they have such a tendency would have to take care to lead a carefully regulated life and avoid abnormal schedules. Thus, shift work, sleep reversal, and irregular hours would increase disease.

Mental Health Timing affects mental health in a great many situations, including periodic illness, stress and disruptions in rhythmicity, insomnia and sleep rhythms, and long-term disruptions caused by the continued process of aging. Each of these must be examined in order to understand the effects of mental health on longevity.

Periodic Illness There are notable periodic illnesses, including cases of periodic hypertension, psychosis, manic depression, and catatonia. German medical researchers have compared the rhythms of body temperature, urinary excretion, and other physiological functions among healthy and ill patients. They noticed that patients who had unusual sleep patterns manifested unusual 12-hour bodily function rhythms, as opposed to the daily patterns of healthy patients (17).

American researchers investigating periodic hypertension have noted a great regularity in the recurrence of symptoms (1). Physicians at Johns Hopkins University credit this to radical and unusual hormonal changes and irregular rhythms. Additionally, people suffering from depression also show abnormal rhythms. They seem to shift quickly from one stage of sleep to another in irregular or fully random patterns.

It has been thought that research on biorhythms and mental health will lead to numerous breakthroughs in psychiatry in the near future. It may well be one method with which to predict epileptic seizures or asthma attacks. However, are not these psychological and physical conditions dependent upon one's environment? Are biorhythms significantly reliable to be used in the determination of one's aging process and promotion of longevity? Only future research will provide the answer.

Summary

Longer life possibilities have exhibited diverse patterns worldwide, but few of these possibilities have proven valid. It is evident that senility is obvious among the total population but the degrees to which it manifests itself vary. Theories for extending life have suggested that senility as well as all other psychological and physical effects of aging may be eliminated.

References

1. Atchley, R. C. "Disengagement Among Professors." *Journal of Gerontology* 26 (1971):476–80
2. Bennett, R. "Social Context—A Neglected Variable in Research on Aging." *Aging and Human Development* 2 (1970):97–116.
3. Birren, J. E. *The Psychology of Aging*. Englewood Cliffs, N.J.: Prentice-Hall, 1964.
4. Blau, Z. S. *Old Age in a Changing Society*. New York: New Viewpoints, 1973.

5. Bruhn, J. G. "An Ecological Perspective of Aging." *The Gerontologist* 4 (1971):318–21.
6. Cain, L. D. *Life Course and Social Structure.* Chicago: Rand McNally & Company, 1964.
7. Clark, M., and M. Mendelson. "Mexican-American Aged in San Francisco." *The Gerontologist* 9 (1969):90–95.
8. Dale, Arbie. *Biorhythm.* New York: Pocket Books, 1976.
9. Dowd, J. J. "Aging as Exchange: A Preface to Theory." *Journal of Gerontology* 30 (1975):584–94.
10. Fower, A. "The Polity." In *Aging and Society,* Vol. 3, pp. 115–54. New York: Russell Sage Foundation, 1972.
11. Gittelson, Bernard. *Biorhythm.* New York: Warner Books, 1978.
12. Granich, M. "Factors Affecting Aging: Pharmacologic Agents." In *Developmental Physiology and Aging,* pp. 607–14. New York: Macmillan, 1972.
13. Gurbium, J. F. *The Myth of the Golden Years: A Socio-Environmental Theory of Aging.* Springfield, Ill.: Charles C Thomas, 1973.
14. Kuypers, J. A., and V. L. Bengtson. "Social Breakdown and Competence: A Model of Normal Aging." *Human Development* 16 (1973):181–201.
15. Laufer, R. S., and V. L. Bengtson. "Generations, Aging, and Social Stratification." *Journal of Social Issues* 30 (1974): 181–205.
16. Maddox, G. L. "Disengagement Theory: A Critical Evaluation." *The Gerontologist* 2 (1964): 80–82.
17. Neugarten, B. L. "Personality and the Aging Process." *The Gerontologist* 12 (1972):9–15.
18. Palmore, E. *Normal Aging.* Durham, N.C.: Duke University Press, 1970.
19. Reichard, S., F. Livson, and P. G. Peterson. *Aging and Personality,* New York: John Wiley, 1962.
20. Riley, M. W. "Social Gerontology and the Age Stratification of Society." *The Gerontologist* 12 (1971):29–87.
21. Schaie, K. W. "Age Changes and Age Differences." *The Gerontologist* 7 (1967):128–32.

22. "Themes and Issues in Sociological Theories of Human Aging." *Human Development* 13 (1970):17–27.

23. Timiras, P. S., ed. *Developmental Physiology and Aging.* New York: Macmillan, 1972.

24. Williams, R. H., and C. G. Wirths. *Lives Through the Years.* New York: Atherton Press, 1965.

PART TWO

Psychosocial Aging

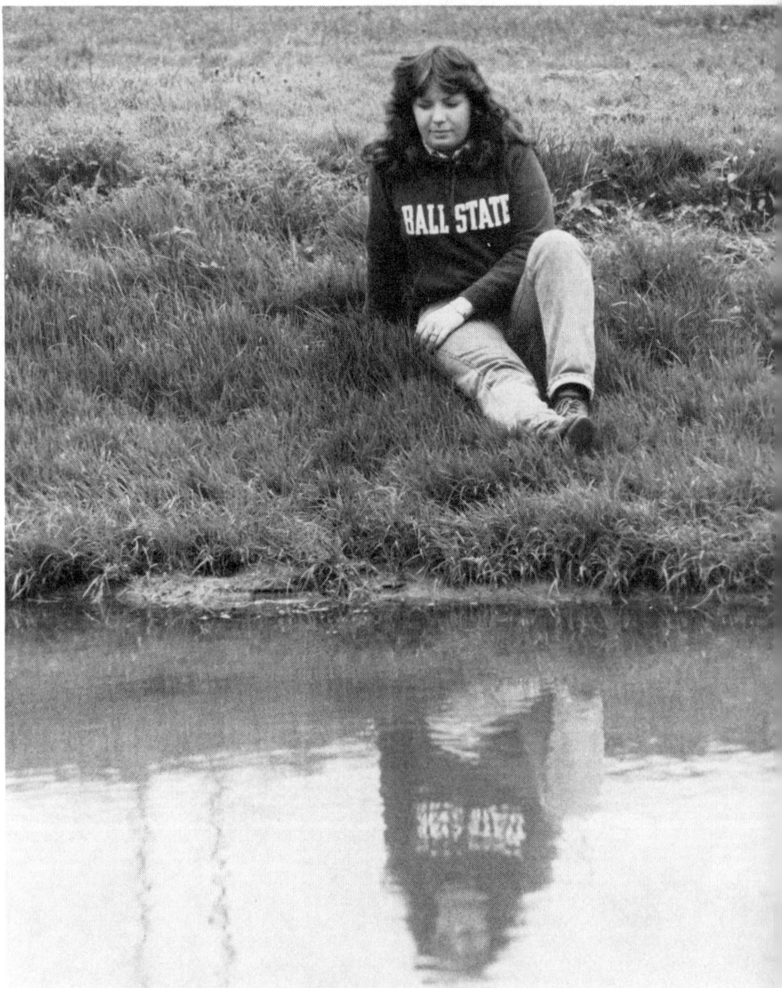
BALL STATE

■ Chapter 4

Positive and Negative Mental Health

Major Concepts

1. Mental health is a continuous process of adjustment to physical and psychosocial factors.
2. Deviations from mental health result from physical or emotional disorders.
3. Prevention and treatment of mental health problems involve a team effort.

Both real and imaginary perceptions, thought processing, and behavioral responses to specific situations describe the component of total health which deals with the mind. This dimension is called *mental health.* Mental health is an entity in itself, but at the same time it is influenced or it influences the social and physical dimensions of total health. From the time infants are aware of their surroundings until death occurs, this aspect of health is always present. Mental health can be positive or negative and it often fluctuates. It is directly related to experiences which occur in life.

People who are judged as being mentally healthy have learned to deal effectively with a variety of familiar and unfamiliar situations. First, mentally healthy people have learned to assess a situation objectively and to identify accurately the degree of threat it poses. Assessment is based upon one's perceptions and past experiences. Second, they identify feasible alternative responses to the situation, weighing the possible consequence of each. In unfamiliar situations they use imagination, intelligence, and common sense. Third, they take action.

Figure 4.1 The mentally healthy person can assess situations, identify reasonable alternative responses, weigh their consequences, and act as need be.

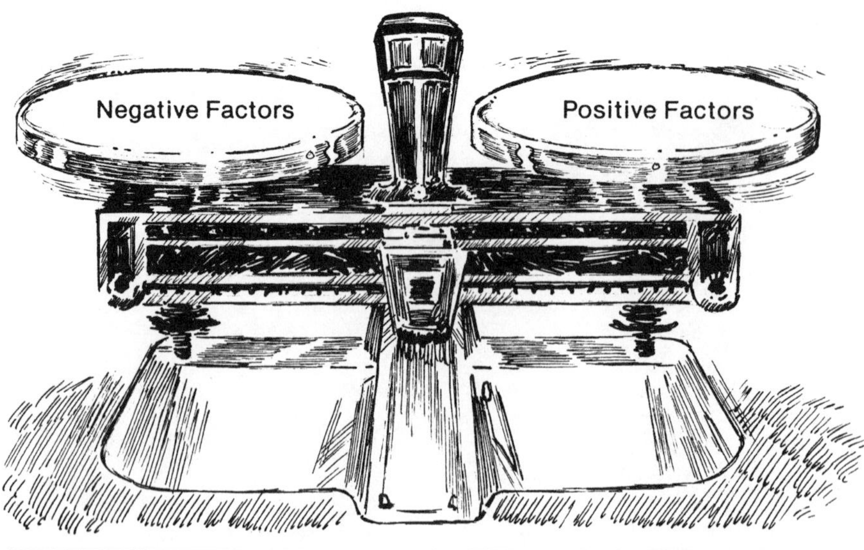

Finally, they assess or evaluate the success or failure of the action taken and store this information for later use. Individuals who do not learn this process, who continually fail and receive little emotional support often experience high levels of frustration, insecurity, low self-concept, low self-esteem, and eventually poor mental health. Mentally healthy people feel good about themselves, are able to meet the demands of life, and feel right about other people (20).

Each stage of life brings new situations requiring new responses. Children, adolescents, and young adults, for example, must respond to such things as beginning school, outstanding achievements, moving to a new school, parental arguing, separation or divorce, illness and poor health, failure in school, changes in parent occupation, and peer relationships.

College students are faced with being away from home for the first time, choosing a field of study, peer relationships, grades, finances, managing time, illness and poor health, and finding a job. These examples briefly illustrate the types of situations which generally are experienced in the early phases of the aging process. This chapter will discuss in detail the vast array of situations facing the middle and older aged individuals as they go through the later phase of the aging process.

The adjustments to the aging process can be categorized as being either physical or psychosocial.

Adjustment to Physical Components of Aging

Living Arrangements The environment in which a person lives can bring about physical and emotional responses and necessitates continuous adjustment. The college student who lives in a dormitory or shares off-campus housing is in constant contact with people. Social contact and making new friends, for most people, is an important part of developing as a person.

Being constantly exposed to other people often makes a person irritable, mentally tired, and tense. The likelihood of contracting a communicable disease is greater. When one is ill, it is more difficult to get the rest and relaxation needed to recover from the illness.

An example of the effects of being in close contact with

people and having no opportunity for privacy was seen in a Midwestern college in the late winter of 1977. The community in which the college was located experienced a severe blizzard. No one was prepared for the blizzard and everything in the community was closed for three days. No one could get in or out and everything came to a standstill. Students of all ages reported severe cases of "cabin fever." Hostility, tensions, and frustration levels increased. Good friends had arguments over trivial matters. The incidence of communicable diseases increased. It took several weeks before the emotional impact of the storm passed.

Reduced income plays a role in one's living arrangements. At the time of retirement many people own their own homes and have developed strong emotional ties to them. Unless individuals have given some thought to and prepared financially for retirement, they will find that the maintenance of a home may put a severe strain on their reduced incomes. According to the U.S. Department of Labor, Bureau of Labor Statistics, the greatest expenditure the retired adult will probably have is housing. In addition, poor health may also reduce the feasibility of remaining in the home. The decision to give up one's home is often painful. Many adults perceive owning their home as independence and there is a great deal of emotional security in being in familiar surroundings with personal possessions (9).

For the adult who lives in urban areas, leaving one's home may be a welcomed relief. The people living in urban areas or central cities frequently reside in substandard, unattractive housing and commonly live with pollution, noise, and social tension.

Older adults, especially in large cities, feel that one of their most serious problems is crime. Aging individuals are easy prey for gangs of youth who burglarize, purse snatch, assault, murder, and rape their victims. In a great many cases, the crimes are committed by youths under the age of 16 who know that if they are caught they will go to juvenile court where the penalty is much less severe than that of an adult court. In many cases, older adults will not identify or testify against their assailants because they fear retribution when the youths are released.

The older adult is afraid. Some have reported that they sleep during the day because they are afraid of being victimized at night. The once enjoyed time of taking walks for exercise and shopping has stopped. They lock themselves in their homes and apartments for protection. A critical time in the inner city is the

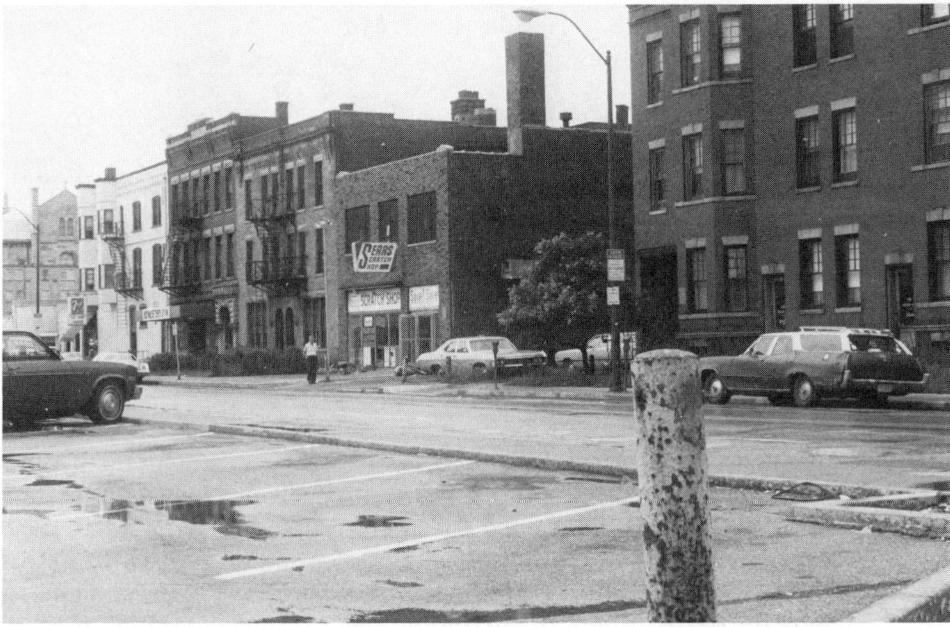

Figure 4.2 Unattractive housing, pollution, noise, and social tension too often characterize urban living.

day the social security check arrives, for that is the day many burglaries, purse snatchings, and muggings occur (29).

Across the country local programs are being implemented in an attempt to help older crime victims. Neighborhood Watch, a program that began in Los Angeles, teaches people to guard against burglaries and other crimes and how to look out for strangers. Wilmington, Delaware, has an automobile escort service. Milwaukee has neighborhood security aides who walk the streets in high-crime areas. New York City has a teen-age escort system. Police units are providing a variety of educational anticrime programs. Most of these programs are operated by volunteers who are concerned about the aged and the crime problem.

Another major problem facing the urban aged is what to do when the city decides to tear down old neighborhoods and rebuild. Without financial means and in the midst of urban renewal, these people are faced with the possibility of relocation.

What are these people to do? Where are they to go? One possibility could be to live with an adult child. In the United States only a few choose this alternative. When a parent who is in good health does choose to live with a family member, generally the arrangement is a successful one. Adult children report no changes in family routines and activities and the mental health of the older adult seems to be maintained. But this is not the case when the parent is over 75 years of age and in need of custodial care. Adult children report changes in family routine and increased strain and tension (19, p. 8).

When custodial care is needed, adult children may make the choice for their parents and place them in a nursing home or home for the aged. As pointed out in Chapter 1, only a very small percentage of older adults actually reside in nursing homes. The concern of both the adult children and the staff at the institution is that socioadjustment takes place and that the parent is able to integrate into and conform with various aspects of the institution. If an aging person does not adjust to the setting, socialization and integration will not occur. The degree of adjustment to this setting depends upon how much social isolation there was before the person entered the institution. Any social isolation appears to impede socialization. If an individual experiences involuntary isolation because of age or decreased health, he or she will feel a much greater degree of isolation when placed in an institution. Conversely, if the individual has lived most of his or her life in social isolation, he or she will feel much less isolation when placed in an institution (2).

Another possibility for the aging person is congregate housing. In the early 1950s the need for public policy on housing the aged became apparent, but no significant gains were made until the 1970s. The Housing and Urban Development (HUD) Act of 1970 authorized financing of congregate housing. The 1974 Housing and Community Development Act specifically defined congregate housing as:

> . . . low income housing (a) in which some or all of the dwelling units do not have kitchen facilities, and (b) connected with which there is a central dining facility to provide wholesome and economic meals for elderly . . . families (16).

The Act also directed the Department of Health, Education and Welfare to provide quality services and management that would meet the needs of the occupants, for example, medical and social services, transportation, and assistance with housekeeping. Most aging people who select congregate housing do so on the basis of how well it will meet their needs.

Congregate housing, unlike a nursing home, allows the participant to remain relatively independent while at the same

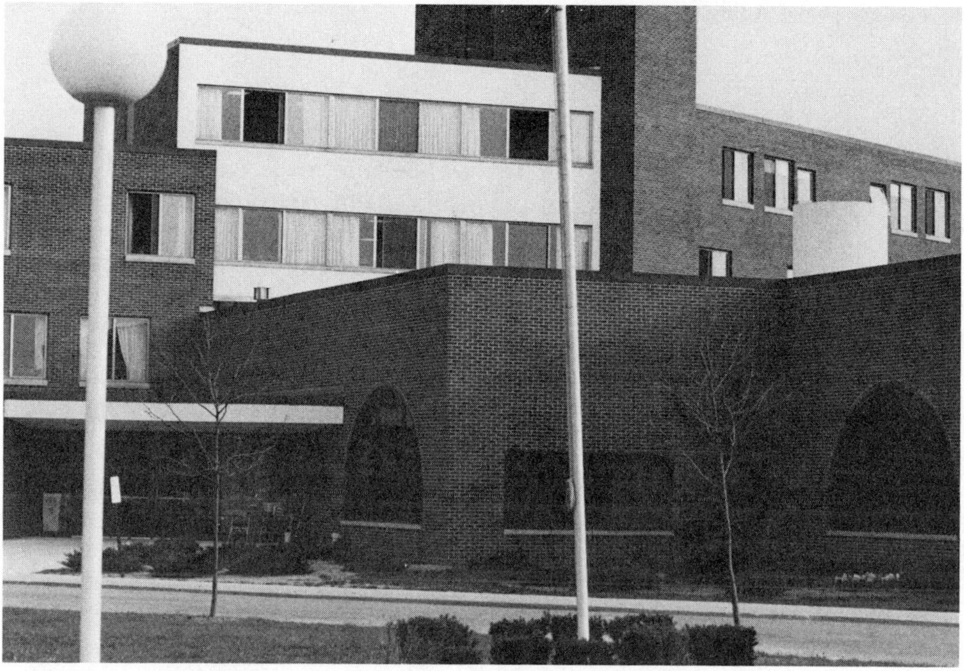

Figure 4.3 Congregate housing can offer the aged relative independence *and* easily accessible services.

time providing easily accessible services. The feelings and the mental health of those living in congregate housing appear to be relatively positive. Residents of such housing report greater satisfaction in being away from other people's children, being with people of their own kind, and being with people of their own age (27). Of course, this does not hold true for all adults.

Whatever the type of institutionalization, providers of human services must consider the possible development of mental skill atrophy. Myths and misconceptions perpetuate the notion that older people suffer memory loss and that they cannot learn. People who suffer brain damage usually exhibit marked memory loss. Not all older people suffer brain damage and/or memory loss. Most experience varying degrees of reduced visual and hearing acuity which affect the rate at which they pick up visual and auditory cues and respond to these cues. Because of the slowness of their responses and because they often lack the motivation or opportunities to use their minds, they are thought to be unable to learn. Educators are beginning to explore the possibilities of continuing education in institutional settings.

In an attempt to help aging adults remain in their homes and keep the cost of heating and repair at a minimum, federal, state, and local agencies have launched a variety of programs.

Funds from Title III of the Older Americans Act, Title I of the Housing and Community Development Act, and the Farmers' Home Administration under Section 504 of the Housing Act are being used to winterize the homes of aging adults. Nebraska, Maine, South Dakota, Wisconsin, and Pennsylvania are among the many states doing such things as insulating homes, installing storm windows and doors, caulking cracks in walls, repairing roofs, and establishing emergency fuel hot lines. Some states are having difficulties because of a lack of funds and the bureaucratic red tape.

Other forms of living arrangements that provide intimacy and bonding among individuals and that may or may not be sexual are neogamous arrangements. This includes cohabitation, polygyny, and communal living.

A small but increasing percentage of college students and young adults are experimenting with cohabitational living arrangements. The rationale for this behavior includes reducing expenses, sharing domestic chores, companionship, and learning about a potential mate before marriage. Those who are proponents of cohabitation feel that it is easier to dissolve this type of arrangement. Those who are against it, including many parents, feel that no useful insights can be gained. They feel that it takes many years of living together in marriage to understand a person.

Cohabitation for aging adults can be practical and at the same time meet emotional and intimacy needs. Older people who live together and are unmarried can maintain maximum social security benefits and widow's pensions, eliminate a child's fear of losing an inheritance, share household jobs, provide opportunities for closeness and sexual outlet for those who choose it, and alleviate loneliness.

Polygyny could help offset the imbalance of the sex ratio in the older population. Although illegal, it could provide the same practical and emotional needs as cohabitation. In addition, some authorities have pointed out other advantages, for example, obtaining group health insurance policies, better care of the sick, improved diets and housing, and the creation of a family network.

Communal living could cut housing and food expenses, better distribute domestic jobs, and provide companionship (8).

It is doubtful that neogamous lifestyles would be acceptable for today's general population of aging adults. First, the value system under which most aged people were raised and have lived with all of their lives would not permit it. Second, societal response to this type of behavior by aged adults would not be supportive. Today's young people may find that in the years to come neogamy may not only be an acceptable way to live but may also be a practical way to meet their physical, mental, and social needs.

Physical Health Impairment of health can be classified as acute conditions, those which are usually temporary, and chronic conditions, those which are long-term and may be permanent or leave disability. Young people most often experience acute conditions, for example, a cold or the flu. Older adults are less frequently afflicted with acute conditions. Most often they are bothered by chronic conditions. The most prevalent chronic health conditions found in the older adult are heart disease, hypertension, cancer, osteoarthritis, cerebrovascular accidents (strokes), and osteoporosis. All of these conditions will be discussed in detail in subsequent chapters. In analyzing the effect of illness in relationship to mental health, it is important to examine the degree of activity restrictions and the attitude of those afflicted with health problems.

As has been previously discussed, being able to maintain independence, to take care of personal needs and to maintain self-esteem and self-concept are extremely important as a person ages. Many adults have grown up believing that they are strong, independent, and productive individuals. The acceptance of illness is difficult and often denial of any health problems relieves the fear of becoming dependent upon someone else.

Activity restrictions are greatest for persons who have cardiovascular illnesses. More males have restrictions due to heart disease, and more females have greater restrictions due to arthritis. In almost all health conditions, activity restrictions increase as age increases.

Restricted activity as a result of a heart condition can be extremely detrimental for the middle-aged male because at this time in his life he is reaching a peak in his career. Our society values work. Work heeds accomplishment and self-identity. If an individual values the work ethic, then the inability to continue activities brings about frustration and anxiety. This is true for the arthritic female when she is less able to carry out her responsibilities at home and at work.

Social level and attitudinal factors are important variables in an individual's personal assessment of health. In the Duke University Longitudinal Study, Maddox reported that the subjective rating of health in two out of three respondents was in agreement with the objective evaluation of medical personnel (13). The remaining one-third of the subjects were not in agreement with medical personnel and were evenly divided between being optimistic and pessimistic about their health. For example, if individuals were viewed as being optimistic about their health, their subjective evaluation was good but their medical evaluation was poor. If they were viewed as being pessimistic, their subjective evaluation was poor but their medical evaluation was good.

In this study, both optimism and pessimism seemed to be related to two factors: (1) social level and (2) attitude. Those individuals who were older, had nonmanual occupations, were relatively active, were male, and had maintained their major lifetime work were rated as optimistic. These factors were not seen in the pessimistic subjects. The optimistic individuals also showed higher morale and an absence of preoccupation with health (14).

Physiological Change Throughout life all people are continuously adjusting to physiological change. The teeth of the infant erupt; later in childhood they are shed and new teeth appear. Although these changes are minor, they do require adaptive behavior of some kind. At adolescence, youth experience sudden spurts of growth that require adjustment to longer arms and legs. At the same time, they experience many other pubescent changes that require some degree of adaptation. As individuals progress through life, various deteriorations occur. For example, hearing acuity begins to decline in the thirties, visual acuity in the forties, and muscular strength peaks in the mid-twenties. Consequently, as specific structures in the body begin to function less efficiently, people develop adaptive behaviors to compensate for the loss. It is apparent that people in each developmental level move, think, and react a little slower than those in younger levels.

By the time a person reaches the sixties and seventies, adaptive behaviors to physiological decline are much more prominent. For example, a person might use one sense to compensate for the loss of another or rely on past experience to fill in gaps of sensory loss. It does take the older person longer to collect sensory data, to interpret data, and to respond accordingly. Most older people are cautious because they do not want to make mistakes. The slowness and cautiousness are often misinterpreted by younger people who label the older people as being mentally rigid, having declining intelligence, being unable to learn, and being senile.

Sleep Patterns and depth of sleep are characterized by: REM (rapid eye movement, characterized by high brain waves), NREM (nonrapid eye movement, characterized by slow brain waves), and stage four EEG (high-voltage, low-wave brain activity, which is considered deep sleep).

During the various stages of sleep the physiological functions of the body are diminished. During sleep the heart beats more slowly, respiration decreases, body temperature declines, nearly all gland secretions diminish, and the muscles relax. In addition to the rest and relaxation sleep produces, sleep is a time of recuperation, repair, growth, and regrowth.

During childhood (ages 5 to 10) the total sleep time changes very little and the proportion of REM to NREM varies between 25% and 30%. During adolescence the total sleep time decreases steeply and the proportion of REMs to NREMs stabilizes at 25%. Stage four EEG, or the deepest sleep, is maximal at age 5, declines slightly in later childhood, and declines steeply during adolescence. The proportion of REMs to NREMs, as well as total sleep time, remains fairly constant between the ages of 20 and 60. Stage four EEG declines by 50% from age 20 to 50.

Spontaneous awakenings are not often seen in childhood and adolescence. During the adult years, beginning about age 40, the awakenings become more frequent and the amount of time in bed spent awake begins to increase. In old age the frequency and time awake are greater than they have ever been. The aging adult will experience sleep interruptions about every hour. In addition, stage four EEG is virtually absent. Poor health, anxiety, and fear can also interfere with the sleep patterns of aging adults. They compensate for the interrupted sleep either by (1) spending more time in bed to achieve the total amount of sleep similar to that of the young adult or (2) by consuming excessive amounts of prescribed sleep medications (28).

Psychosocial Components of Mental Health

Psychosocial aging deals with social and psychological factors. It includes feelings about age, marriage and widowhood, employment and retirement, crime, prejudice, sexuality, and stress.

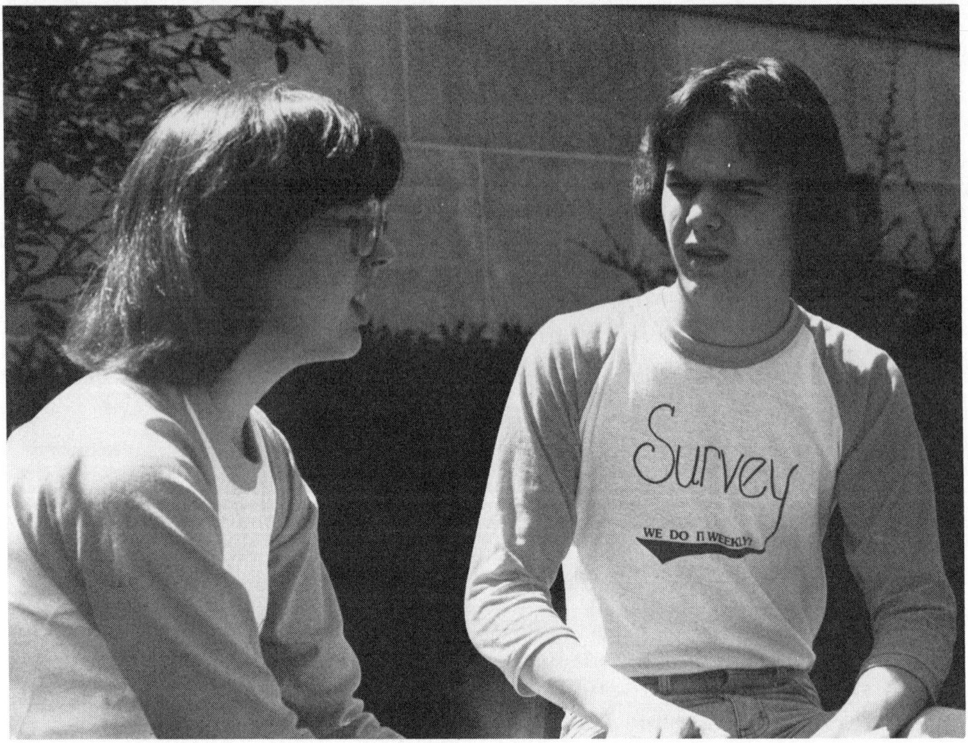

Figure 4.4 Adolescents must adjust to new freedoms and new responsibilities governed by their own decision-making.

Throughout life continual adjustment to chronological age occurs. In the early years children are told "act your age." The child dutifully responds, "Yes, Mommy," but does not really know what "act your age" means. In adolescence, values are developing and teen-agers are beginning to seek independence. There is rebellion against parental authority. Statements such as "Don't you trust me?" and "I'm old enough to do that!" are heard frequently. In young adulthood people are establishing patterns that will eventually become their life behaviors. They are consciously or unconsciously seeking a mate, deciding on a career, marrying, and having families. No longer are they at an age at which parents make all of the decisions. They are at an age which necessitates independent decision making. Up until age 35 or 40 most people have been continuously adjusting to age-related situations. For the most part, a child, adolescent, or young adult has no concrete thoughts about being old. Life is a daily experience; there are plans for the future and a long life. Most realize that they will someday be "old," but this is generally an abstract idea.

Middle Age The realization of aging generally occurs in the period called middle age. Middle age is generally considered to be between the ages of 40 and 60. It is the time in life when the body begins to change and different social roles and societal expectations of the middle-aged person occur.

There are innumerable outward physical changes that begin to be noticed in middle age. The body's metabolism begins to slow down and unless the individual monitors his or her caloric intake and energy expenditure the "middle age spread" becomes quite noticeable. Many men and women find it frustrating when their physical selves do not keep pace with their mental abilities. Skin changes become apparent as wrinkles develop around the eyes and on the neck. Hair begins to turn grey and sometimes to thin. When the eyes begin to fail, glasses are required.

All of these changes are a normal part of the aging process. Some people find the changes devastating and turn to the many products on the market which cream the face, improve the body, cover the grey hair, and so forth. The marketplace is abundant with legitimate, as well as questionable, products which are supposed to enhance a youthful appearance. Other people accept their physical changes as inevitable and are not bothered to any great extent.

Even though in American Society the denial of death is pervasive throughout life, during the middle years an individual becomes aware that life is approaching its end. Death becomes more of a real possibility. Peers, friends, and parents are dying and the individual frequently realizes that he or she may be next in line. Death is more often in the minds of men since they usually die earlier than women do. Females tend to be more concerned about the possibility of their husband's death.

Roles and expectations begin to change. Children become adults and leave home. Although one will always be a mother or father, once children become adults the parental role changes. Some women sit home and wonder what to do with themselves while other women go back to school or get a job and assume a new life role. Men, however, are often reaching a plateau in their careers and begin to think positively or negatively about retirement. Some are nervous and fearful about retirement while others look forward to it and begin to plan for it.

Society expects each age group to behave in specific ways in accordance with its age. For example, it is acceptable for middle-aged people to jog three miles a day, but it is less

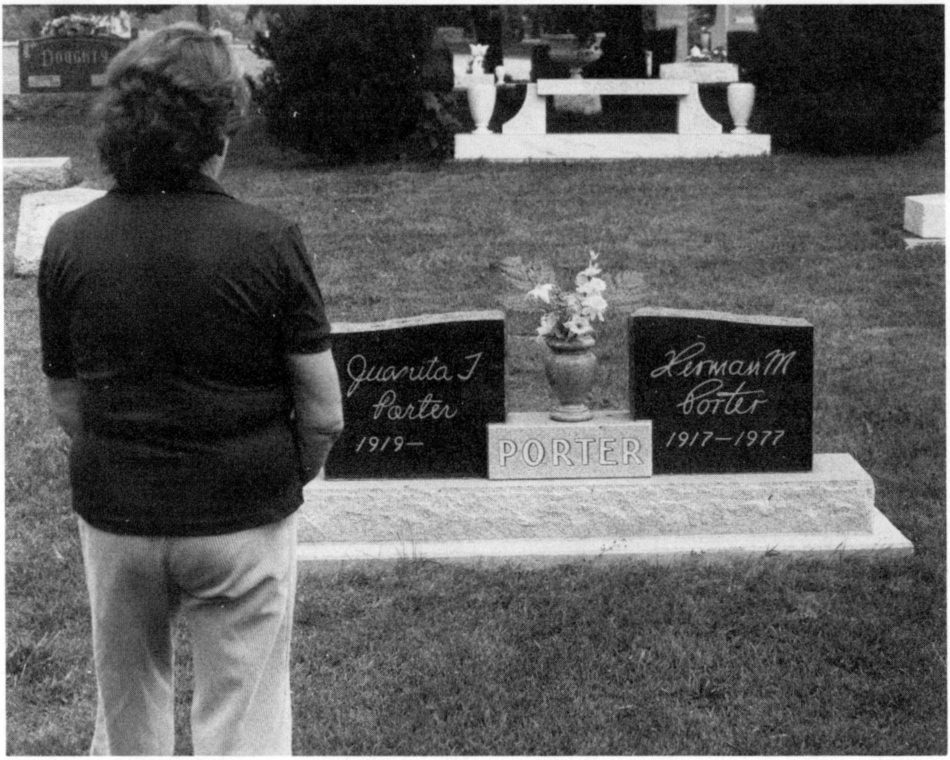

Figure 4.5 Death is the undeniable end of the aging process.

acceptable for them to go to the local discothèque and perform the latest dance. In all likelihood, jogging and dancing will improve both the physical and mental aspects of health, but disco dancing is generally considered an activity of youth, not of middle age. Middle-aged people often find themselves conforming with society's expectation rather than risking ridicule and embarrassment by doing what they enjoy.

Some people become overwhelmed when they realize that their parents are aging and that they might be called on to provide assistance. It is difficult for some because they still perceive their parents as being dependable instead of dependent. In some cases, adult children resent and are openly hostile to parent dependence and this leads to guilt.

Middle age is also the time when men and women take stock of their lives and evaluate marriage, career, personal relationships, and long-standing values. It is not uncommon to see drastic changes in the lives of the middle-agers. In the 1970s these drastic responses were labeled the *mid-life crisis* (15).

Mid-life crisis is associated with the climacteric. Female mid-life crisis is associated with multiple factors. It is the postparental period during which children leave home and it is the time when husbands are busy with their careers. It is not uncommon for a woman in her mid-forties to early fifties to experience severe bouts of depression and feelings of purposelessness. To compound her mental discomfort, menopause and all of its myths signal the end of youth. She may feel old, ugly, and sexually unappealing.

The symptoms of menopause are both subjective and objective and fall into three categories:

1. Autonomic and vasomotor symptoms: "hot flashes," chills, sweats, and hypertension.
2. Neurological and psychosocial symptoms: headaches, dizziness, irritability, emotional and nervous instability, impairment of memory, loss of a sense of well-being, and periods of depression.
3. Somatic symptoms: changes in the reproductive system, disturbances of joints and bones, diabetes, changes in skin especially on the neck and face, and greying and drying of the hair.

A general understanding of menopause, along with medical supervision and sometimes supplementary hormone therapy, helps to alleviate the physical and mental discomfort during this period of life. Middle-aged women going through menopause generally have a more positive viewpoint toward it than younger women who are not experiencing it (21). In other words, once a female begins to experience menopause, she begins to accept it and the changes that go along with it. Chapter 5 will discuss in greater detail the physiological aspects of menopause.

Middle-class women often find new roles to substitute for old ones, for example, more education or a new career. Lower-class women may not experience the same emotional upheaval that her middle-class peer does because less is expected of her in terms of establishing her own identity. In all likelihood, she will not expect intimacy with her husband and may have closer relationships with grown children and grandchildren (21).

Male mid-life crisis is also associated with the climacteric. Men do not experience the degree of physiological and hormonal changes as do women. The climacteric of the male is mostly an attitudinal and psychological change rather than a physical change. There are several contributing factors. For example, most

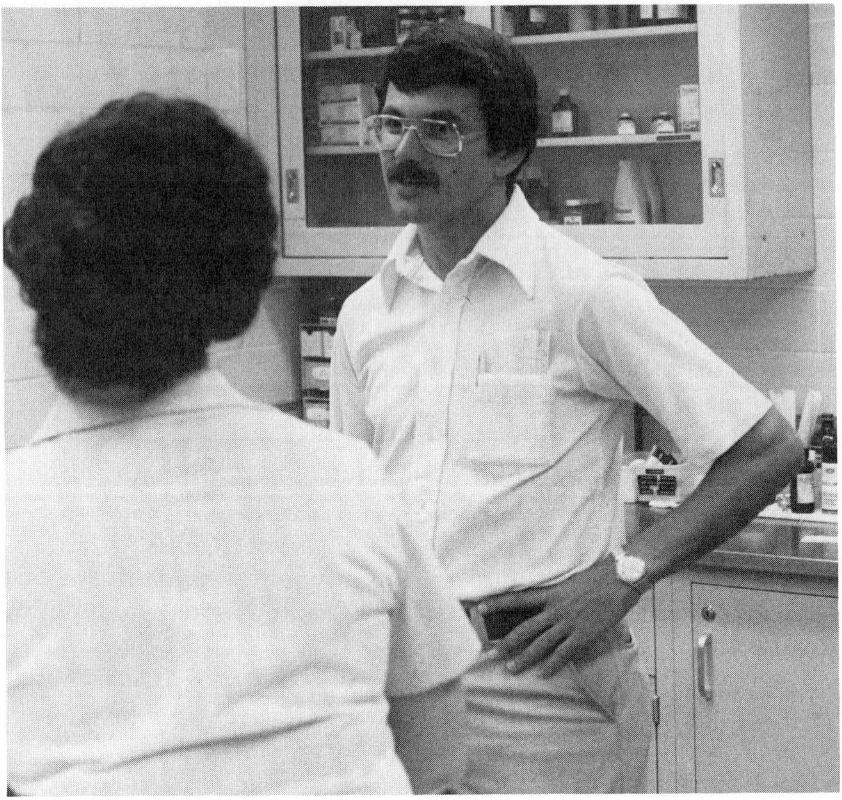

Figure 4.6 An understanding of menopause, along with medical supervision and sometimes supplementary hormone therapy, can help to alleviate the physical and mental discomfort during this period of life.

men have reached a peak in their careers and realize that any occupational movement will be either lateral or a demotion. Some are called "old fogies" by younger workers. The middle-age man may suspect that his younger counterparts are eager for his job. Sometimes a younger and better educated man is given more opportunity than the older worker with all of his years of experience and past accomplishments.

The home situation may also add to the male mid-life crisis. The middle-age man may see himself as the "forgotten male." He may feel that he is being taken advantage of. He frequently is forced to interact with a menopausal wife who is having her own problems and may no longer devote as much time to his needs.

Any number of reactions may take place during this time. The male may take stock of his life, feel negative about it, leave his position, family, and everything familiar to him, and start a new life. Some men blame their wives for their own shortcomings and failures. Her faults, real or imaginary, are blown out of proportion and she may no longer be attractive to him. The male who has always thought of himself as having sexual prowess may, as his sexual performance begins to diminish, seek a younger woman. To protect his ego and restore his perceived sexual prowess, he invariably selects a female 10 to 20 years younger than himself and one from a lower socioeconomic level who thinks he is a "good catch" (7). Of course, not all men respond in the above ways, but statistics increasingly indicate that this behavior is becoming more frequent in our society. Many men evaluate their lives, adjust to and accept them, and continue to live the best they can.

Marriage, Widowhood, and Remarriage The adjustment to marriage in later life seems to be very difficult to assess objectively. The literature is filled with contradictory findings that provide few definite conclusions. Analysis of research since the early 1950s indicates that there are two schools of thought on later-life marriage. One analysis suggests that following the initial years of marriage there is a gradual decline in marital adjustment throughout the life cycle. Another analysis suggests that there is a decline in marital adjustment following the initial years, a leveling off, and then increased adjustment during the postretirement years.

All authorities agree that adjustments to marriage occur throughout marital life. Typical factors which require adjustments for the aging adult are retirement, relationship changes from romance and passion to companionship, reduced income, decreased levels of health, and decline in sexual activity. The degree to which these and other factors influence marital adjustment appears to be strongly influenced by the personal makeup of each individual. Therefore, it is impossible to suggest specific steps that can be followed to achieve successful adaptation to marriage in later life.

In any marriage it is inevitable that one partner will have to adjust to widowhood. Women tend to assume this role more frequently than men. For years women mentally rehearse for this role. Most of them know that they will outlive their husbands, and with the death of a friend's spouse they go through a mental process of how they will feel, of making funeral arrangements, and so forth. However, nothing can prepare them for the real experience. When their husbands die, they typically experience grief, loneliness, depression, insomnia, and irritability.

There are three patterns of adjustment to widowhood. One pattern of adjustment is seen in the woman who has a history of social involvement, who is involved in many activities, has developed problem-solving skills, and has flexible social roles. She can usually reexamine her lifestyle and goals and reorient her activities into personally gratifying areas. A woman who has relatives and peers or who has many neighborhood friends can usually continue these relatonships with little change. This is especially true of the lower-class urban woman and suburban woman who has lived in a sex-segregated environment and has never developed multifaceted relationships with her husband.

A second pattern of adjustment to widowhood is seen in the woman who has been passive most of her life, has relied upon her husband, and has not developed any interests and circles of friends of her own. This woman generally becomes socially isolated. This pattern can also be seen in widowers. There are, however, some differences between men and women. Men generally are financially more secure and seem to have a better chance of finding a new partner. Some men seem to become more dependent upon their wives for personal needs and do not establish a circle of friends in whom they can confide. Instead, they confide in their wives. Women usually confide in several female friends as well as in their husbands.

The third pattern of adjustment to widowhood is remarriage. Many men and women will choose to remarry after being widowed for a while. They most often give their reasons for remarriage as needing companionship, alleviation of anxiety about poor health, or to avoid dependence upon their children. Additional reasons cited by women are a desire to take care of someone and the need for intimacy (17).

The success of remarriage depends upon several factors. The approval of children and friends is very important. Children will readily give their approval if they are sure that their parent is acting prudently and if there is no concern over a loss of inheritance. Another important factor is the length of time the couple has known each other. McKain (17) found that the couples in his study had known each other at least 11 years prior to their marriage. Many times couples knew each other socially during their first marriages. Sufficient income, especially if both can contribute something, also adds to successful remarriage.

Finally, each must be reasonably adjusted and feel comfortable with his or her life. Today more and more couples are making the choice to remarry rather than live alone.

Sexual Adjustments "Grow old along with me, the best is yet to be," wrote Robert Browning. How true this could be for every aging man and woman. At last they have reached the age when the fear of interruption by a child, fatigue from a hard day's work or the everyday stresses and strains of making a living, providing transportation for the children, and finding "enough time to do everything" are history. This is the ideal time of life to renew the fun and pleasure derived from an intimate sexual relationship. Society, however, with its stereotypical attitudes, continues to reinforce the notion that the aging adult is asexual, unable, and uninterested. Cartoons, jokes, and slogans continue to perpetuate this idea.

Over the past few years research has given us enough information to dispell the myths about sexual activity in later life. In the late 1940s Kinsey pioneered research in this field. Although his sample included few older adults, he concluded that most men in their sixties were sexually capable and that there was little evidence that showed sexual decline in women until very late in life (11, 12). As a result of the Duke University Longitudinal Study, researchers found that the sexual drive remained constant throughout life. In other words, if the sex drive was strong in youth, it was also strong in old age. The researchers found that the degree of activity began to decline in the sixties but interests did not decline until after age 75. Marital status had little effect on activity and interest in aging men. Unmarried women reported little to no activity, but 20 percent still remain interested. In general, men appeared to be interested and had a greater degree of activity than women, regardless of marital status. Both men and women attributed the cessation of sexual intercourse to males, with the median age for stopping being 68 for males and 60 for females (22).

In 1969 a pilot study was conducted to determine the attitudes of different age groups of adults toward each generation's sexual knowledge, desire, skill, capacity, attempts, opportunities, access, and frequency. The results showed a stereotype with no variation among the age groups. The aged saw themselves as below average in all areas of sexuality, the middle aged saw themselves as average, and the young saw themselves as high average in sexual knowledge and desire and average in other sexual aspects (6).

The research clearly indicates that interest, desire, and activity remain relatively high in older age groups but the attitude or feelings of all age groups remain negative. It is not uncommon for physicians or other medical personnel to see aging persons who are suffering high levels of guilt and anxiety because they still have sexual thoughts and interests. These negative feelings are the result of continuous reinforcement of the negative attitudes of other people. For example, adults who live with their children or in institutionalized settings are provided with no privacy or are segregated by sexes or are told "don't make a fool of yourself' or called "a dirty old man" or "dried up old maid."

Authorities know that in most instances there is no physiological reason for the cessation of sexual intercourse until perhaps very late in life or unless persistent health problems exist. The physiological changes and the implications for continued sexual activity will be discussed in Chapter 5. In this section the concern is with the mental adjustments to this aspect of life.

Self-concept, self-esteem, and sex are closely related. In order to maintain self-concept, self-esteem, and sex, and consequently mental health, doctors, nurses, social workers, and any other personnel working with aging adults must change any negative attitudes of their own and then seek ways to assist older people in dealing with their own fears, apprehensions, and lack of knowledge. It is hoped that these health personnel can then dispel the guilt and apprehension that aging people often experience. If they can accomplish this, the aging adult may possibly live a more fulfilled life.

Mona Wasow has prepared a booklet specifically for the aging adult in which she clearly discusses the various aspects of sexuality in later life (28). The booklet concludes with the following statement:

> This book was written for those of you who would like to use it, and enjoy. Sex should be a pleasure, not a chore (31).

Employment and Retirement Continued full-time employment in the labor force by older workers presents advantages and disadvantages to society and the economy of the country. Some of the advantages are listed below:

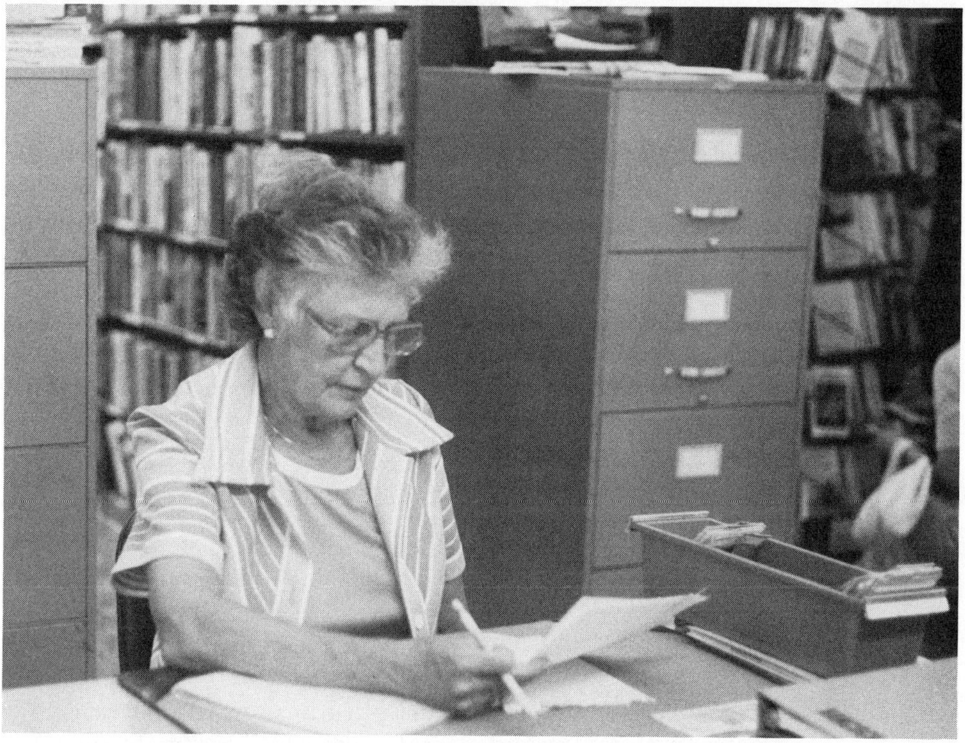

Figure 4.7 Continued full-time employment of older workers involves both advantages and disadvantages (see text).

1. Continued employment provides relief to the social security system and younger workers who help support the rapidly increasing older population.
2. Continued employment helps to reduce the retiree's feelings of living a life that has no meaning, of uselessness, and of despondency, which consequently lead to poor health.
3. Continued employment provides gains in national product in added labor force participation by older workers.

Large corporations argue that having a fixed retirement age helps them when they need to remove older workers whose job performance is unproductive and that it provides the opportunity to promote younger workers so that they will not seek other jobs. In the next few years economic, social, and financial forces will insist that the government and business world change the mandatory retirement age.

The person who retires today has an average of from 10 to 15 productive years remaining. As the rate of inflation and cost of living continues to escalate, retired workers, even those who have social security and private pensions, run the risk of nearing the poverty level.

Did You Know?

- that the social security benefit formula provides a retiring worker who has earned (each year) a benefit amount equal to the median wage with a retirement benefit equal to about 46% of earnings just prior to retirement?
- that if a worker has a nonworking spouse, the replacement rate jumps to almost 70%?
- that the median earnings before retirement are based on an average for workers at all stages of their earning career (i.e., for all age groups) and that average was about $8800 in 1976? (It is not based upon the average $12,000 median income of a 1976 retiree.)
- that a recent social security study showed that private pension funds provided male recipients a 25% or more replacement of earnings pension and females 20%?
- that the replacement rate for a two-worker couple could easily fall below 40%?
- that the higher earnings of a two-worker couple are not replaced proportionally by higher social security benefits?
- that if a single worker takes an early retirement, the social security replacement rate drops to about 26%, that the rate drops to about 45% for a one-worker couple, and to less than 45% for the two-worker family?
- that the private pension supplement which boosts the replacement rate is not available to all people? (26)

If you answered yes to all of the above questions, you did better than many administrators of social security programs and most all of the prospective retirees. The social security system is constantly changing in an effort to keep pace with the changing economy.

Not all prospective retirees dread retirement. Many look forward to a time when they can choose how to spend their time, whether it is beginning a second career, fishing, building furniture, or volunteering their time to help someone else. In 1977 people under age 72 receiving social security benefits could work part-time and earn up to $3000 a year without losing their full benefit payment. For every $2 above the $3000 maximum, $1 of social security payment was deducted. If a person earned less than $250 in one month, he or she was eligible for the full monthly social security benefit payment.

There are many ways that aging adults can earn money and maintain their self-esteem and self-concept. The U.S. Department of Labor allocated $15.2 billion in 1977 to state governors for 3800 part-time jobs for low-income persons over 55 years of age. Another example is a program authorized under the Older Americans Comprehensive Services Amendment of 1973 called Senior Companions. The purpose of the program was to provide needed services to people living in institutions and to disabled people living in their own homes. It also was aimed at involving aging adults in meaningful roles in the community while supplementing their incomes.

To qualify as a companion, the participant has to be sixty and have an income of not more than $3157 if single or $4107 if married. The participant works about 20 hours a week and earns $1670 a year plus lunch, transportation, and a medical exam. Participants report positive feelings because they are able to help others. A survey of 1000 participants who evaluated the program revealed that as a result of their involvement 80% were happier and 85% felt financially secure.

Another example of resourcefulness in retirement is Vic Peterson. He had always been interested in trees, especially evergreens. Knowing that the average Christmas tree would take up to eight years to grow, he planted seedlings seven years before his retirement in 1958. In 1971, at the age of 74, he personally cut, loaded, and sold 400 trees. By 1973 he owned a plantation of 20,000 trees. Mr. Peterson was confronted by his brother who called him an "old fool" and asked why he planted the trees at age 76 when in all likelihood he would never live to market them. He replied that he was well aware of that but while still alive he could watch the trees grow and that was the "greatest and most satisfying reward one has a right to expect" (32).

Discrimination and the Aging Female Vital statistics indicate that women outlive men and that older women have lower incomes, have poorer housing, are more often widowed, are less frequently employed, have lower paying jobs, and more frequently live alone. Only a few women have been able to rise above these facts and dispel the ever-perpetuated discrimination that most women experience. Helena Rubinstein, Grandma Moses, Martha Graham, Helen Hayes, Lucille Ball, and Maggie Kuhn are examples of women of various ages who for one reason or another are viewed as exceptional. The vast majority of women have low visibility and only when something newsworthy happens does their plight become known.

The media have perpetuated discrimination against aging women. Advertising has shown aging women promoting products for vitamin deficiency, constipation, or products that make her job easier at home. The logical conclusion is that age brings vitamin deficiencies or constipation. Television programs generally are directed at younger women and seldom do writers and producers present programs that realistically portray the aging woman, especially the woman of any class other than the middle class.

Two important factors contribute to the media picture. First, the American public spends many hours watching television. For some, television is a means of escaping from the realities of their own lives. Television is a good escape because the viewer is seldom required to think about what is being viewed. In any case, most of them do not want to be confronted with the negative realism of life. Second, advertisers pay exorbitant fees to advertise their products on national television. Why should they realistically portray the plight of the aging female and risk angering the American public which purchases the products being advertised?

The emotional impact of and the response to this discrimination vary. If a negative, stereotypical picture is presented for a long enough time, women will believe what they see. Thus, women often discredit themselves. If women are described as obedient, asexual, unemployable, and unintelligent, then society, and especially women, will believe it. In an attempt to change this picture and maintain a feeling of self-worth, women will respond in several ways. Some will dress and behave as their younger counterparts in an attempt to recapture youth. Others, lacking male companionship, will compensate by idolizing their sons or grandsons, competing with other females for the remaining males, or expressing their jealous feelings by becoming troublesome mothers-in-law. Some women turn to religion and others join clubs and charities.

Representatives of television and other forms of media are

not unaware of the problem. The University of Michigan–Wayne State University Institute of Gerontology 26th Conference on Aging dealt with the topic of aging women in America. Representatives of the media indicated that television producers were eager for materials and ideas that could be used for programs.

This gradual metamorphosis was seen in *All in the Family's* female character, Edith, who gradually changed from a passive, subservient, and unthinking wife into a woman who began to think for herself and occasionally speak out. Bea Arthur played the role of Maude, an outspoken middle-aged female. Commercials are beginning to show women in positive family situations, riding motorcycles, and being "on top" of contemporary issues. These represent only a small number of changes. It seems inevitable that the media and commercial advertisers will have to change their approach and programming if they are to attract the older viewing audience who will, in the next 30 years or so, comprise the majority of viewers and consumers.

Stress The stress state is a response to a physiological or psychosocial event or stressor. It is obvious that the aging adult experiences a wide variety of stressors. The degree to which these stressors stimulate the stress state depends upon individual personality factors and the degree of threat perceived.

Research over the last few years indicates that any kind of change, whether it is positive or negative, results in a degree of the stress state. The higher the stress state and the longer the duration, the more likely it will negatively influence physical and mental health. According to an article in *The New York Times,* widows and widowers die ten times more frequently during the first year of widowhood than do others their age. The grief and bereavement are too stressful (4, 10). The illness rate for divorced persons is 12 times greater in the year following divorce than for married persons (4).

The Social Readjustment Rating Scale lists 43 life events or stressors (see Table 4.1). The scale was constructed by having people of different ages, cultures, and walks of life rank the relative amount of adjustment necessary for various life events (19). This instrument can estimate the likely amount of stress for various life events, but it cannot take into consideration the differences in stress tolerance.

As discussed earlier in this chapter, the mentally healthy

Table 4.1 Stress Associated with Change

Events	Scale of Impact
Death of spouse	100
Divorce	73
Marital separation	65
Jail term	63
Death of close family member	63
Personal injury or illness	53
Marriage	50
Fired at work	47
Marital reconciliation	45
Retirement	45
Change in health of family member	44
Pregnancy	40
Sex difficulties	39
Gain of new family member	39
Business readjustment	39
Changes in financial state	38
Death of a close friend	37
Change to different line of work	36
Change in number of arguments with spouse	35
Mortgage over $10,000	31
Foreclosure of mortgage or loan	30
Change in responsibilities at work	29
Son or daughter leaving home	29
Trouble with in-laws	29
Outstanding personal achievement	28
Wife begins or stops work	26
Begin or end school	26
Change in living conditions	25
Revision of personal habits	24
Trouble with boss	23
Change in work hours or conditions	20
Change in residence	20

Table 4.1 *(continued)*

Events	Scale of Impact
Change in schools	20
Change in recreation	19
Change in church activities	19
Change in social activities	18
Mortgage or loan less than $10,000	17
Change in sleeping habits	16
Change in number of family get-togethers	15
Change in eating habits	15
Vacation	13
Christmas	12
Minor violations of the law	11

Source: T. H. Holmes and R. H. Rahe, "The Social Readjustment Rating Scale," *Journal of Psychosomatic Research, 11* (1967), 213–18.

person has learned to assess a situation, choose a way to respond, act on the choice, and then evaluate the success or failure of the action. This mentally healthy person also uses the same process in coping with various physical or psychosocial stressors. The inability to cope with stress is probably the result of a lifelong pattern.

Many mechanisms are used to ease the discomfort of the stress state. Alcohol is one. It is difficult to determine the exact number of men and women who become addicted to alcohol in later life. It is known that some adults will turn to alcohol because of grief, depression, boredom, pain, or loneliness. Residents of a nursing home can easily become addicted to alcohol when family members bring it to them either openly or in disguised containers. Sometimes staff members can be bribed to get drinks for their patients.

Because young people outnumber older people, their misuse of drugs receives much more publicity and attention. There prevails an image of what older people are supposed to be like and few perceive the older person as having a drug problem.

Drug misuse in the older people is described as ". . . a

departure from rational therapeutics, an unwholesome reliance on drugs as the solution for all problems . . ." (13). Advancing age brings changes in physiological function and abilities of the body and changes in social relationships. Thoughts very often turn toward body changes and decreasing health. The need for medical assistance and drug prescriptions increases with age. It is within this context that drugs are often misused by the older person.

Most of the time drug misuse is unintentional. Multiple health problems require multiple medications, that create a problem because there are differences in absorption, distribution, metabolism, and secretion of a drug and because there are alterations of action at receptor sites (23). Lack of knowledge about the drugs being taken and the importance of proper intake pattern and the risks of deviating from the prescription influence the unintentional misuse of drugs.

Little research has been done to conclusively establish the reasons for the intentional misuse of drugs in older people. It is supposed that the stresses of getting old, the loss of status, the feelings of uselessness, and the loss of health are all contributing factors (25).

The most common and usually inadvertently misused prescription drugs are anti-anxiety drugs like Equanil, sleeping pills, and pain pills. Deliberately misused over-the-counter drugs include such things as aspirin, laxatives, and bromides (25).

Because available data on the older drug misuser are limited, providers of health services are confronted with the issues of early identification and treatment of drug problems, including alcohol, in the older population. For further information on drug problems in the older age group, the reader is directed to specific readings listed at the end of this chapter.

Suicide is another way to cope with perceived unsurmountable stress. Suicide ranked ninth as a cause of death in 1976. The rate for white males surpassed that of females of both white and other races, as well as males of other races. The highest rate of suicide is found in the 75 to 84 age group (18). Vital statistics indicate that the suicide rate for the older adult is higher than for any other age group (30). The elderly are much more effective at committing suicide than are the young (1, 3, 24). Depression and failing health are probably the most common reasons for suicide in later life.

Common Emotional Problems

Family and friends seem to attribute the peculiar behavior of aging to senility. In some cases this is true. But, as with all other stereotypes, it is unfair to generalize that all aged people whose behavior is unusual are senile. Poor mental health is caused either by functional disorders or by organic brain disorders. These disorders are discussed in the following pages.

Functional Disorders Functional disorders are generally diagnosed as being either neurotic or psychotic. A neurosis is a condition that is characterized by anxiety brought on by unresolved, unconscious emotional conflict. Although neuroses are common in later life, they are not necessarily inevitable. A psychosis is a condition that is characterized by delusions, hallucinations, inappropriate behavior and attitudes, and reduced ability to control impulses.

Neurotic disorders are seen in people of all ages. In many cases, a neurosis in later life is simply an extension of behavior that was overlooked when the person was younger.

Psychosomatic Disorders. The psychophysiological disorders, also called *organic neuroses,* result in physical symptoms caused by emotional events. Common symptoms of organic neurosis in adults are itchiness of the skin, psychogenic rheumatism, frequency of urination at night (nocturia), cardiac neurosis with fear of sudden death, irritable colon, and hyperventilation.

Hypochondriasis. When an individual is overconcerned about his or her emotional or physical health and frequently has bodily complaints for which there are no physical basis, the individual is said to be a *hypochondriac.* There are no physical problems to be treated, but there is a need to determine and treat the emotional factors that created the need for the complaints. People of all ages use hypochondriasis as a way of avoiding problems. Butler and Lewis described the functional use of hypochondriasis as a way to interact with other people, to displace anxiety, relieve guilt through personal punishment, to punish others, and to regulate relationships with others (5, p. 64).

Depression. Factors that contribute to chronic depression in later life are declining physical health, physical disabilities that interfere with communications, and the loss of social roles resulting from changes in the family structure and retirement.

Depression, which is the most common mental health problem in later life, is characterized by feelings of guilt, boredom, and loneliness. In severe cases of depression other symptoms include hypochondriasis, loss of appetite, insomnia, constipation, and impotence.

Anxiety. An exaggerated sense of trouble or danger, nameless dread, or a sense of threat are characteristics of anxiety. Feelings of dependence, worthlessness, abandonment, and anger can increase anxiety. The symptoms of anxiety are also manifested in physiological responses such as impotence, rapid heart beat, excessive sweating, restlessness, and muscular tenseness.

Psychotic problems include paranoia, manic-depressive illness, involutional melancholia, and latelife schizophrenia.

Paranoia. Isolation, disfigurement, blindness, and deafness are the primary factors in the development of paranoia. Paranoid states usually result from feelings of grandioseness or persecution and they may be observed in changes and disturbance of mood, thinking, and behavior. Severe arthritis and the decreased ability to discriminate visual and auditory stimuli can precipitate paranoia in aging men and women.

Manic-depressive Illness. Women tend to experience manic-depressive illness more frequently than do men. It is characterized by severe swings or shifts in mood from elation to depression. During the elation or manic period the individual experiences elation, self-assertive aggression, and grandiose delusions. The most extreme response in the manic phase is violence toward others. In the depressive stage the individual may experience either agitated depression characterized by sustained tensions, overactivity, despair, and apprehensive delusions or retarded depression characterized by slowed or reduced activity, feelings of sadness, dejection, self-depreciation, and self-condemnation. The extreme response to depression is suicide. Manic and depressive states may be mixed in a single phase or alternate regularly.

Involutional Melancholia. This is generally observed between the ages of 48 and 60 when signs of aging become apparent. It is observed more frequently in women, especially after the menopause. Symptoms include insomnia, restlessness, loss of appetite and sexual desire, worries about health, and feelings of worthlessness, self-condemnation, and guilt. Both involutional melancholia and manic-depressive illness are classified as affective psychoses.

Table 4.2 Types and Descriptions of Schizophrenia

Simple	Gradual reduction in external relationships and interests. Shallow expression of emotion. Thinking tends to be simple and on concrete things rather than abstractions.
Hebephrenic	Inappropriate emotional reactions, silly or bizarre behavior, delusional beliefs and perceptions in the absence of the usual stimuli (hallucinations).
Catatonic	Striking changes in body movement. Extreme compliance, mutism, and loss of all voluntary activity are common. Sometimes inactivity may be interrupted by episodes of excessive movement and excitement.
Paranoid	Unrealistic, illogical, and hallucinatory thinking and bizarre delusions of being persecuted or of being a great person. Usually seen in later life.
Schizo-affective	Characterized by moods of elation and depression not usually seen in other forms of schizophrenia.
Undifferentiated	Behavior and thinking are disturbed but not sufficiently distinctive.
Pseudoneurotic	Predominant neurotic behavior but with brief psychotic episodes.

Adapted from "Psychoses," in *Encyclopaedia Brittanica,* 15th ed. (1974), Volume 15, p. 174.

Late-life Schizophrenia. Schizophrenia is characterized by signs of withdrawal from the environment. Two developmental patterns may be seen in the aging adult. One pattern is called *chronic schizophrenia.* It usually develops when the person is young and it continues into later life. The other pattern, called *late-life schizophrenia,* usually develops in conjunction with chronic brain syndrome. Table 4.2 outlines the seven types of schizophrenia.

Organic Brain Disorders Organic brain disorders are of two types. Acute brain syndrome is a secondary condition brought on by some other generally correctable problem. Acute brain syndrome is also known as *reversible brain syndrome* (RBS). Chronic brain syndrome (CBS) involves those problems which affect the brain and are irreversible.

Acute Brain Syndrome. In this classification of brain disorders the levels of awareness fluctuate, ranging from active delirium to mild confusion. Other characteristics may include:

1. Visual hallucinations
2. Anxiety
3. Uncooperativeness
4. Restlessness
5. Dazed expression
6. Aggressiveness
7. Disorientation
8. Mistaking one person for another
9. Delusions of persecution

Many factors contribute to reversible brain syndrome. Diabetic acidosis results from the shortage of effective insulin. Symptoms include nausea, vomiting, reduced blood serum and carbon dioxide levels, shallow and rapid respiration followed by deep overbreathing, and finally coma. Circulatory collapse can result from dehydration and salt depletion. If the acidosis is not corrected in time, the result is that the reduced oxygen to the brain temporarily creates confusion, disorientation, and other symptoms of mental impairment.

Emphysema, a lung disease in which the tissue loses its contractability and elasticity, can result in an ineffective exchange of oxygen and carbon dioxide. Consequently, the blood contains low levels of oxygen. When the brain is deprived of oxygen, disorientation, confusion, and unconsciousness can occur.

Congestive heart failure results in the heart's declining ability to pump adequate amounts of blood. Consequently, the lack of sufficient oxygen, as well as nutrients, to the brain causes a state of mental confusion.

In a cerebrovascular accident (CVA) a temporary lack of blood supply results in an inadequate supply of oxygen to the brain. The effects of the CVA depend upon the length of time the brain is without oxygen and the particular location in the brain where the oxygen supply is decreased. The effects of a CVA range from acute confusion to the loss of speaking ability, paralysis, or death. "Little strokes" commonly occur before a major stroke occurs. Symptoms are passing confusion, nausea, vomiting, dizziness, and numbness of the extremities.

Improper or prolonged use of prescribed medications can produce both reversible and irreversible brain disorders. The steroids, for example, can bring on manic or depressive moods. Health conditions such as declining kidney function may react negatively to even small amounts of drugs. Thiazides, used as diuretics, may lead to dehydration and a confused mental state. Certain drugs used for Parkinson's disease and arthritis can result in psychotic behavior. Some anesthetics, for example, halothane and methoxyflurane, may affect the liver or kidneys resulting in dehydration and mental confusion (5, p. 80).

Chronic Brain Syndrome. Chronic brain syndrome (CBS) is irreversible; that is, once there is brain damage, the individual is left with a permanent mental disability. CBS has been called senility by many laymen. Any unexplained mental deterioration, including conditions of acute brain syndrome, has been inappropriately labeled senility. The two most common types of CBS are senile dementia, also called senile psychosis, and psychosis associated with cerebral arteriosclerosis.

The major characteristic of senile dementia is a very gradual decline in brain function. In the early stages apathy, lack of interest, inability to think abstractly, error in judgment, and decline in personal care are commonly seen. As the condition worsens, the individual becomes disoriented as to time, place, and people, hallucinates, has rambling incoherent speech, and frequently is restless and unable to sleep. Paranoia may develop. Ultimately, senile dementia is fatal, usually taking five years but occasionally taking up to ten years.

Unlike the gradual decline of senile dementia, cerebral arteriosclerotic psychosis is an erratic downward decline of brain function. Cerebral arteriosclerotic psychosis is attributed to the vascular damage that occurs as a result of arteriosclerosis and atherosclerosis. Men more frequently experience this type of psychosis, and the average age of onset is 65.

The onset of symptoms can be either gradual or sudden. In the beginning dizziness, headaches, decreased mental and physical vigor, and vague physical complaints are most common. Intellectual disability does occur but it is gradual. Impairment of memory is sporadic. A typical pattern is difficult to describe because each case is different. Other health problems such as heart conditions can greatly change the symptoms of those who also have cerebral arteriosclerotic psychoses.

■ Mental Health Services

One of the main concerns of mental health personnel is the prevention of mental health problems before they start. Public and private schools are beginning to implement mental health curricula at all grade levels. The public broadcasting system (PBS) is making its contribution by producing public awareness programs. Grants from large corporations have provided funding for mental health programs such as the *Inside/Out* film series for upper-elementary students and the *Self-Incorporated* film series for junior high school students. Both series have been designed to assist young people in developing life-coping skills. These programs may help the future generation, but the immediate problem is identifying the millions of adults who are in need of mental health services and establishing programs to meet their needs.

Identifying individuals who need help, especially those in the middle or older age group, presents several problems. Social service employees generally have very high caseloads, and working with impaired aged adults demands a large amount of the caseworkers' time. Little time is left for identifying others in the community who are in need of help.

The attitudes of caseworkers and other personnel also inhibit the identification and treatment of aged adults. For example, if the caseworker fears growing old, it will be difficult for him or her to work with the aged, infirmed adult. Or the caseworker may be unable to resolve a conflict with his or her own aging parents. Some personnel feel that they are wasting their time working with aged people because they will not live very much longer. To complicate the matter, many aged adults do not want help. Many were raised in an era in which accepting help from the government was not socially acceptable. They resist mental health intervention because they fear losing their independence, they fear change, and they are often suspicious of such services.

One of the goals of the mental health services for aged adults is to keep them in their home environment. It has been

Table 4.3 Resources for a Community Multidisciplinary Team

Nursing Services	Registered nurse Licensed practical nurse Home health aides Visiting Nurse Association
Therapeutic Services	Physical therapists Occupational therapists Speech therapists
Nutrition Services	Food Stamp Program Meals-on-Wheels Group Dining Title VII Nutrition Programs
Health Services	Medical doctors and specialists Dentists
Social Services	Social workers Clergymen Policemen Government officials Volunteers Paraprofessionals

suggested that the best way to accomplish this is by using a multidisciplinary team to deliver a variety of services. It is essential that there be a team coordinator so that maximum benefits and services can be given to those who need them. Table 4.3 lists a variety of services and personnel found in most communities who could work on a multidisciplinary team.

Another valuable community resource is the vast array of programs that utilize the services of the aging adult. By using aged adults two things can be accomplished. First, the participants in the programs experience a sense of fulfillment in being able to help others less fortunate than themselves. Second, the programs provide the community with needed manpower at no local expense because the programs are federally funded. Table 4.4 outlines seven volunteer programs and describes the purpose of each program.

It is inevitable that some people who have functional and organic brain syndrome will require institutionalization. However, recent reports from the U.S. National Institute of Mental Health indicate that in the last 20 years mental health personnel and the

Table 4.4 Volunteer Programs for the Elderly

Volunteer Program	Purpose
RSVP (Retired Senior Volunteer Program)	Funds for volunteer program in public and nonprofit institutions; volunteers reimbursed for travel and meal expense
VISTA (Volunteers in Service to America)	Volunteers for one to two years in community projects in United States; small salary to cover living expenses
SOS (Senior Opportunities and Services Programs)	Services in programs to meet the needs of older people: nutrition, consumer education, outreach, employment, information, and referral
Green Light	Community service
Senior AIDES	Community service
Senior Community Service Program	Community service
Senior Community Service Aides	Community service

general public have recognized the need for outpatient psychiatric services and the importance of keeping the patient in a home environment. In 1955, 74% of those needing treatment obtained it in inpatient facilities. By 1975 the percentage had dropped to 28 (see Table 4.5).

Through the combined efforts of social services, government programs, advisory groups, and community residents, many aged people can be identified and helped and still remain at home.

■ Summary

Maintaining mental health requires a continuous balance of positive and negative situations. The aging adult adjusts to the physical components of mental health, such as living arrangements, impaired health, physiological changes, and changes in sleep patterns and to the psychosocial components of mental health, such as middle age, marriage, widowhood, remarriage, sex, employment, retirement, discrimination, and stress.

Table 4.5 Percentage of Patient Care Episodes [1] by Type of Treatment Facility for 1955 and 1975

Inpatient Services Mental Hospitals	1955	1975	Outpatient Services	1955	1975
Total	77.4	27.9	Total	22.6	72.1
State and County	48.9	9.3	Community Mental Health Centers [5]	N/A	24.7
Private [2]	7.3	2.6	Other	22.6	47.4
General [3]	15.9	8.8			
VA [4]	5.3	3.3			
Community Mental Health Centers [5]	N/A	3.9			

Source: U.S. National Institute of Mental Health, *Utilization of Mental Health Facilities,* 1971, Series B, No. 5 and unpublished data.

[1] Patient care episode is defined as the number of residents in inpatient facilities or as the number of persons on the rolls of outpatient facilities, plus the total additions of both types of facilities during the year.
[2] Includes estimates of episodes for care in residential treatment centers for emotionally disturbed children.
[3] Hospitals (non-VA) with psychiatric inpatient units.
[4] Veterans Administration.
[5] Federally funded.

The inability to cope with these changing components and/or physiological changes in the brain result in functional or organic disorders.

The prevention, detection, and treatment of mental health problems require a multidisciplinary approach that takes advantage of the expertise of many people. The trend today is to keep the mental patient in the home environment.

■ Selected References on Drug Problems

Books

1. Exton-Smith, A. N., and Overstall, P. W. *Guidelines in Medicine—Geriatrics.* Vol. I, Chapter 16. Baltimore: University Park Press, 1979.

2. Kayne, R. C. "Drugs and the Aged." In *Nursing and the Aged,* edited by I. M. Burnside. New York: McGraw-Hill, 1976.

3. Kayne, Ronald C., ed. *Drugs and the Elderly.* Berkeley, Calif.: The Ethel Percy Andrus Gerontology Center, University of California Press, 1978.

4. Mishara, Brian L., and Kastenbaum, Robert. *Alcohol and Old Age.* New York: Grune & Stratton, 1980.

5. Peterson, David M., Whittington, Frank J., and Payne, Barbara P., eds. *Drugs and the Elderly Social and Pharmacological Issues.* Springfield, Ill.: Charles C Thomas, 1979.

Periodicals

1. Beardon, William O., Mason, J. Barry, and Smith, Edward M. "Perceived Risk and Elderly Perception of Generic Drug Prescribing." *The Gerontologist* 19 (1979):191–95.

2. Bender, A. D. "Pharmacodynamic Principles of Drug Therapy In the Aged" *Journal of the American Geriatric Society* 22 (1974):296.

3. Cohen, S. "Drug Abuse in the Aging Patient." *Journal of Studies on Alcoholism* 37 (1975):1455–60.

4. Freeman, J. T. "Some Principles of Medication in Geriatrics." *Journal of the American Geriatric Society* 22 (1974):289.

5. Glassock, Janet Ashton. "Rehabilitating the Older Alcoholic." *Aging* (Sept.–Oct., 1979):19–24.

6. Krupka, Lawrence R., and Vener, Arthur M. "Hazards of Drug Use Among the Elderly." *The Gerontologist* 19 (1979): 90–95.

7. Melmon, K. L. "Preventable Drug Reactions—Causes and Cures." *New England Journal of Medicine* 284 (1971):1361–67.

8. Peterson, David M., and Whittington, Frank J. "Drug Use Among the Elderly: A Review." *Journal of Psychedelic Drugs* 9 (1977):25–36.

9. Schuckit, Marc A. "Geriatric Alcoholism and Drug Abuse." *The Gerontologist* 17 (1977):168–74.

10. Snyder, Phyllis K., and Way, Ann. "Alcoholism and the Elderly." *Aging* (Jan.–Feb., 1979):8–11.

■ References

1. Atchley, Robert C. *The Social Forces in Later Life*. Belmont, Calif.: Wadsworth, 1972.
2. Bennett, Ruth. "Social Isolation and Adjustment in a Home for the Aged." In *Research on the Mental Health of the Aging*, p. 1. Washington, D.C.: National Institute of Mental Health, U.S. Department of Health, Education and Welfare, 1977.
3. Benson, R., and Brodie, D. "Suicide by Overdoses of Medicine Among the Aged." *Journal of the American Geriatric Society* 23 (1975):304–308.
4. Brody, Jane. "Doctors Study Treatment of Ills Brought on by Stress." *New York Times*, 10 June, 1973.
5. Butler, Robert N., and Lewis, Myrna I. *Aging and Mental Health*, 2nd ed. St. Louis: C. V. Mosby, 1977.
6. Cameron, P. C. "The Generation Gap: Beliefs About Sexuality and Self-Reported Sexuality." *Developmental Psychology* 3 (1970):2.
7. Cohen, Frederick. *Understanding Human Sexuality*, pp. 57–58. Englewood Cliffs, N.J.: Prentice Hall, 1974.
8. Dressel, Paula L., and Avant, W. Ray. "Neogamy and the Older Person." *Alternative Lifestyles* 1 (1978):13–36.
9. Hamovitch, M. B., and Peterson, J. E. "Housing Needs and Satisfactions of the Elderly." *The Gerontologist* 9 (1969): 30–32.
10. Kastenbaum, Robert J. *Death, Society and Human Experience*, pp. 241–65. St Louis: C. V. Mosby, 1977.
11. Kinsey, A. C., Pomeroy, W. B., and Martin, C. R. *Sexual Behavior in Human Male*. Philadelphia: Saunders, 1948.
12. ———. *Sexual Behavior in the Human Female*. Philadelphia: Saunders, 1953.
13. Krupka, Lawrence R., and Vener, Arthur M. "Hazards of Drug Use Among the Elderly." *The Gerontologist* 19 (1979): 8–11.
14. Maddox, George L. "Self-Assessment of Health Status." Normal Aging—*Reports from the Duke Longitudinal Study*,

1955–1969, pp. 350–62. Durham, N.C.: Duke University Press, 1970.

15. Mayer, Nancy. "The Male 40's: A Turmoil of Doubt and Discontent." *The Washington Star,* 11 June, 1978.
16. McFarland, M. Carter. "The Emergence of a New Concept—Congregate Housing for the Elderly. *Aging* (Feb.–March, 1976):8.
17. McKain, W. C. *Retirement Marriage.* Storrs, Conn: Storrs Agricultural Experiment Station, University of Connecticut, 1968.
18. *Monthly Vital Statistics Report, Final Mortality Statistics, 1976.* Washington, D.C.: U.S. Department of Health, Education and Welfare, 1978.
19. Morgan, James N. "Effects of Aging on Housing and Living Arrangements." *Research on the Mental Health of the Aging.* Washington, D.C.: U.S. Department of Health, Education and Welfare, 1977.
20. National Association for Mental Health. "Mental Health Is 1,2,3." New York, n.d.
21. Newgarten, B. L., Wood, V., Kraimes, R. J., and Loomis, B. "Women's Attitudes Toward Menopause." *Middle Age and Aging,* pp. 195–200. Chicago: University of Chicago Press, 1968.
22. Palmore, Erdman, ed. *Normal Aging Reports from the Duke Longitudinal Study, 1955–1969,* pp. 277–303. Durham, N.C.: Duke University Press, 1970.
23. Peterson, David M., Whittington, Frank J., and Payne, Barbara P., eds. *Drugs and the Elderly Social Pharmacological Issues.* Springfield, Ill.: Charles C Thomas, 1979.
24. Pfieffer, E. "Psychopathology and Social Pathology." In *Handbook of the Psychology of Aging,* edited by J. Birren and E. Schaie. New York: Van Nostrand Reinhold, 1977.
25. Schuckit, Marc A. "Geriatric Alcoholism and Drug Abuse." *The Gerontologist* 17 (1977):168–174.
26. Schulz, James. "Pension Adequacy and Pension Costs." *Aging* (Jan.–Feb., 1978):15–21.

27. Sherman, S. R., et al. "Psychological Effects of Retirement Housing." *The Gerontologist* 8 (1968): Part I.

28. Timiras, P. S. *Developmental Physiology and Aging*, pp. 520–21. New York: Macmillan, 1972.

29. U.S. Department of Justice. *Myths and Realities About Crime.* Washington, D.C.: U.S. Government Printing Office, 1978.

30. U.S. Public Health Reports, National Center for Health Statistics. *Final Mortality Statistics* 25 (1977):14.

31. Wasow, Mona. *Sexuality and Aging.* Madison, Wisc.: School of Social Work, University of Wisconsin, 1976.

32. ———. "W E Retiree, 76, Has Career in Live Christmas Trees." *Aging* (Jan.–Feb., 1973):5.

PART THREE

Physiological Aging

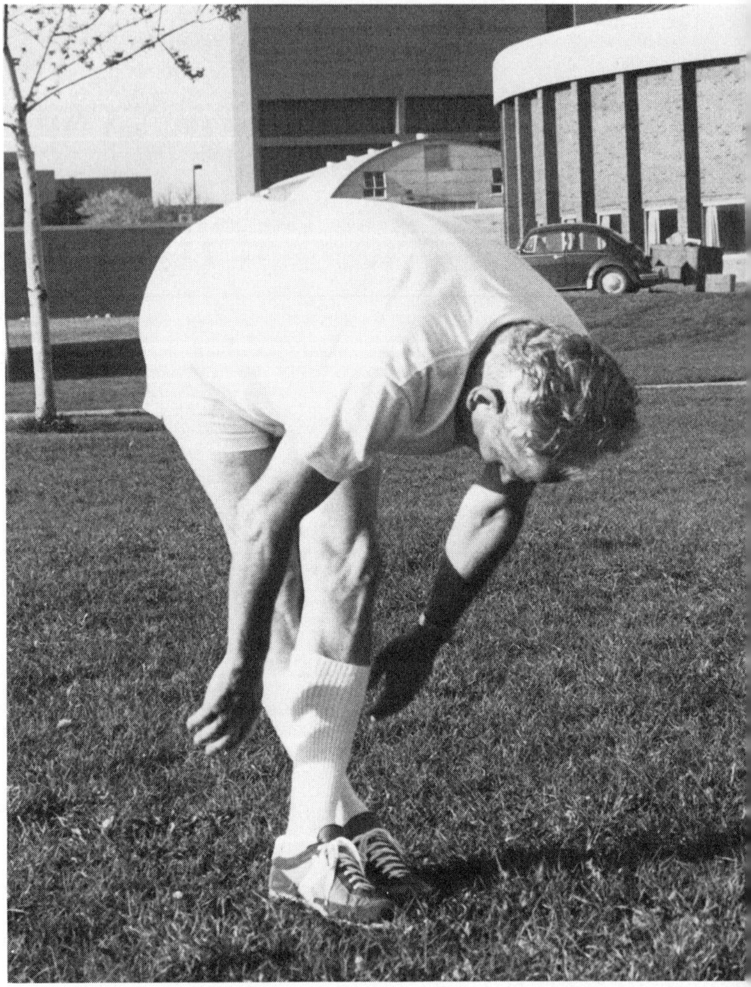

■ Chapter 5

Body Changes

Major Concepts

1. Physiological degeneration and changes take place in most body organs and systems.
2. Certain physiological changes may not be totally related to chronological age.
3. Regardless of preventive measures, various physiological changes are inevitable.

Nowhere to Go But Old

I'm old
And I'm going to get older.

O my God,
Seriously,
It just hit me.
All along I've been acting as if old age were the flu.
Or a sprained ankle,
Painful, inconvenient, but something I'd get over
Which is not a bad way to act.
But I can't act that way any more.
Because I'm suddenly struck, laid low and weighed down
With the truth.
I'm old and I'm going to get older.
There is no alternative.
There is nothing that can be done about it.
So I don't have to look for alternatives.
I don't have to try to do something about it.
A liberating thought,
If you look at it that way.
Help me to look at it that way.
Help me to rejoice in the freedom of letting You run the show.

Anonymous

Concern with problems surrounding recent medical advances continues to mount within the medical profession and the lay community. Organ transplants have contributed sharply to the level of interest in the prolongation of life and the degeneration process. Nonetheless, radical surgical interventions are only one of a large number of medical advances that have extended the physicians' control over the degenerative process and eventual self-destruction. In turn, greater control over life and death has increased the number of decisions that doctors have made on the prolongation and termination of life and on the allocation of medical resources. Moreover, changes in the degenerative

Figure 5.1 Some individuals become confused about life direction.

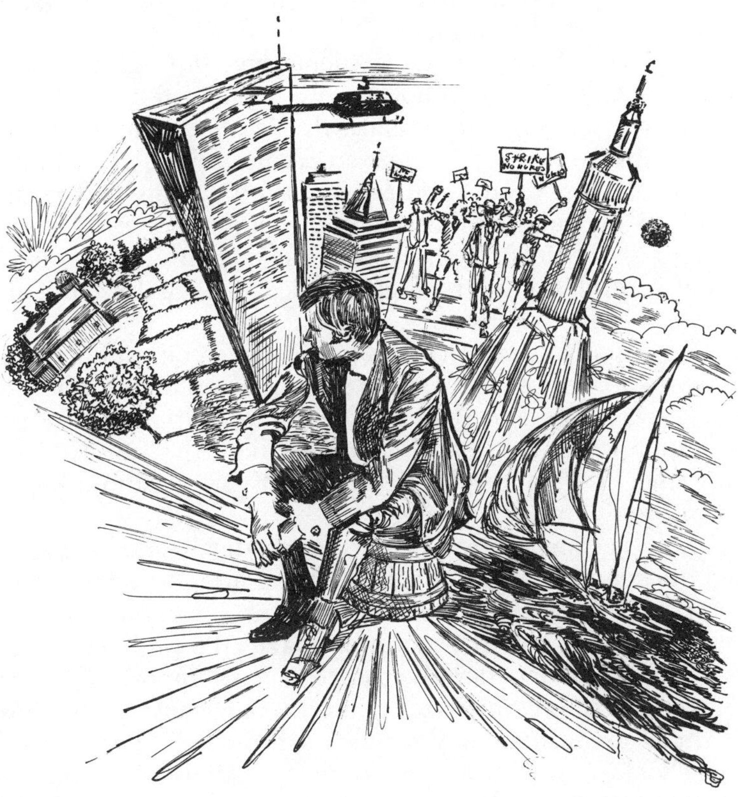

process from disease have meant that more individuals are now surviving for long periods with terminal conditions. Is life not terminal?

A gradual change in social values is also related to the attention now paid to the issues that surround the medical care of the ill. Although there has not yet been any definitive documentation, it seems fairly apparent that western society has gradually become increasingly humanitarian in its outlook. Suffering is no longer believed to have significant religious value. A decline in the belief of an afterlife has meant that the importance of this life is magnified. These factors have contributed to the concern for the quality of the human body.

There has been a change in social attitudes toward human intervention, at both the beginning and end of the aging process. Today the aging process need not be blindly accepted by human beings. Consequently, humans are in the midst of developing new ethics on their own aging.

A 12-year-old study on accidents and the aging process hypothesized that the psychologically maladjusted have a poor capacity for coping with hazards in the environment. Susceptibility to serious illness can result from a proneness to illness on the part of maladjusted aged individuals that reduces their physiological immunities to the aging process. These illnesses may manifest themselves as use of improper medications, alcoholism, and failure to seek medical advice for obvious symptoms of chronic diseases.

The opposite concept, "life proneness," could also become a thing of the future. For example, some people diet when they gain a few pounds and they smoke in moderation. These people have responded to medical discoveries about the causes of heart disease and lung cancer by decreasing their consumption of fats and by giving up smoking.

There is some evidence that the medical establishment is being questioned. Allied health leaders are becoming less research oriented and are becoming more concerned for their patients' welfare. This reorientation makes the problems involved in aging and the degenerative process more important because the new approach emphasizes people and because disfunctional individuals are prone to the more serious complications of disease. Society is moving toward more equitable health care for individuals of all social classes and economic backgrounds. This direction should produce further awareness in the recognition of degenerative diseases and the resources allocated to combat the process.

In the past, scientists undertook only minimal research on the aging process and its relationships to the youth of today. An explanation of what can be expected to occur and how and to what degree the various systems of the body will be affected by the aging process should be given at this point.

Health was once considered the state of complete physiological, psychological, and social well-being and not only the absence of disease. When young people become ill, it is most often as a consequence of exogenous factors and frequently of infectious disease. The courses such illnesses follow are often traumatic and have a definite onset, crisis, and limited aftereffects. Later in life the causes of various illnesses change, that is, they become essentially nonspecific. They are chronic in nature, develop slowly, have no marked crisis, and tend to linger. In contrast to acute illnesses, chronic illnesses usually involve a number of bodily functions and cannot be attributed to a single cause. Chronic illness sometimes creates a situation in which the physician and patient become antagonistic toward each other because, unlike the illnesses of youth, the pathological conditions of the later years seem to be progressive and degenerative; thus they offer little hope for total recovery and those afflicted must redefine health.

Recent investigations have indicated that advances in medicine may leave future generations of older individuals free from many of the degenerative diseases of today. Nevertheless, medical researchers continue to view disease as a factor of the aging process and a process that may not be altered regardless of future medical developments. This view is based upon the assumption that once one disease condition responds to treatment, a new set of physiological impairments will arise. Whether or not this is the case, one's health status in the aging process represents the dynamic interplay of phenomena that are continually subject to change. One means of achieving a better understanding of an individual's health status and the aging process is to look at the ways in which the human body changes with chronological age.

Physiological changes are often detected with greater frequency with advancing chronological age, but these changes are not totally related to chronological age. Such changes are tissue deterioration, retarded cell division, reduced rate of cell oxidation, cellular atrophy, reduced tissue elasticity, decreased neuromuscular speed, and impaired cell homeostasis.

■ Skeletal System

Aging affects the skeletal system through the increased loss of calcium and increased porosity and erosion. Bones become more brittle and tolerate less stress. There is also a deterioration of articulating surfaces and supports. This deterioration may contribute to an arthritic condition. Arthritic ailments have become second to heart disease as the most common reason for disabilities during the total aging process and have accounted for 20% of the total impairments during the life cycle. However, these rates seem to be genetically related and higher among women. Arthritis is less frequent among nonwhites than among whites.

Arthritis may be categorized in two broad categories: osteoarthritis and rheumatoid arthritis.

Osteoarthritis The demarcation between natural involution of bone material and osteoarthritis is not clear (24). Osteoarthritis is caused by a gradual demineralization of bone structure in the lower back and in joints where the harder outer surface of bone wears away most rapidly. Probable causes of this physiological change have been attributed to dietary insufficiencies, alterations in bone metabolism, physiological wear and tear, and variances in physical environments. Most significant seems to be a change in collagen structure which is assumed to allow an alteration. It allows bones to rub together, causing noticeable pain.

Rheumatoid Arthritis Rheumatoid arthritis is less frequently found in the elderly and it cannot be termed a disease of later years in the aging process, since it often occurs after infancy. The greatest number of cases develop during early adulthood, but because of the disease's chronic nature, few cases are diagnosed until later life. Rheumatoid conditions are found primarily in smaller joints where the membranes lining the joint cavity wear thin. This allows the ends of the bones to scrape against one another. In its active phase the bone marrow may also become involved, resulting in marked atrophy and muscular deterioration. The role of the body's defense mechanisms in the breakdown of connective tissue and the development of rheumatoid arthritis has been the most widely studied in the field of arthritis.

Generally, as the individual ages, muscles and joint tissue atrophy in mass, lose cells, accumulate water and nonactive mass, decrease vascularly, decrease in elasticity, and decrease in stress latitude (36).

Some of the most difficult aspects of arthritis to predict are the various directions or courses in which the disease may progress. Although considered a chronic progressive disorder, there are examples of intermittency with remissions or relapses.

After debating over the difficulties of arriving at a definite diagnosis of arthritis, the subcommittee of the American Rheumatism Association has set forth the following criteria that indicate an individual has arthritis:

1. Morning stiffness
2. Motion tenderness in a specific joint
3. Swelling in a joint
4. Additional swelling in an unrelated joint
5. Bilateral joint swelling
6. Nodules over bony surfaces

Osteoporosis Osteoporosis, commonly known as bone loss, is an insidious disease that strikes millions of postmenopausal women. The disease takes from 10 to 20 years to manifest itself and, unfortunately, by this time, those who have the symptoms are unable to replace calcium in the bone.

Perhaps as many as 10 million women already face chronic pain, disability, sexual problems, and in the case of severe hip fractures, a possible early death. And there are an estimated 10 million more who are showing evidence of bone demineralization to a lesser degree.

The disease shows up in the bones of the legs, arms, and spine. It can lead to an ailment known as the "dowager's hump." Statistics show that there are about 200,000 hip fractures annually and most of them occur in osteoporotic women. In addition to the personal suffering, these fractures cost the nation about $800 million annually.

Once a woman has gone three years without sufficient amounts of estrogen, she has already suffered an amount of calcium loss, and calcium is irreplaceable. Up to that point, estrogen (low dosage) therapy can put a patient in a positive calcium balance. If started after that time, it will prevent any further calcium depletion (25).

It has been shown that women who are quite active create a stress on bones and this stress results in a significant calcium-spurring effect (25). A real concern is the young women who have both ovaries removed because of infection, abscess, and other gynecological problems. If estrogen therapy is not started, they may have osteoporosis at a significantly younger age and be subject to all the associated fractures and discomforts.

■ Muscular System

The body's mass of muscular tissue is reduced with age. In part, this is related to changes in connective and circulatory tissue, a loss of neurons, and a decreased capacity for transmitting nerve impulses, as well as a reduction in physical activity. Muscle reflexes become less efficient as a result of neurological changes. Individuals in their latter years adjust to such alterations by taking a longer time to complete a task. They should be cognizant of their physical capabilities and pace their activities accordingly. Muscular weakness along with arthritic changes and joint stiffness might make learning to use canes, crutches, and walkers a little more difficult.

Exercise is important because it helps to increase blood flow and thus keep tissues healthier. It is imperative for minimum loss of muscular strength that one exercise to the fullest capabilities. The smooth muscles surrounding the blood vessels and the intestines do not tend to lose their strength with age.

Muscular weakness can have an effect on the efficient functioning of various other body systems. Decreased strength of the muscles involved in respiratory activity is an important factor in age-associated changes in the respiratory system. Also, the reduced muscularity of the bladder leads to partial emptying of the bladder and thus more frequent urination for older persons.

■ Reproductive System

The reproductive system is characterized by a number of age-specific changes in physical integrity and function. Very few age-specific disorders are associated with this system. The problems associated with the reproductive system and its relationship to sexuality are more important to the majority of the elderly than the actual pathologic condition reported. Most of the problems surrounding changing sexuality with age are social and psychologic.

Male Reproductive System The male reproductive system produces a male sex hormone (testosterone) until death. Concentration of production gradually declines, but it is maintained at a higher level longer than estrogen production is maintained in women. The decrease of testosterone has definite effects on older men. It contributes to a decline in both the muscle tautness and the number of viable sperm produced. The waning of sexual desires may be related to decreasing testosterone, but other physiologic changes such as decreased sensitivity of the genitalia may be more responsible for the decline (25).

With age, a number of physical changes occur. The size and firmness of the testes decrease, and the seminiferous tubules thicken and decrease in diameter. The prostate gland enlarges and its contractions become less forceful. Diseases of the prostate or corrective surgery associated with pathologic conditions of

Figure 5.2 The male reproductive system.

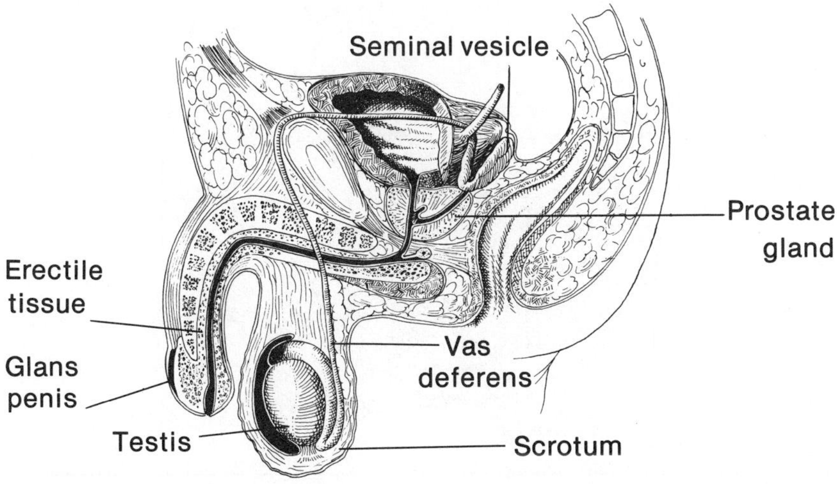

the prostate gland may lead to impotence as well as psychologic problems. Other changes which may occur include reduced force of ejaculation and a reduced volume, viscosity, and general quality of the seminal fluid. Ignorance of these conditions may be cause for personal concern and possibly may affect sexual activity (25).

Female Reproductive System The female reproductive system becomes less efficient with age. Two possible explanations for this reduced efficiency include less frequent ovulation and the declining ability of the oviduct to provide an unobstructed passage to the uterus.

A great number of physical changes take place in the female genital tract. The vulva develops less pronounced folds, and the skin becomes thinner. Vascularity and elasticity decrease, and the area becomes more susceptible to tissue trauma and the development of pruritis. The glands decrease in number and amount of secretion, and general atrophy leads to shrinkage and drying of the area. The vaginal wall becomes thinner, has less vascularity, and is easily irritated by bacteria and various foreign

Figure 5.3 The female reproductive system.

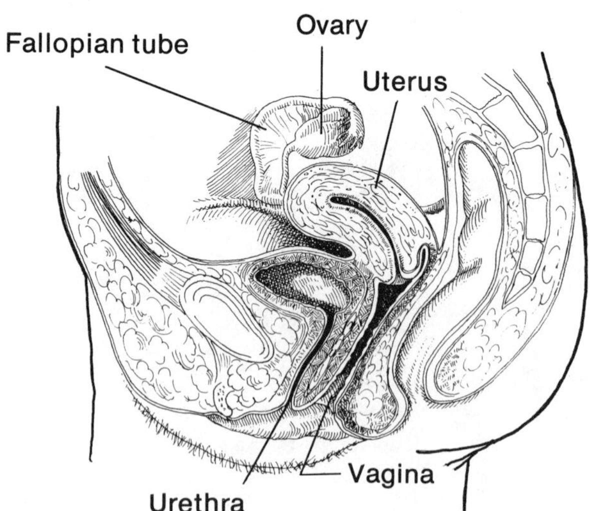

substances. The uterus decreases in size, becomes more fibrous, and has fewer endometrial glands. The cervix is reduced in size, but less so than the uterine body, and the cervical canal decreases in diameter. The oviducts become thin and constricted, and the ovary takes on an irregular shape. The ovary secretes less progesterone and experiences failure of ovulation and estrogen production (16).

■ Gastrointestinal System

The gastrointestinal tract is the product of biocultural evolution. The human evolved from primate ancestors who were primarily vegetarian but who had the capability of omnivorous alimentation. The nature of the human helped it expand and evolve to fit a wide variety of ecologic conditions. Judging from the development of a great variety of cultural traditions with their dissimilar eating customs, it seems that the human gastrointestinal tract has served the species well.

Because humans are subject to the aging process, there are general and specific changes in the gastrointestinal tract. These changes include atrophy of the secretion mechanisms, loss of strength and tone of the muscular tissue and its supporting structures, changes in neurosensory feedback on such things as enzyme and hormone release, innervation of the tract, and the diminished response to pain and internal sensations. Although the indisputable evidence for the relationship between these changes and aging is still not overwhelming, there is certainly enough circumstantial evidence to consider the possibilities. The magnitude of the changes and the possible preventive, rehabilitative, and supportive measures to effectively deal with them remain to be determined (24, 16).

Gastrointestinal symptoms such as indigestion, heartburn, and epigastric discomfort increase with age. Many symptoms are caused by normal physiological changes of the tract that may be accepted as "normal" aging. Gastrointestinal symptoms become a matter of great concern. Threat or fear of cancer often associated with gastrointestinal symptoms can place a great deal of psychologic pressure on individuals of all ages. This pressure affects not only the mental health of the individual but it can also affect other body symptoms, causing or complicating problems such as hypertension and chronic respiratory disease (16).

■ Cardiovascular System

It has been thought that the degeneration of the cardiovascular system may be caused by factors other than physiochronological factors. During the aging process one may expect a decrease in cardiac output, increased blood pressure, increased arhythmia, decreased stress latitude, decreased blood formation, increased atherosclerosis, increased blood vessel irregularity, increased vulnerability to rupture and clots, and increased vein varicosity with impaired blood transport (14, 15).

Myocardial and Valvular Degeneration Cardiovascular "disease," including myocardial and valvular degeneration, hypertension, and atherosclerosis, surpass all other disorders in terms of incidence in industrialized societies. In fact, cardiovascular problems are so common in the third and fourth decades of life and beyond that until recently they were thought to be part of the onset of the aging process. In addition to the dehydration of bodily tissue, the normal aging cardiovascular system shows an accumulation of subpericardial fat and lipofuscin plus thickened, less efficient valves with marked atrophy. The left atrium becomes larger with age, and the heart configuration is somewhat altered (19). This has a causal effect with the cardiac output declining at about 1% per year past the chronological age of 23 (35).

There is a loss of reserve capacities and with it the cardiovascular system's ability to respond rapidly under psychological stress. Although the specific etiology of later-life myocardial degeneration remains a question, the so-called "disease" is manifested by progressive deposits of fatty substances and loss of heart muscle flexibility. These physiological changes are functional as well as structural, thereby bringing about an eventual infarction as a consequence of platelet buildup in vessels or of a biochemical process. The result is oxygen imbalance and oxygen deprivation of the active tissue. The most common symptoms are pain, breathlessness, and irregular rhythms. There also seems to be psychological confusion when blood pressure is diminished (35).

Recent studies indicate that cardiovascular problems are responsible for approximately 60% of fatalities in North America, Scandinavia, and the United Kingdom. Cardiovascular incidents were particularly apparent in younger males during the 1970s. There is some conjecture that females are protected due to some hormonal secretion lost at menopause. This theory accounts for the higher incidence of cardiovascular problems in women over 50.

Epidemiological investigations suggest that cardiovascular problems are closely linked to affluent socioeconomic populations found in most industrialized countries. Can it be that sociological conditions determine physiological aging? There are implications that high-calorie diets and low-activity levels may heighten the risk of cardiovascular problems.

Statistics show that nonwhites are more prone to cardiovascular dysfunctions than are whites. The same risk factors exist in both groups, but a corresponding lower level of medical services reverses the trend; thus, socioeconomic factors may redistribute mortality and disability factors. However, there is no substantial evidence indicating an increase or decrease in cardiovascular degeneration based upon race.

Atherosclerosis Atherosclerosis is characterized primarily as a hardening of the interior walls of major blood vessels and is considered the leading precursor of other retrogressive coronary changes. Americans have the highest cardiac mortality rates in the world (4). As do other innate aging cardiovascular diseases, atherosclerotic conditions discriminate on the basis of sex. The incidence among American males is about three times that among similarly aged females. It has been said that if one lives long enough, the condition will be 100% terminal.

Over the past 70 years there have been numerous theories on the causes of atherosclerosis. To date, however, no theory has been totally accepted. The appearance of fatty streaks in the inner wall of the arteries during the first decade of life has prompted investigators to conclude that the blood deposits fatty substances that are absorbed into the vessels, reducing the actual blood flow of the artery. Since the artery is a living form of connective tissue, damage begins immediately. Thus, this condition begins with initial intake of nutritive substances. Which factor actually initiates the damage is a debated topic among physiologists, but it is agreed that certain preventive steps may

Figure 5.4 The progression of atherosclerosis.

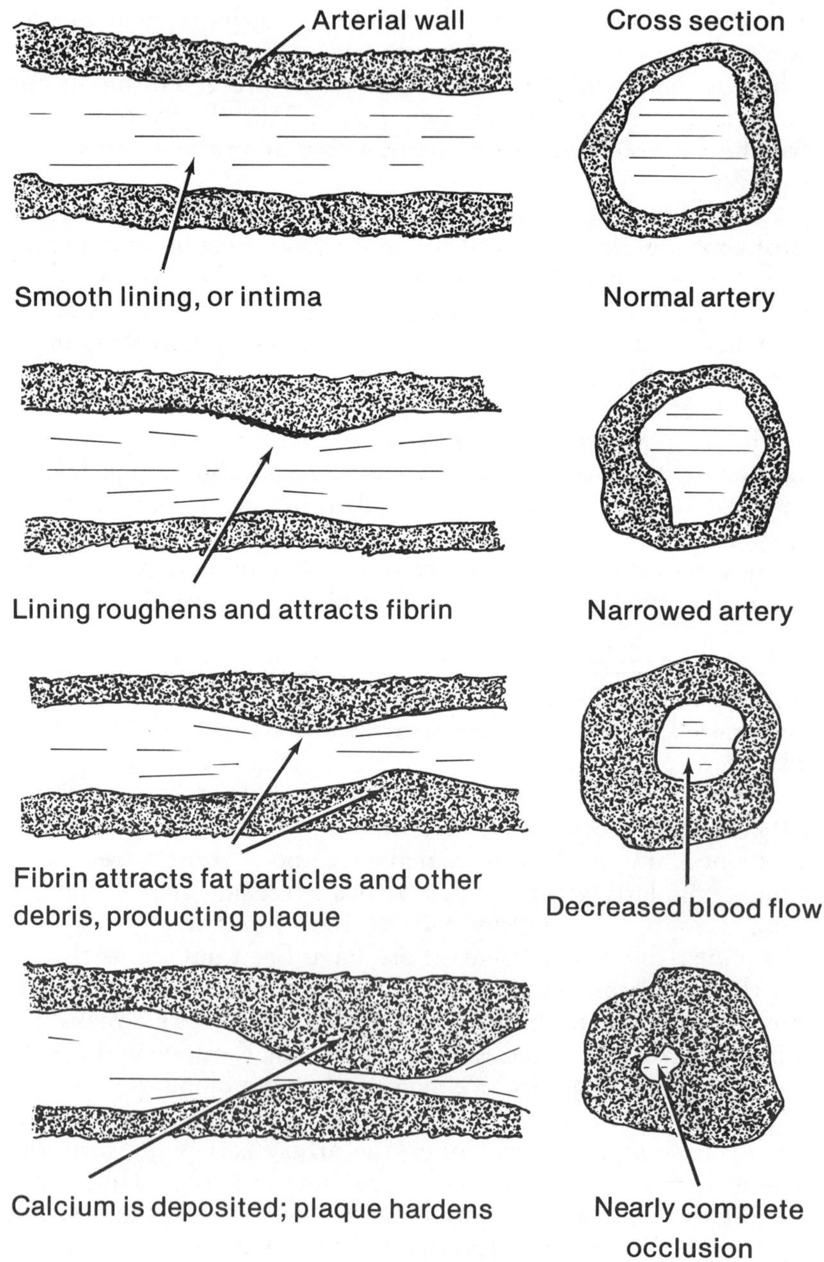

inhibit this development in the aging process. However, nothing can be done about reversing the effects until the process is more fully understood.

Hypertension Hypertension, most commonly referred to as high blood pressure, affects approximately the same percentage of individuals in their third decade of life as do other cardiovascular problems. Blood pressure is affected by the presence of other illnesses, fever, obesity, and air temperature. In turn, hypertension may cause other bodily homeostatic functions to become unbalanced, thus indirectly contributing to terminal situations. However, personal history and family background are important factors that must be taken into account as precursors in the aging process and hypertension.

Figure 5.5 Hypertension is often associated with overwork!

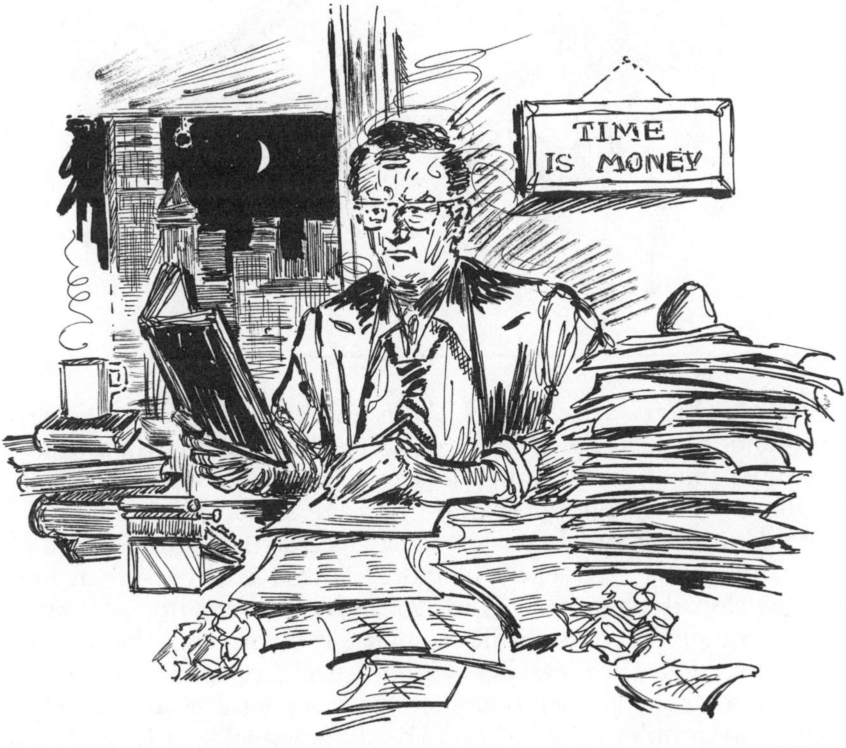

Figure 5.6 General anatomy of a *stroke,* a sudden paralysis with total or partial loss of consciousness and sensation, caused by the breaking (*hemorrhage*) or obstruction of a blood vessel in the brain.

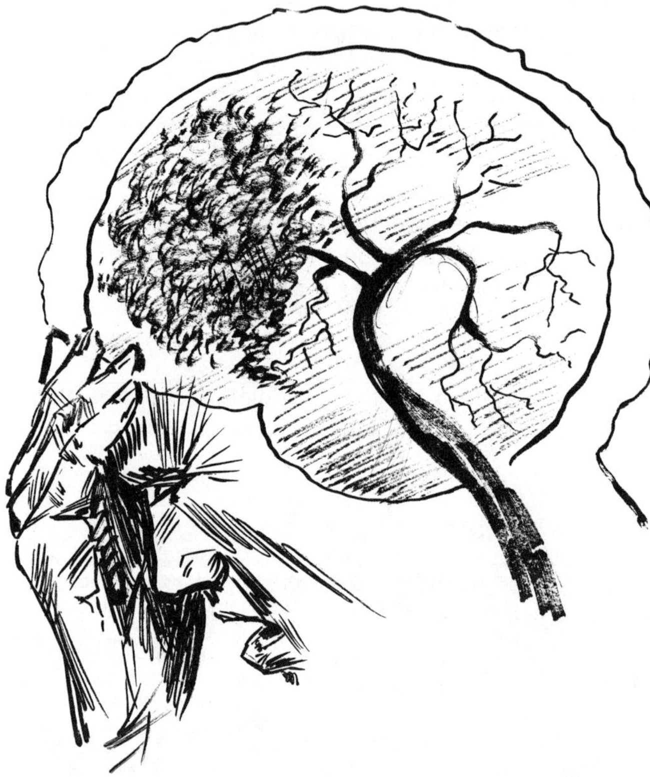

Stroke Every year strokes claim approximately one-quarter of a million lives in the United States and leave many times that number impaired. Although a number of events can cause brain damage at any age, most brain damage is due to circulatory problems. Epidemiological studies suggest that strokes tend to occur more frequently in industrialized countries than in undeveloped countries. Thus, sociophysical conditions may substantially dictate cardiovascular problems and the aging process. Most all researchers agree that cigarette smokers impose a greater risk on themselves in terms of strokes and other coronary problems than those who do not smoke. It is significant to note that many of the cerebral conditions are developed in the second and third decades of life but only manifest themselves during stressful episodes during later decades or when other accidents occur.

During the past century, when pathology began to play a significant role in medicine, degenerative vascular disease was considered an aging phenomenon, and it is still thought to be so today. Judging by the accomplishments of the past three decades, it appears that a return to the neglected area of relating the aging process directly to degenerative vascular disease will be in vogue for years to come.

■ Respiratory System

As the individual ages, the ability to exercise and work decreases. Much of the capacity to enjoy life rests upon an ability to be

Figure 5.7 The respiratory system.

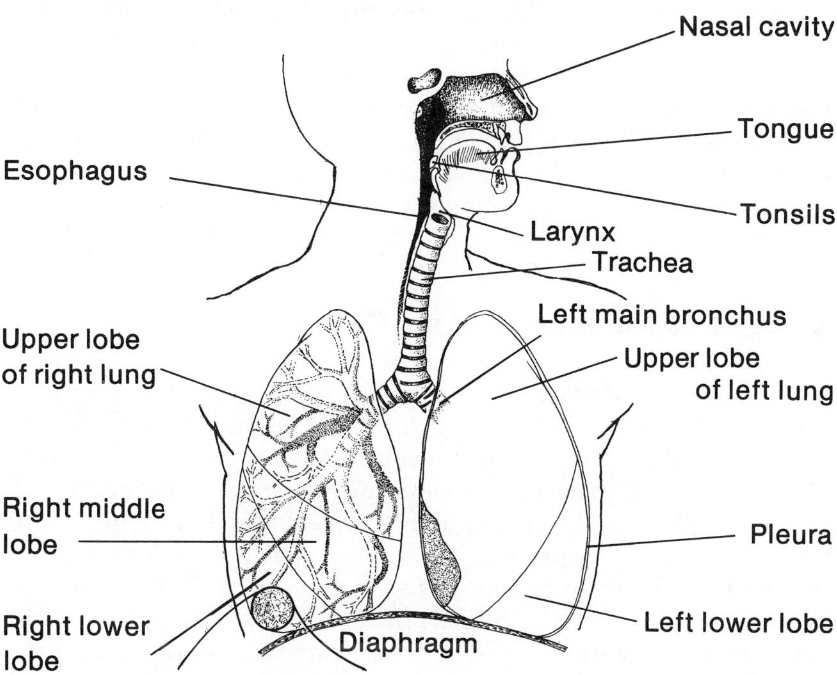

physically active. And this ability to be physically active depends upon the respiratory system. Following the second decade of life, an individual may expect lowering vital lung capacity, lowering of maximum breathing capacity, lowered diffusion and absorption, and decreased diaphragm action. The decreased function of the diaphragm is theoretically linked to skeletal postural changes in the same time period.

The cumulative impact of various environments on the aging process and on the respiratory system often results in numerous diseases. Of all factors influencing respiratory disease in the second and third decades of life, smoking is by far the most significant. It is the major cause of chronic bronchitis and it is linked to cancer. Habitual smokers have lowered ventilatory performance, often evidenced by reduced air flow rates, although the residual lung volume may be moderately elevated above predicted norms (37).

It is therefore difficult to separate the impact of a lifetime of living from that of lifelong smoking. In addition, distinct structural alterations such as squamous metaplasia, loss of cilia, and alveolar septal damage occur as a result of smoking.

As mentioned earlier, the severity of emphysema seems to increase progressively with increasing decades and it is presumed that the causal factors have a cumulative effect over consecutive decades. Other forms of lung destruction that produce extensive scarring and distortion of the remaining normal lung tissue, as in healed inactive tuberculosis, may be a cause of dyspnea, respiratory failure, and possible death. Such degenerative processes are not limited to any decade in the life cycle (37).

■ Central Nervous System (CNS)

Significant neurological changes take place during the aging process. Most notable is the pace of various functions with age. Although this change in pace occurs independently of disease, disease does enhance the process. Since cells in the central nervous system do not reproduce themselves, when neurons are lost, they are not replaced. Therefore, cell destruction could reduce the efficiency of the brain's functioning. There is also some indication that the human brain decreases in weight with age, but investigations from a significant population are not available.

Figure 5.8 A simplified view of the brain and the spinal cord, which make up the central nervous system.

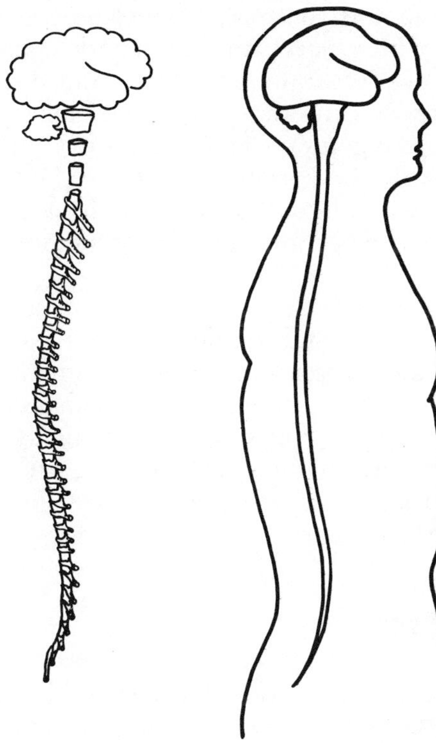

This slowing of the central nervous system with chronological age becomes most apparent in tests of reaction time. Reaction time involves a number of aspects of the central nervous system functioning, but it is not clear whether the slowing occurs only in some of the processes or in all of the processes. This slowing may occur in the transmission of the neural impulse and may reduce neural excitability.

An interesting theory about the change in the central nervous system with age states that there is a disturbance of the impulse resulting from interference in neural transmission. This is shown in a decrease in one's noise reaction. The decrease may result because there are fewer active cells and it might result because there is greater random activity within the central nervous system. The exact nature of these changes in neural activity is not known, but in the next decade it may be possible to treat these changes with an assortment of drugs to reduce the neurological changes with age.

Additional factors that may have some effect on the central nervous system with progressing age include changes in hormones that affect the level of brain excitability and the production of proteins and enzymes that affect the efficiency of the central nervous system. Oxygen deficiency resulting from cardiovascular diseases is probably the best theory. It may be possible that the changes involved in adaptation to high altitudes resemble those changes that take place during the aging processes of the central nervous system.

The effects of central nervous system changes are more likely to be widespread and to influence a wide range of behaviors in the behavior and motor skill areas. In general, regardless of the basic cause of central nervous system changes with age, all behaviors mediated by the central nervous system can be expected to show the characteristic slowing with advancing age. Perhaps the most noticeable indicators are the functionings of the sensory organs.

■ Sensory Organs

As people age, they will undoubtedly show declining acuity in at least four of the five senses. It is not clear how much of this decline in acuity is from the aging process alone. In general, with increasing age, an individual may require higher levels of stimulation in vision, audition, taste, and smell for the sense receptors to perform with intense acuity. Such declines in acuity, especially in vision and hearing, are important because they not only influence the individual's ability to function in the physical environment, but they may also create a social isolation that may have significant psychological and social effects.

Vision Many aspects of vision decline with age. Visual acuity reaches its maximum during the teen years and remains generally constant until the fourth decade of life when it gradually begins to decline. Approximately 10% of this population have less than 20/30 vision. Toward the sixth decade of life, 50% of the population have poorer than 20/80 vision. In addition, the threshold for adaptation to darkness increases with age. Generally, this is shown in the inability of light to penetrate the lens

Figure 5.9 The loss of senses that often accompanies aging can be dangerous!

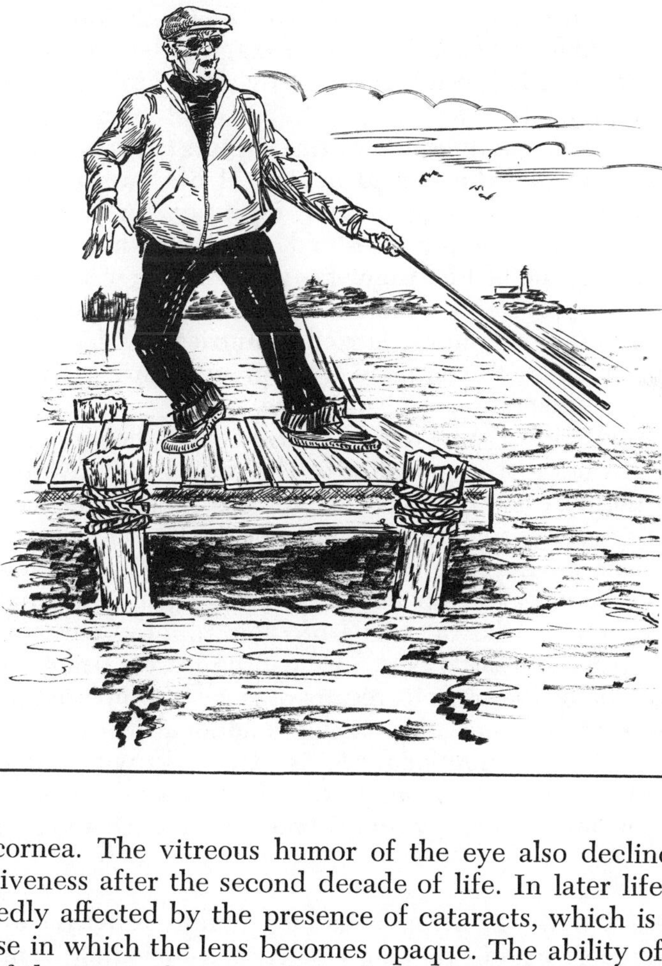

and cornea. The vitreous humor of the eye also declines in effectiveness after the second decade of life. In later life it is markedly affected by the presence of cataracts, which is an eye disease in which the lens becomes opaque. The ability of the lens of the eye to focus on close objects decreases from the first decade of life at a fairly constant rate. However, the cumulative aging process shows itself in later years. By the time they reach age 50, many people need bifocals. A bifocal is a lens adjusted to two different focal lengths: one for close focus and one for distant focus.

Hearing Many replicated logical and physiologic studies have indicated a marked loss of hearing among individuals in the fifth and sixth decades of life. Hearing is one of the most valuable of the senses. When hearing becomes impaired, people are at a tremendous disadvantage. Long-term exposure to noise and lowered sensitivity of the auditory receptors are significant factors. Current estimates suggest that 7% of individuals in the fifth decade suffer hearing losses of a magnitude that hinders social interaction. It is estimated that by the middle of the sixth decade the percentage has jumped to 50% of all men and 30% of all women. Most young adults can hear pure tones in the high frequencies. Around the second decade of life, presbycusis, an age-related loss of the ganglion cells necessary for conduction, causes erosion of the upper threshold and diminishes threefold in the seventh decade of life. Conversely, low-range tones do not appear to be appreciably affected by age. The increasing amount of noise pollution in industrialized countries has led many authorities to predict even more widespread hearing difficulties among future generations of Americans.

From all indications, the declining acuity shown in testing conditions is not a true indicator of the total loss individuals suffer. Although many of the changes are a consequence of retrogressive alterations, diseases of the inner ear, vascular difficulties, or environmental assaults, other variables such as sex or intelligence are also implicated. Across the life span, women and those people who by virtue of their training pay close attention to speech patterns experience the least hearing loss as they age. One of the obvious results of severely impaired hearing is the sense of isolation and possible emotional distress. It has been noted that the emotional upsets may occur with reduced reality testing and that paranoid ideational states develop if impairments are sufficiently severe and continue for a long period of time (40).

Taste and Smell There are some degenerative changes in smell and taste receptors, but they may be caused by variances in the individual's threshold for taste and smell. Sensory perception generally becomes less efficient, requiring higher levels of stimulation in older people than in younger people. This loss in sensory perception may be partly responsible for the clinically noted increase in complaints about food among older people.

Kinesthetic Sensitivity Kinesthetic sensitivity refers to a person's total awareness of his or her body's spatial location. Sensitivity is dulled by receptors in muscles, joints, and the apparatus of the inner ear. The simplest way to explain kinesthetic sensitivity, without going into great detail, is to give an example. Individuals in the first decades of life know when they are either vertical or prone, but many older people are unable to control body position or movement because the loss of kinesthetic sensitivity has left them vulnerable to accidental falls and postural instability. The sense of movement, touch, and position depend in part upon receptors located in the muscles, joints, and skin and is in direct correlation with one's kinesthetic sensitivity.

Fluid balances in the semicircular canals of the inner ear help maintain spatial orientation. Each of the three canals extends in a different plane and each contains a liquid and activated receptors that transmit a message to the cerebral cortex and thalamus whenever the equilibrium is disturbed. For various reasons, the dizziness, or vertigo, reported by many individuals in the fifth to eighth decades of life is attributed to dysfunctions in these areas. The specific causes of kinesthetic malfunctions are not yet known.

Pain The clinical impression is that sensitivity to pain may decrease with aging, perhaps because many older people so frequently experience pain from chronic disease. This decrease in sensitivity to pain is partly because the threshold for physical stimulation may increase with chronological age. However, various studies have not validated this theory. Perhaps the normal threshold for pain sensitivity is offset by a lowered tolerance to pain; again, this is only a theory.

Reaction and Motor Responses Degenerating sensory acuity and the concurrent slowing of behaviors involving the central nervous system are seen most clearly in motor performance of individuals beyond the fifth decade of life. This relationship is by no means simple and direct. The speed at which impulses travel accounts for only a small fraction of the delay in reaction times. Reaction time is defined as the lag between stimulation and initial response. It is important to remember that when scientific test results are translated into realistic daily performances, it is almost impossible to draw sensible conclusions. Evidence indicates that when there is no time pressure, the older individual is capable of reacting almost as quickly as a younger person. Whether or not this is always true in fact depends as much upon personality and emotional variables as upon psychomotor skills. It is thought that reaction time lengthens when the individual is in a lethargic or depressed mood. However, heightened activity levels may stimulate possible improvements but within minor limits. Deterioration of the circulatory system, depressed cerebral metabolism, and suppressed brain rhythms also tend to correlate with slower reaction times and lessen mental functioning. The tendency toward cardiovascular problems may also be a retardation factor that older individuals cannot overcome regardless of their physical exercise levels.

Memory A myth that should be destroyed is that individuals in later life cannot learn. They can and they do. It has been hypothesized that individuals of all ages might be able to improve their memory skills if given the opporunity and under optimal situations. If given a chance to refresh their skills or to acquire new techniques for organizing materials, they might be able to improve their performance.

The distinction between learning and memory is confusing because learning involves retrieving data from the memory bank. Where learning leaves off and memory enters the picture is unclear. If something is to be remembered, it must be consciously recognized. Memory consists of incidental memories and intentional memories.

Age-related memory deficiencies have been widely reported in the media and in professional writings. Short-term recall seems to decay with age, perhaps as a consequence of poor sorting strategies, but long-term recall does not show similar changes. Why people forget depends upon the complexities of social, psychological, and physiological influences. Some chemists tend to favor RNA coding as the source of memory, and enzyme agents as the cause of forgetting, but there is no conclusive evidence in this area. Some psychologists say that people remember things that affirm their contemporary self-images and that unpleasant things are conveniently forgotten. An extreme example may be evident in the development of a psychological disorder that enables a person to block out particularly stressful events.

In addition, since society expects old people to suffer a loss of memory, many old people give in and do not even try to remember things.

Figure 5.10 The decay of short-term recall with age: "I used to *remember* all your names!"

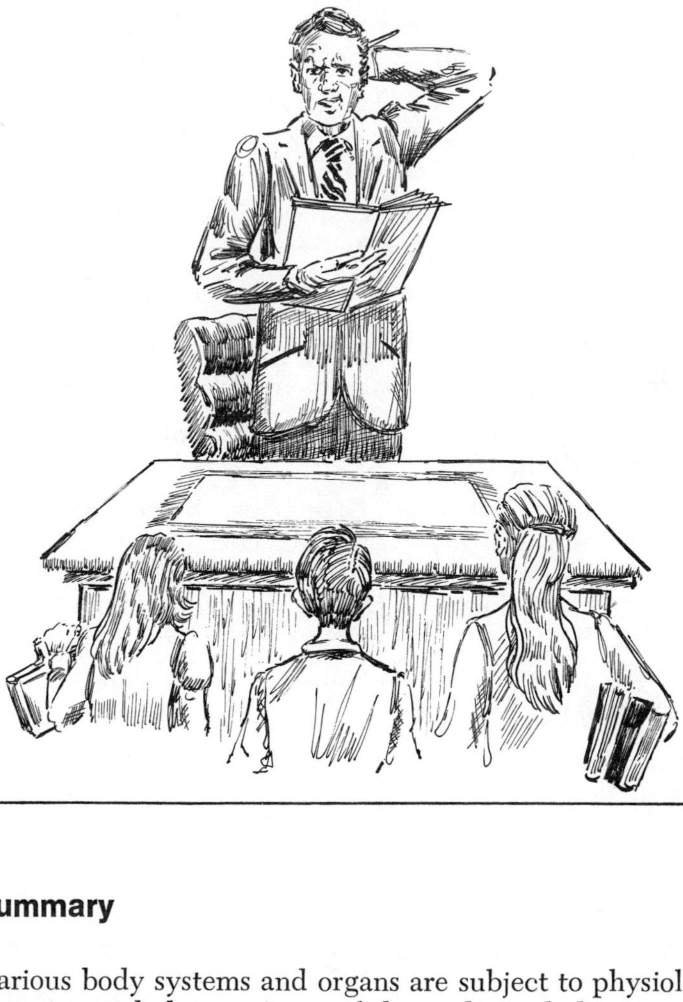

■ Summary

The various body systems and organs are subject to physiological degeneration and change. Some of these physical changes may be directly related to chronological age, and regardless of preventive measures, are inevitable. Myths about the sensory organs and their reactions to the aging process abound. Abnormal degenerative processes notwithstanding, people will undoubtedly suffer a combination of organ dysfunctions and joint malfunctions in their lifetime.

References

1. Alffram, P. "An Epidemiologic Study of Cervical and Trochanteric Fractures of the Femur in an Urban Population." *Acts Orthopedic Science* 65 (1964):1–109.
2. Bartler, F. "Bone as a Target Organ: Toward a Better Definition of Osteoporosis." *Perspectives on Biological Medicine* 16 (1973):215–31.
3. Barzel, U., ed. *Osteoporosis.* New York: Grune & Stratton, 1970.
4. Birren, James E. "Behavior Theories of Aging." In *Aging: Some Social and Biological Aspects,* edited by Nathan W. Shock, Publication No. 65. Washington, D.C.: American Association for the Advancement of Science, 1960.
5. —— *The Psychology of Aging.* Englewood Cliffs, N.J.: Prentice-Hall, 1964.
6. ——, Butler, Robert N., Greenhouse, Samuel W., Sokoloff, Louis, and Yarrow, Marian R., eds. *Human Aging. A Biological and Behavioral Study.* Publication No. (HMS) 71–9051. Washington, D.C.: U.S. Government Printing Office, 1963.
7. Bjorksten, J. "The Limitation of Creative Years." *Scientific Monthly* 62 (1946):94.
8. Botwinick, Jack. *Cognitive Processes in Maturity and Old Age.* New York: Springer, 1967.
9. ——. *Geropsychology. Annual Review of Psychology* 21 (1970):239–72.
10. Brody, Harold. "Organization of the Cerebral Cortex. III. A Study of Aging in the Human Cerebral Cortex." *Journal of Comparative Neurology* 102 (1955):511–56.
11. Bromley, D. B. *The Psychology of Human Aging.* Baltimore: Penguin, 1966.
12. Clark, H. "Osteoarthritis: An Interesting Case?" *Neurology Clinic of North America* 11 (1976):199–206.
13. Coley, B., and Sharp, G. "Pagets Disease. A Predisposing Factor to Osteogenic Sarcoma." *Archives of Surgery* 23 (1931):918–36.

14. Comfort, Alex. *Aging: The Biology of Senescence.* New York: Holt, Rinehart & Winston, 1964.

15. Cristofalo, V. J. "Metabolic Aspects of Aging in Diploid Human Cells." In *Aging in Cells and Tissue Culture,* edited by E. Holeckova and V. J. Cristofalo. New York: Plenum, 1970.

16. Curtis, Howard J. *Biological Mechanisms of Aging,* Springfield, Ill.: Charles C Thomas, 1966.

17. Dennis, Wayne. "Creative Productivity Between the Ages of 20 and 80 Years." *Journal of Gerontology* 21 (1966):1–8.

18. Dent, C. "Idiopathic Osteoporosis." *Royal Society of Medicine* 48 (1955):574–78.

19. Dovenmuehle, Robert H. "Aging Versus Illness." In *Normal Aging,* edited by Erdman Palmore. Durham, N.C., Duke University Press, 1970.

20. Granick, Samuel, and Patterson, Robert D., eds. *Human Eleven-Year Follow-Up Biomedical and Behavioral Study Publication* (HMS) 71–9037. Washington, D.C.: U.S. Government Printing Office, 1971.

21. Himwich, Williamina A., and Himwich, Harold E. "Neurochemical." In *Handbook of Aging and the Individual,* edited by James E. Birren. Chicago: University of Chicago Press, 1959.

22. Hotcin, John, and Sikora, Edward. "Long-Term Effects of Virus Behavior and Aging in Mice." *Proceedings of the Society for Biology and Medicine* 134 (1970):204–209.

23. Johnson, L. K. "Memory Loss with Age: A Storage of Retrieval." Paper presented at the meeting of the Gerontological Society, San Juan, Puerto Rico, December, 1972.

24. Kohn, R. R. "Human Aging and Disease." *Journal of Chronology* 27 (1963):5–21.

25. Laws, R. M. "Patterns of Reproductive and Somatic Aging in Animals." In *Aging in Relation to Developmental Reproduction,* edited by George A. Sacher. Argonne, Ill.: Argonne National Laboratory, 1971.

26. Lehman, Harvey C. *Age and Achievement.* Princeton, N.J.: Princeton University Press, 1978.

27. Lehman, H. C., "The Creative Production Rates of Present Versus Past Generations of Scientists." *Journal of Gerontology* 17 (1962): 409–17.

28. ——. "The Psychologist's Most Creative Years." *American Psychologist* 21 (1966):363–69.

29. Mead, Margaret. "Long Living in Cross-Cultural Perspective." Paper presented at the meeting of the Gerontological Society, San Juan, Puerto Rico, December, 1972.

30. Myers, G. C., and Pitts, A. M. "The Demographic Effects of Mortality Reduction on the Aged Population of the U.S." (Some baseline projections.) Paper presented at the meeting of the Gerontological Society, San Juan, Puerto Rico, December, 1972.

31. National Center for Health Statistics. "Binocular Visual Acuity of Adults," U.S., 1960–62." *Vital and Health Statistics,* Series 11, No. 3. Washington, D.C.: U.S. Government Printing Office, 1964.

32. Papalia, D. E., True, M. and Salverson, S. "The Status of Mass Weight and Volume Conservation Ability During Old Age." Paper presented at the meeting of the Gerontological Society, San Juan, Puerto Rico, December, 1972.

33. Reed, Homer, B. C. Jr., and Reitan, Ralph M. "Changes in Psychological Test Performance Associated with the Normal Aging Process." *Journal of Gerontology* 18 (1963):271–74.

34. Riley, Matilda White, Foner, Anne, and Associates. *Aging and Society.* St. Louis: C. V. Mosby, 1968.

35. Spieth, Walter. "Cardiovascular Health Status, Age and Pathological Performance." *Journal of Gerontology* 19 (1964):277–84.

36. Strehler, Bernard L. *Time, Cells, and Aging.* New York: Macmillan, 1962.

37. Timiras, P. S. *Developmental Physiology and Aging.* New York: Macmillan, 1972.

38. U.S. Bureau of the Census. "Some Demographic Aspects of Aging in the United States." *Current Population Reports,* Series P29, No. 41. Washington D.C.: U.S. Government Printing Office, 1977.

39. Walford, Roy L. *The Immunologic Theory of Aging.* Baltimore: Williams & Wilkins, 1969.

40. Weiss, Alfred D. "Sensory Functions." In *Handbook of Aging and the Individual,* edited by James E. Birren. Chicago: University of Chicago Press, 1959.

41. Weissman, August. *Essays on Heredity.* Oxford, England: Clarendon Press, 1891.

42. Welford, Alan T. "Psychomotor Performance." In *Handbook of Aging and the Individual,* edited by James E. Birren. Chicago: University of Chicago Press, 1959.

43. Wetherick, N. E. "Changing an Established Concept: A Comparison of the Ability of Young, Middle-Aged and Old Subjects." Paper presented at the Gerontologic Association, 1965.

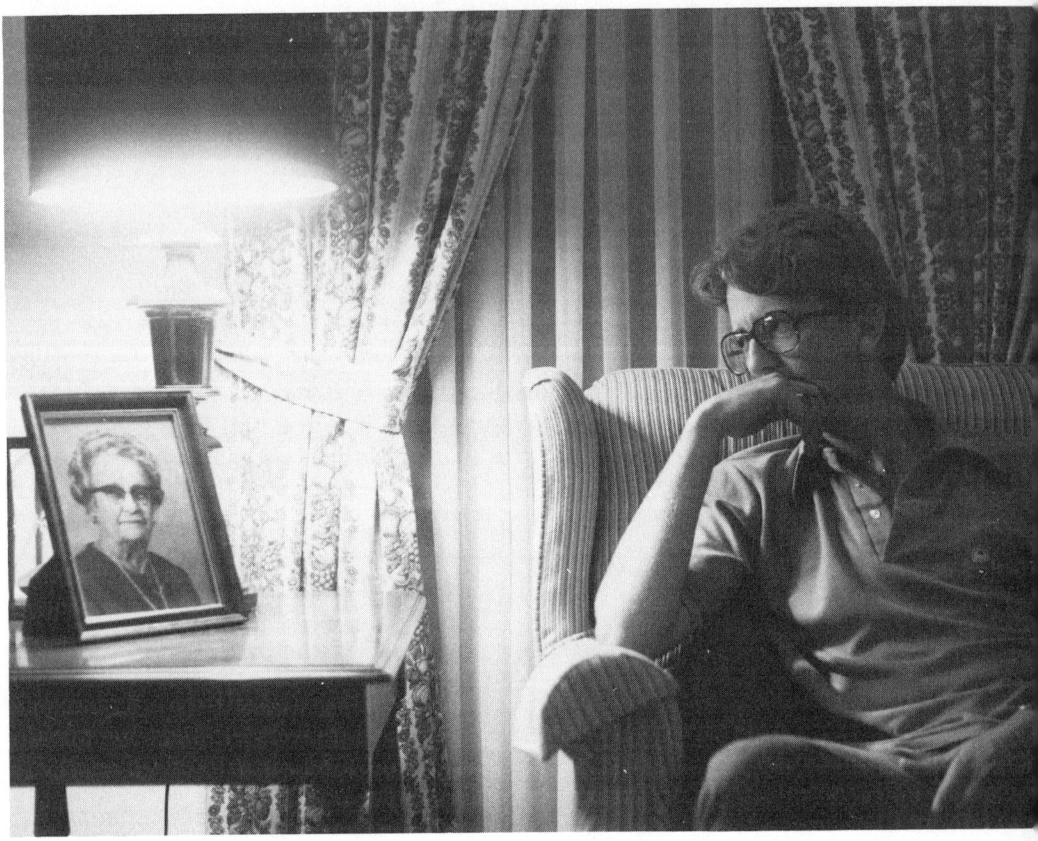

■ Chapter 6

Cosmetic Changes

Major Concepts

1. Changes in the skin, hair, and oral cavity occur as a natural part of aging.
2. Many causes are responsible for changes and diseases in the integumentary system.
3. Income, body changes, and the ability to select and purchase clothing are factors that contribute to a positive or negative appearance.

■ Physiology of the Skin

Everyone experiences changes in the integumentary system (skin, hair, and teeth), but the rate and degree of change depend upon hereditary factors, environmental factors, and disease process.

The skin is divided into two layers called the epidermis and dermis. The epidermis is the outer layer. It is made up of layers of dead cells that are compacted to form a tough, outer protective cover. This layer is formed as new cells are produced in the deeper layers of the skin and old cells begin to die and migrate to the outer surface where they eventually are sloughed off.

The dermis is the layer just under the epidermis. It contains hair follicles, glands, nerves, and blood vessels. The two types of sweat glands are the eccrine glands, which secrete water containing some salt and minerals which has no odor, and apocrine glands which release a scented material. The sebaceous glands are located at the base of the hair follicles and on hairless surfaces of the lips and inside of the cheeks. They secrete an oily substance that lubricates the hair and skin. There are numerous

Figure 6.1 The structure of the skin.

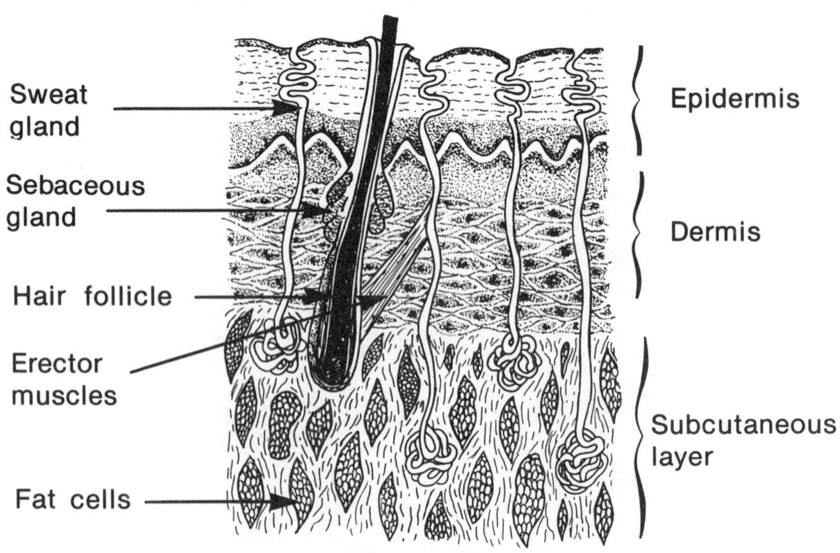

blood vessels in the skin and they work along with the eccrine glands as a body-cooling system. Nerves are located throughout the skin to enable sensory contact with the environment.

Between the dermis and epidermis are melanocytes, special cells that produce pigment called melanin. Melanin protects the skin from solar radiation. Fair-skinned people have less pigment than dark-skinned people, but both skin types have the same number of melanocytes.

Below the dermis is the subcutaneous tissue, which contains fat cells and connective tissue made up of collagen and elastin fibers. These give the skin a certain amount of flexibility, suppleness, and shape.

■ Skin Changes

Effects of the Sun The ultraviolet rays of the sun have both positive and negative effects on the skin. On the positive side, ultraviolet rays convert chemical substances in the skin to vitamin D. On the negative side, excessive ultraviolet rays damage the skin and cause skin cancer.

During the spring and summer months males and females of all ages proudly display their tanned skin. Occasionally this tan is preceded by a sunburn or redness of the skin. The redness and pain of a sunburn are caused by a change in molecular structure, coagulation of some of the substance of the epidermal cells, and enlargement of the small blood vessels beneath the epidermis. Years of sunbathing will result in dry, wrinkled skin, changes in skin pigmentation, and skin cancer.

A tanned appearance occurs two to three weeks after a sunburn and after repeated exposure to the sun. A tan is the result of the darkening of melanin in the epidermis and the stimulated production of new pigment.

Ultraviolet rays inhibit the formation of DNA and RNA. These rays also inhibit protein synthesis in the skin, which limits the skin's regenerative capacity. Decreased regeneration of elastin fibers causes the skin to lose its normal elasticity. The epidermis becomes thin, wrinkled, and irregularly pigmented.

Lentigenes and Keratoses Accumulative exposure to the sun can also result in the development of lentigenes and actinic keratoses. Lentigenes are small brown spots that resemble large

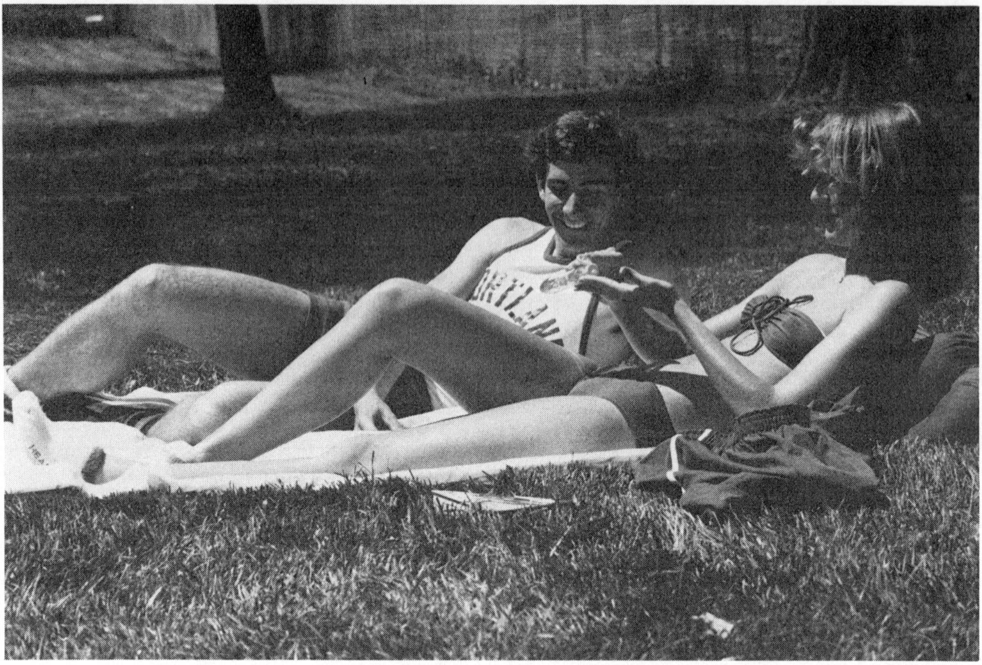

Figure 6.2 The ultraviolet rays of the sun can have both positive—the beauty of a tan—and negative effects on the skin.

freckles but have distinctive characteristic differences from a freckle. The epidermal cells over the spot thicken and may be up to an inch in diameter. Small injuries to the skin that result in hemorrhaging may add to their development. Lentigenes are commonly called "liver spots" or senile lentigenes because they are more frequently seen in older people.

Actinic keratoses usually develop on areas of the skin that are constantly exposed to the sun and wind. They look much like a wart with small raised spots that have a grey, brown, or yellow appearance. There may be some reddening of the skin around the area. Often these spots are called precancerous lesions because many progress into a squamous cell carcinoma (11, pp. 12–13).

Skin Cancer Squamous cell carcinoma is not as common as basal cell carcinoma. Squamous cell carcinoma has potential for metastasis and the lesions generally result from exposure to the sun or as a progressive development of an existing actinic keratoses. This type of carcinoma is a flesh-colored nodule that may ulcerate. Generally, it is seen in people in their late sixties.

Basal cell carcinoma is the most common type of skin cancer. Individual susceptibility may be a contributing factor, but most authorities believe that it develops as a result of sun exposure. This lesion starts as a small nodule that has a raised pearly border. As the lesion enlarges, it tends to ulcerate in the center. It generally does not have the potential for metastasis and is seen in people in their fifties (11, pp. 13–16).

Other Skin Problems Trapped natural oils in the outer layer of skin results in a condition called seborrheic dermatitis. It is an inflammatory condition that affects areas of the scalp, the eyebrows, the sides of the nose and cheeks, around the ears, and on the sternum of men.

Rosacea, a chronic inflammatory disorder of the sebaceous gland, is usually localized to the middle half of the face. It is always accompanied by redness and inflammation (erythema).

A very common skin lesion is seborrheic keratosis. The lesion is not malignant and it seldom becomes inflamed. Seborrheic keratoses develop in two locations and have both similar and different characteristics. Those that develop in areas of low sebaceous gland activity are dry and light in color. Those that develop in sebaceous areas such as the face, neck, and upper chest are dark and greasy in appearance. Both types seldom exceed one inch in diameter and they have a "warty" surface made up of many fingerlike projections. This type of lesion results in a negative cosmetic effect about which the older adult frequently complains.

The skin of the older person tends to be dry and it chaps more easily. This results in itching skin. In addition, the use of soap has an alkalinizing effect that aggravates the condition. Occasionally reactions to drugs will cause itching. Severe itching can also be a symptom associated with advanced liver or kidney disease, thyroid dysfunction, gout, and malignancies (11, p. 9, 17, 22).

Vitamin deficiencies can also result in specific skin-related changes. A lack of vitamin A causes phrynoderma, a dry skin condition. Fissured lips and sore tongue result from vitamin B deficiency. Horniness around hair follicles and skin hemorrhage often occur because of a vitamin C deficiency.

Preventing and Correcting Skin Problems One of the surest ways to help prevent premature aging of the skin and the development of an array of lesions is to protect the skin from the ultraviolet rays of the sun. The dark-skinned person is less inclined to get sun damaged skin than the light-skinned person. However, any prolonged sun exposure will damage any type of skin. Individuals who have sun-sensitive skin should consider using a product that contains a sun screen or sun block. Most authorities agree that products containing PABA (para-aminobenzoic acid) are the best to use. Other effective screening agents include digalloyl trioleate, cinnamates, anthranilates, pyrones, and salicylates. Sunbathers should reapply lotions if they swim or if they perspire heavily. People who sunburn easily should also consider using effective screening lotions in the winter.

Any unusual changes in the skin should be watched carefully and reported to the family physician. Conditions such as seborrheic dermatitis and rosacea require frequent shampooing with special tar-based, sulphur-based, and salicytic acid-based shampoos. Other helpful control methods are drying, peeling, and topical medicinal application regimens, local steroid preparations, and systemic antibodies.

If itching is the problem, then medical diagnosis is essential. Only trained personnel can determine if the itching is resulting from prescribed medications, a disease process, or just dry skin. Itching which results from dry, chapped skin can be helped by substituting an alkalinizing soap with a superfatted soap. Bath oils make the bathtub slippery, potentiate accidents, and should not be used by older people. Applying oil, such as baby oil, to the skin is generally satisfactory.

Either improved dietary practices and/or supplementary vitamins that have been recommended by a doctor can alleviate skin problems associated with vitamin deficiency.

Normal Changes with Age It is known that the prolonged exposure to the sun has damaging effects on the rate at which the skin ages and on the development of other physiological changes. Sometimes it is difficult to differentiate between normal changes in the skin and those induced by extrinsic factors. Generally, it is believed that the following changes occur as a result of normal aging:

1. The skin becomes thinner, especially in the dermal layer.
2. There are fewer elastin fibers and they are less elastic.
3. Fat deposits directly under the skin diminish.
4. Muscles decrease in size.

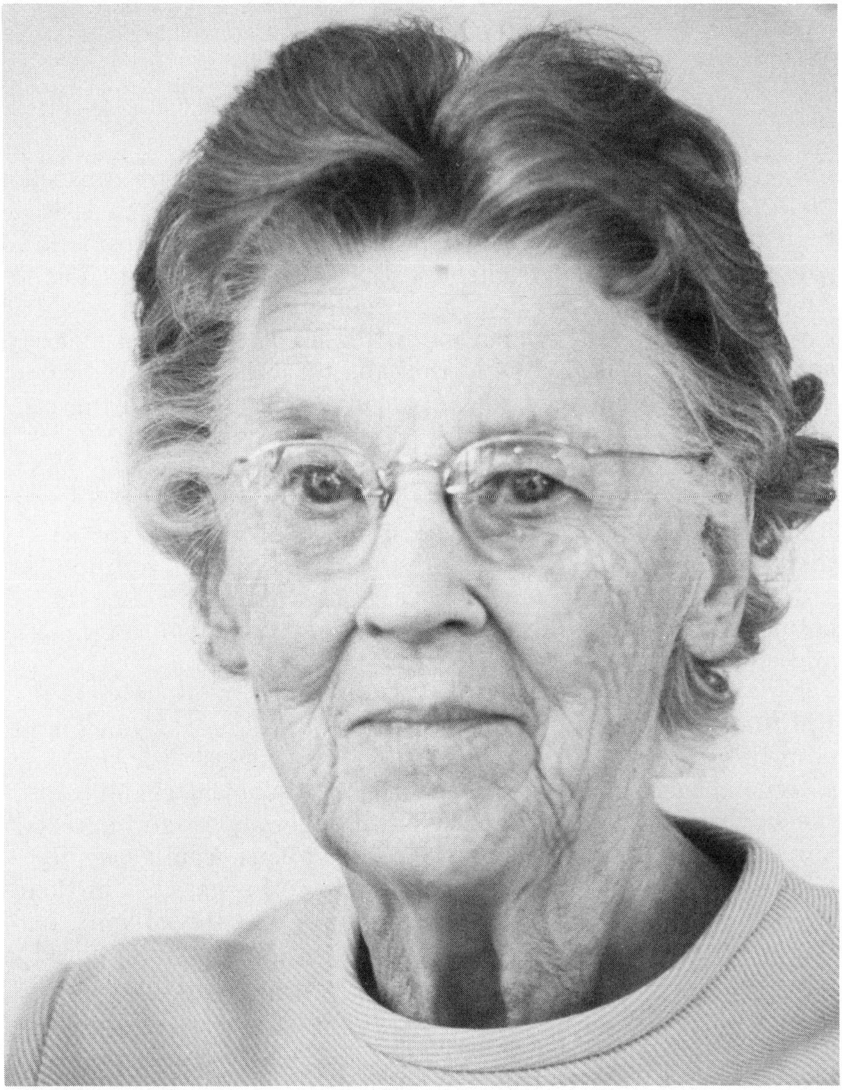

Figure 6.3 Certain changes in the skin occur as a result of normal aging (see text).

As these changes occur, the blood vessels show through loose, translucent skin, and wrinkles, grooves, and fissures appear on the face and neck.

■ Surgical Search for Youth

Cosmetic or esthetic surgery is a relatively new specialization of plastic surgery borne out of the human's psychological fear and anxiety of aging. In its infancy, cosmetic surgery catered to the jet set and movie personalities, but today surgeons are seeing men and women from all walks of middle-class life. In less than ten years the number of individuals receiving cosmetic surgery has increased tremendously. New York, Miami, Los Angeles, Brazil, and Mexico have become the centers for cosmetic surgery. In the past women more frequently sought cosmetic surgery, but a consensus of leading plastic surgeons has indicated that the number of men seeking changes has tripled in the last five years (3).

There are no statistics on the exact number of people who obtain cosmetic surgery. Unless there is a definite health reason for cosmetic surgery, private insurance will not pay for it; therefore, insurance statistics are of limited use. In addition, a great many physicians who have limited their practice to cosmetic surgery perform their operations in private hospitals and clinics.

Rationale for Surgery Many reasons have been given for cosmetic surgery. Most of them deal with perceived physical and emotional inadequacies. The normal physiological changes in the skin do not begin to appear until generally around age 30, although variations may be seen in individuals. Young people who seek cosmetic surgery generally do so for changes in their noses or to remove facial scarring from severe cases of acne. In the mature adult we see that the image of grandma and grandpa has changed over the years. Today's older people retire earlier, and are ". . . living longer and maintaining good health longer, they're doing things that only young people used to do, . . . they feel good and want to look as good as they feel" (4).

Job Security. Some cosmetic surgeries are related to job security. For example, one woman said that she wanted surgery because she did not want her employer to know her age so that she could keep her job. She was 70. A top executive showing premature signs of aging was incorrectly thought to be an alcoholic (2). Men feel that they fare better in daily job competition if they look young and fresh (3).

Marital Security. Martha was anxious and fearful that her husband was no longer interested in her. She was beginning to show signs of aging which bothered her. Her children were grown and had left home. Her husband, a college professor, was engrossed in his career and a female graduate assistant whom he described as "sharp and all fired up over teaching." His enthusiasm and constant talk about the graduate student only confirmed Martha's fears that her marriage was beginning to fail because she looked old. She sought and was refused cosmetic surgery from a trained medical specialist. As her frustration and anxiety mounted, she turned to a lesser trained physician who agreed to her surgery.

At first, her surgery seemed successful, but after several months her eyelids drooped unevenly and she looked far worse than before her surgery. At this point she finally admitted to her husband her fears about his interest in younger women. Martha's husband insisted that she was wrong and took her to meet the graduate assistant who turned out to be Martha's age. The graduate student told Martha that she had had the same feelings about her children's leaving home, her husband being busy with his career, and her own feelings about her age changes, and so she had decided upon a second career. With the support of her husband, Martha obtained help from a trained specialist to correct the botched surgery. She then reassessed her life and went back to school (13).

This is only one example. Hundreds of other surgeries are performed on both men and women because they fear loss of interest of a spouse and marriage failure because they are beginning to look older. Men who marry much younger women often seek cosmetic surgery in hopes of improving their marriage.

Societal Attitudes. Many adults fear the bags, sags, wrinkles, and double chins which often accompany age. As the gerontological literature points out, we seem to be currently living in a youth culture. Some obtain facial remodeling in order to conform to society's attitude toward being "young and beautiful." Undoubtedly, divorce rates are higher than ever before. In order to make a good "catch" for a second or third marriage, some feel they have to look younger.

Physician Concerns Medicare or private insurance will cover the expenses for cosmetic surgery if there are justifiable medical reasons for the surgery. Most generally, this includes such things as a divided nasal septum, impaired vision, or catastrophic injury. This means that the thousands of men and women who are having cosmetic surgery are paying for it themselves (Table 6.1).

Most physicians are concerned about the physical and mental well-being of their patients. They obtain complete

Table 6.1 Types and Cost of Cosmetic Surgery

Type	Description	Cost
Rhytidoplasty (Face lift)	The tightening and lifting of excessive skin which has lost its elasticity producing sags and wrinkles. Usually done under a general anesthetic. Most common type of surgery sought.	\$1000–\$5000
Blepharoplasty (eyelid lift, brow lift)	The tightening and removal of excessive skin on the eyelid or eyebrow.	\$1000–\$2000
Submandibular lipectomy	The removal of excessive skin from the neck and chin.	\$1000–\$2000
Full face lift	A combination of the rhytidoplasty, blepharoplasty, and submandibular lipectomy.	\$2000–\$5000
Full body contour	Removal of excessive fat from the hips and thighs.	\$5000
Rhinoplasty	Removal of unwanted nasal bone and cartilage.	\$1000–\$1500
Hair transplants	Small plugs of hair growing skin are removed from the back of the head and reimplanted in the front.	\$15 per plug
Mammioplasty	Reduction or enlargement of the breasts.	\$1500, depending on whether there are complications

Source: Gertrude Lang, "Facing the Facts About Face-Lifts," *Retirement Living,* (February, 1978), 74. Matt Clark et al., "The Plastic-Surgery Boom," *Newsweek* (January 24, 1977), 26.

medical histories of their patients and discuss with them the reasons why they want to have cosmetic surgery. Most of the time a patient is refused surgery when one of the following situations exists (12):

1. Another person has encouraged the surgery.
2. No obvious problem exists.
3. The person feels that his or her marriage will improve.
4. The person is a surgery seeker.

5. The person feels that cosmetic surgery will solve his or her personal problems.
6. The person is under psychiatric care.

Perhaps the most serious concern of the physician is with breast enlargements using silicone. Physicians report that about 60% of the cases will develop one or several of the following complications (5, 6):

1. Siliconomos (excessive scarring in fatty layers of breast tissue)
2. Silicone lumps
3. Migration of silicone to other parts of the body which result in disfigurement
4. Severe infection
5. Gangrene
6. Mastectomies

One physician in San Diego reported 400 breast complications between 1967 and 1974. Twenty percent of them resulted in breast removal (5, 6).

For the most part, cosmetic surgery will not make a person look younger. What it does do is make an individual look less tired and more refreshed. Surgeons report that the effects of cosmetic surgery only last from five to ten years before excessive skin begins to show up again. Cosmetic surgery does not eliminate other characteristics of aging such as changes in body contour, hands, skin tone, voice, and posture.

One man had cosmetic surgery when his wife did. When he was asked if he would have it done again when it was needed, he said that he wouldn't because his original motivation for having it done was to carry him over into retirement and that had been fulfilled and because it would be too expensive on a retirement income. He also said, "Sooner or later we all reach an age where we're willing to *be* our age" (12).

■ Body Hair

The hair on the head, eyelashes, eyebrows, hair on the inside of the ears and nostrils, and hair around the urogenitals serve as protection. Other body hair has no useful purpose.

Hairs are produced by follicles attached to the epidermis at the surface and extend into the depths of the skin. Body hair grows to a specific length peculiar to a particular part of the body. The exception to this is the hair on the scalp and face. Follicles become dormant after a hair is mature. When the follicles become active again, new hair is constructed and works its way to the surface of the skin. The old hair loosens and is shed. Hair varies in contour, diameter, color, amount, and distribution depending upon hereditary characteristics and the type of melanin pigment in them. Hair grows about one-third of a millimeter per day.

Hair Color Change in hair color is a universal occurrence as a person ages. The rate at which hair becomes grey or white depends largely upon heredity. It is believed that changes in hair color result from a general atrophy of the hair cells and reduction in the number of melanin pigments. Stories of people whose hair turned white overnight are myths. Since hair normally grows about one-third of a millimeter per day, it would take several days before the effects of hair color change would be visible on the surface.

Hair Loss Scalp hair appears to be the only hair which is lost with increasing frequency in aging men and women. Baldness (alopecia) is a systemic involution of hair follicles in which there is a lack or loss of hair. There are two types of baldness: permanent hair loss and temporary hair loss.

Permanent hair loss results from destruction or regression of the hair germ centers. Pattern baldness, which is most common, results from hereditary factors, age, and male sex hormones acting on genetically predisposed follicles. Baldness may start after puberty. The hair begins to recede at the temples and thin over the crown. In pattern baldness the follicles are not destroyed but gradually regress to the stage of producing lanugo hair. Permanent hair loss can also be the result of scar-producing injuries and diseases, inborn lack of hair development, or exposure to chemical or physical agents that severely injure the hair germ center.

Temporary loss of hair, called alopecia areata, can result from X-rays, drugs such as anticoagulants, malnutrition, some inflammatory skin diseases, chronic wasting diseases, endocrine disorders of the adrenal cortex, pituitary, thyroid or gonads, and illness accompanied by a high fever.

A temporary hair loss can also occur and is characterized by sharply outlined patches of baldness for which there is no known cause. Disorders of the hair shaft, fungus infections, or mechanical damage can cause the hair shaft to break off close to the skin, which gives a bald appearance.

Preventing Hair Loss Nothing can be done to prevent hereditary baldness. Avoidance of chemical agents that damage the hair root and avoidance of potential accident situations that could result in permanent damage could serve as preventive measures. There have been some claims that excessive oiliness and dandruff result in hair loss, but scientific studies have shown no relationship between these variables and hair loss.

Normal Changes with Age Usually hair loss and hair change occur by age sixty in both sexes. Patterns of hair loss are classified as full loss, early W-shaped, late W-shaped, U-shaped, and O-shaped. The greatest number of men experience U-shaped hair loss. Women generally are seen with early W-shaped loss (1). The amount of facial hair in older adults increases and most report little to no change in eyebrow hair or hair on the extremities. Hair in the external auditory canal of men generally becomes quite coarse (9).

■ Teeth and Gums

The development and eruption of the teeth occur in a fairly predictable manner, but great variation based upon familial patterns can be seen. The formation and calcification of the incisors, cuspids, and molars begin in the fifth and sixth month of fetal development. The eruption of the deciduous teeth begins about the fifth month after birth and continues until the twentieth and thirtieth months. The shedding of the 20 primary teeth begins at about the sixth year and continues until about the thirteenth year. The eruption of the secondary or permanent teeth is completed when the third molars appear between the seventeenth to twentieth years (8). The adult has 32 permanent teeth.

Figure 6.4 The structure of a human tooth (see text for details).

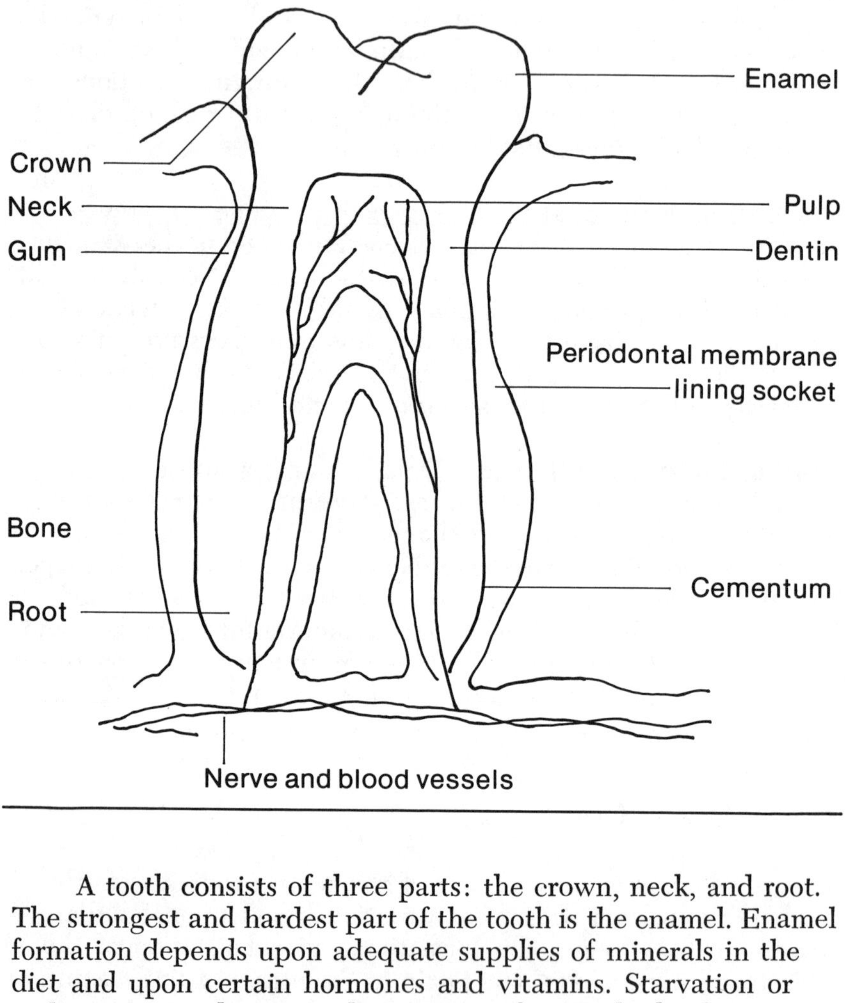

A tooth consists of three parts: the crown, neck, and root. The strongest and hardest part of the tooth is the enamel. Enamel formation depends upon adequate supplies of minerals in the diet and upon certain hormones and vitamins. Starvation or malnutrition and certain diseases interfere with the formation of enamel.

Dentin is more elastic than enamel and it is less highly mineralized. Dentin can regenerate itself and it develops from the pulp.

Specialized cells of the dental follicle form the cementum which is layered on the surface of the root. The cementum provides anchorage for the fiber bundles of the periodontal membrane. Cementum is also capable of regenerating itself.

In the central cavity of the tooth is the pulp. Pulp is made up of cells, a framework of fibers, blood vessels, and nerves. The pulp provides nutrition for the dentin.

The tooth is held in its socket by a fibrous tissue called the periodontal membrane. This membrane contains blood vessels and sensory nerve endings. The membrane is attached to the aveolar bone by fiber bundles.

Dental Problems Dental problems include dental caries, periodontal disease, and necrotic ulcerative gingivitis, all of which have an effect on the overall health of an individual.

Dental Caries. Tooth decay, or dental caries, is considered a progressive bacterial disease. In order for dental caries to occur, there must be a susceptible tooth, bacterial plaque, and fermentable carbohydrates. The enamel of the tooth is first decalcified by the acid which forms as a result of the bacteria fermenting the carbohydrates. If left untreated, the enamel continues to be decalcified and the dentin becomes affected. As the disease progresses, the pulp is exposed and undergoes decomposition.

Dental caries is an extremely prevalent health problem in the United States. Recent figures show that 50% of all three-year-olds have an average of one decayed deciduous tooth. The average increases to three decayed teeth by age 5 and to seven teeth which are decayed, missing, or filled by age 16. Sometime between the ages of 15 and 24 one person out of 100 will be edentulous (7, p. 159). As age goes up, the incidence of dental caries and missing teeth goes up. Women tend to have a slightly higher incidence of dental caries and edentulousness than do men.

Periodontal Disease. Periodontal disease affects the gums and surrounding tissues, including the periodontal membrane, cement, alveolar bone, and gingiva. The first stage is called gingivitis and the symptoms generally include red, swollen, and tender gums which tend to bleed easily if pressure is applied. There may be several causes of gum disease including:

1. Malocclusion
2. Faulty restoration
3. Epilepsy
4. Blood diseases

5. Nutritional deficiency, primarily the vitamin B complex and vitamin C
6. Improper use of a toothpick or digging into the gums with an object
7. Mouth breathing
8. Soft diet
9. Poor brushing and flossing techniques
10. Bacteria
11. Lodged food particles
12. Excess tartar (hard deposits around the neck of the tooth) (7, p. 161)

Middle- and older-aged persons can develop periodontal disease as a result of the following health conditions:

1. Hyperparathyroidism
2. Cushing's syndrome
3. Diabetes mellitus
4. Osteomalacia
5. Syphilis
6. Postclimacteric hormonal deficiencies
7. Disease that causes faulty protein metabolism
8. Vesiculation of herpes zoster
9. Pigmentation of Addison's disease
10. The peeling of desquamative stomatitis (11, pp. 345–346)

If left untreated, the second stage, called periodontitis, develops. As the bacteria invade the gums, the gums become more inflamed and begin to recede from the teeth, leaving a pocket in which bacteria, pus, and food particles collect. Tartar adds to the recession and irritation. The infection spreads to the periodontal membrane and alveolar bone and if left untreated causes extensive bone loss. The tooth becomes loose and either comes out by itself or must be extracted. Periodontitis may involve one tooth or all of the teeth.

Periodontal disease is found in all age groups. At least 50% of all elementary children and an even higher percentage of adolescents have it. In the older population, 65 and over, 58% of the males and 36% of the females have periodontal disease (10).

In addition to preventing extensive gum destruction, patients and dentists should be concerned about the development of bacterial endocarditis. This condition can develop as a result of severe oral or respiratory infection which invades the tissues of the heart. The development of bacterial endocarditis is *not* a common occurrence in old age.

Necrotic Ulcerative Gingivitis. Other names for this condition are NUG, trench mouth, and Vincent's infection. The exact cause is not known, but it is believed that important contributive factors in its development are lowered resistance of the body and tissues of the mouth and unhygienic conditions of the mouth. The symptoms include ulcerations along the gum margins, greyish color of the gums, swelling, tender gums that bleed easily, soreness making chewing and brushing the teeth painful, malodorous breath, throat infections, poor appetite, and illness causing swollen lymph glands and fever.

In most cases, individuals past retirement and on social security, private pensions, or Medicaid find that the rising costs of medical care, including dental care, have far exceeded their limited budgets. Consequently, as age goes up, fewer people seek dental care (Table 6.2).

Changes with Age As people age, there are changes in the teeth, gums, and oral cavity.

The Teeth. The teeth of older adults show a great deal of attrition or wearing down. Teeth become harder as a result of increased calcification. Older adults also lose a considerable amount of moisture in their mouths. Cracked and stained teeth are common and cusps often break off. Generally, there is an increase of fluorides which give the teeth a stained, yellowish color. With age, the pulp cavity decreases in size and the pulp becomes more fibrous, less cellular, less vascular, and less sensitive.

The Gums. Because of age and neglect, the periodontal tissue becomes fibrous. Connective tissue fibers replace much of the normal gingiva. Reduced blood flow makes the tissue pale and metabolic exchange is retarded. Injury or surgery to the gums heals very slowly. Due to the hypovascularization of the tissues, the gingiva recedes painlessly and exposes the root.

Oral Cavity. The lining of the cheeks (mucous membrane) is normally a thin, delicate epithelial lining. In older people this lining is thinner and less vascular and has a shiny appearance. The epithelial cells pile up, resulting in a whitish keratoses.

Table 6.2 Dental Visits for Males and Females in 1975

Sex and Age of Patient	Dental Visits (millions)
Total visits	341
Males	153
Females	186
Visits per person	1.6
Males	1.5
Females	1.7
Under 6 Years	.6
6–16	2.0
17–24	1.8
25–44	1.7
45–64	1.8
65+	1.2

Source: U.S. National Center for Health Statistics, *Vital and Health Statistics,* Series 10, 115, 1975.

Sometimes benign white lesions called leukoplakia develop. These result, partially as a result of vitamin A deficiency. Other greyish lesions which develop may be cancerous.

The gums of people who have heart and lung disease are cyanotic or pale if there is anemia. The dentist treating an older patient should obtain a complete medical history before doing any corrective work. It is particularly important to be aware of heart conditions and hypertension and any medications the patient is currently taking. It is not necessary for the dentist to be an expert on heart conditions, but he or she should be aware that if a patient complains of a toothache in a left posterior mandibular tooth, it could be a warning symptom of impending angina pectoris. The dentist should also be concerned about excessive stress and fatigue while treating a heart patient. Patients who have hypertension should not be given anesthetics that leave a high content of vasoconstrictor because this raises the blood pressure even more.

Older people who still have their teeth should be encouraged to practice good oral hygiene because it helps to reduce tooth decay and periodontal disease. Those who have dentures should be encouraged to eat with their dentures.

However, with increasing age the gingiva recedes and dentures no longer fit properly and so many choose to eat without their dentures. In this case, they should be encouraged to eat solid foods cut into small pieces instead of eating all soft foods. In addition, poorly fitting dentures irritate the gums. Dentures may be removed at night to relieve the pressure on the gums and the gums should be massaged daily to improve circulation. People who have dentures should be encouraged to wear them not only for cosmetic reasons but also to improve the morale.

Preventing Dental Problems A relatively high percentage of dental decay can be prevented through proper toothbrushing and flossing. Ideally, teeth should be brushed every time one eats, but if this is not possible brushing should be done at least once a day. The outer, inner, and biting surfaces should be brushed thoroughly and the position of the toothbrush should be changed frequently. The American Dental Association recommends that the toothbrush be replaced often. A worn-out toothbrush does not clean the teeth properly.

Flossing provides additional cleansing of the teeth by removing dental plaque and tiny food particles from between the teeth, on the surface of the tooth, and in the gingival margin.

Scientists believe that each individual inherits a degree of resistance to tooth decay. Some people have more resistance than others. In addition, the size and position of the teeth and the depth of the grooves and pits are also inherited. The deeper the grooves or the more irregularly the teeth are positioned, the greater the likelihood that dental plaque and food particles will become lodged in these locations.

A balanced diet is necessary not only for good health but also for good dental health. The diet should be restricted in sugar content and abundant in foods high in vitamins, minerals, and protein.

■ Overall Appearance

The healthy, active individual continues to maintain personal appearance throughout life. Those who lose interest in life also lose interest in their appearance. A great many of today's young people choose a casual manner of dress. Parents who purchase clothing for their adolescent children are often dismayed at the casualness of dress as well as the high cost of clothing. As adults stereotype youth by their appearance, so do youth stereotype adults by their appearance.

The typical stereotype of the older adult is of a "dumpy," straggly haired, wrinkle faced slovenly dressed person. Several factors contribute to this physical appearance. A fixed, low income limits the possibility of purchasing up-to-date clothing. Nothing ages a person more than wearing old-fashioned, ragged clothing. As a person gets into the seventies and eighties, footing sometimes becomes less secure. Therefore, well-fitted shoes are necessary. Older women should not wear spike-heeled shoes but this does not mean that they have to wear unattractive, old-fashioned shoes.

As body metabolism changes, older people are more acutely aware of climate changes. In colder weather they should wear warm clothing and in warmer weather they should wear light-weight clothing.

Visual acuity lessens with age. As a result, the older person is often not aware of stained or wrinkled clothing, buttons not buttoned, and tears. Careful grooming becomes more difficult. Makeup is not placed properly, hair is unkempt, and shaving may be incomplete. Whenever possible, family members should assist the older person when a garment needs cleaning, repairing, or pressing or when personal hygiene needs improving.

Most people feel good when they look good. Everyone should be encouraged to purchase new clothing, and as often as possible they should select their own clothing. Jewelry, colorful scarves, colorful ties, cuff links, and regular visits to the beauty salon or barber shop can boost the morale of almost everyone.

■ Summary

Although many physiological changes take place as a person ages, the most noticeable changes have to do with cosmetic changes. General changes in the skin include thinning, loss of elasticity, and decreased muscle size. The ultraviolet rays of the sun do extensive damage to the skin which results in wrinkling and the development of lentigenes, keratoses, and skin cancer. Other skin changes are related to poor hygiene, diseases, and nutritional deficiencies. Increasing numbers of men and women are turning to cosmetic surgery to improve their appearance, but plastic surgery only temporarily reduces the changes. As people age, they can expect changes in hair color and hair loss.

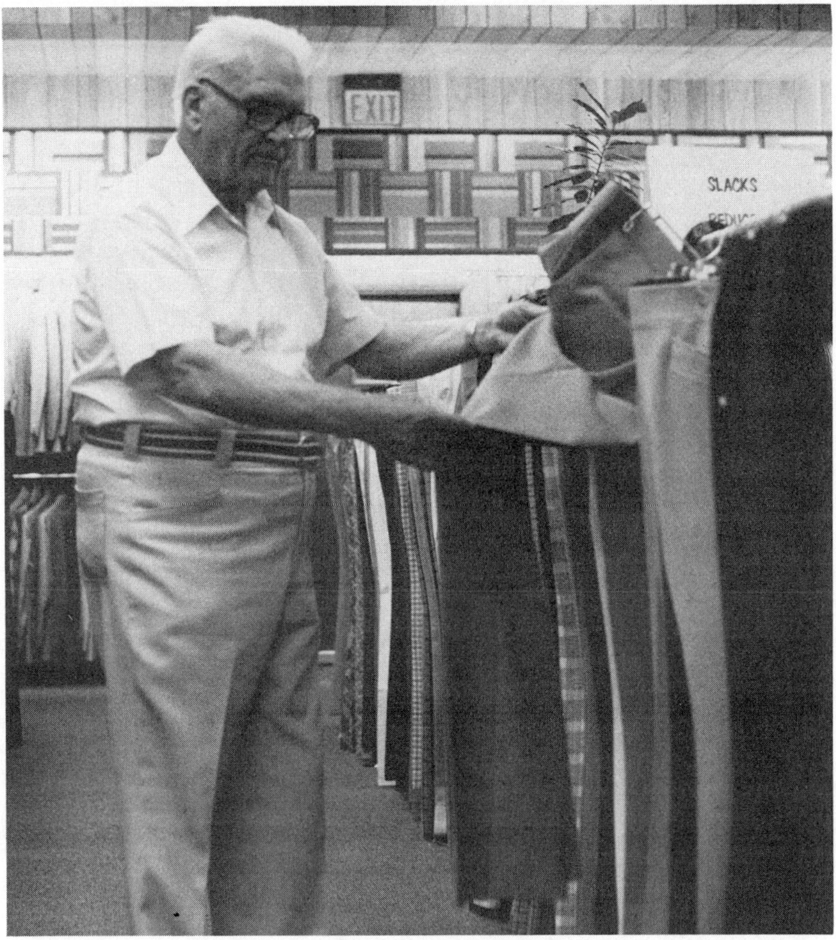

Figure 6.5 As often as possible, shop for and purchase your own clothing—you generally feel good when you look good.

The most prevalent health problem in all age groups involves the teeth and gums. Dental caries and periodontal disease are most frequently seen and have multiple causes.

A good physical appearance has an influence on morale. How a person looks depends upon such things as income, reduced visual acuity, changes in body metabolism, style of clothing, and the use of cosmetics.

References

1. Beek, C. H. "A Study on Extension and Distribution of the Human Body Hair." *Dermatologica* 101 (1951):317.
2. Clark, Matt, Shapiro, Dan, Jaffe, Andrew, and Gram, Dewey. "The Plastic Surgery Boom." *Newsweek,* 24 January, 1977.

3. Kelly, James. "Cosmetic Lib for Men." *New York Times Magazine,* 25 September, 1977, p. 120.
4. Lang, Gertrude. "Facing the Facts About Face-Lifts." *Retirement Living,* February, 1978, p. 25.
5. Larned, Deborah. "A Shot or Two or Three in the Breasts." *MS,* September, 1977, pp. 55, 86.
6. Nashner, Marjorie, and White, Mimi. "Beauty and the Breast." *MS,* September, 1977, pp. 53–54.
7. Nemir, A., and Schaller, W. *The School Health Program.* Philadelphia: Saunders, 1975.
8. Timiras, P. S. *Developmental Physiology and Aging,* p. 202. New York: Macmillan, 1972.
9. Tindall, J. P., and Smith, J. G. "Skin Lesions of the Aged and Their Association with Internal Changes." *Journal of the American Medical Association* 186 (1963):1039.
10. U.S. Department of Health, Education and Welfare. *Health United States,* pp. 595–97. Washington, D.C.: U.S. Government Printing Office, 1975.
11. U.S. Department of Health, Education and Welfare. *Working with Older People—A Guide to Practice,* Public Health Service, Volume IV. Washington, D.C.: U.S. Government Printing Office, 1974.
12. Vernon, Nick. "Face-Lifts for Two." *Retirement Living.* February, 1978, pp. 24–25.
13. ———. "The Face-Lift That Flopped." *Good Housekeeping.* March, 1978, pp. 22–34.

PART FOUR

Physiological Change and Disease

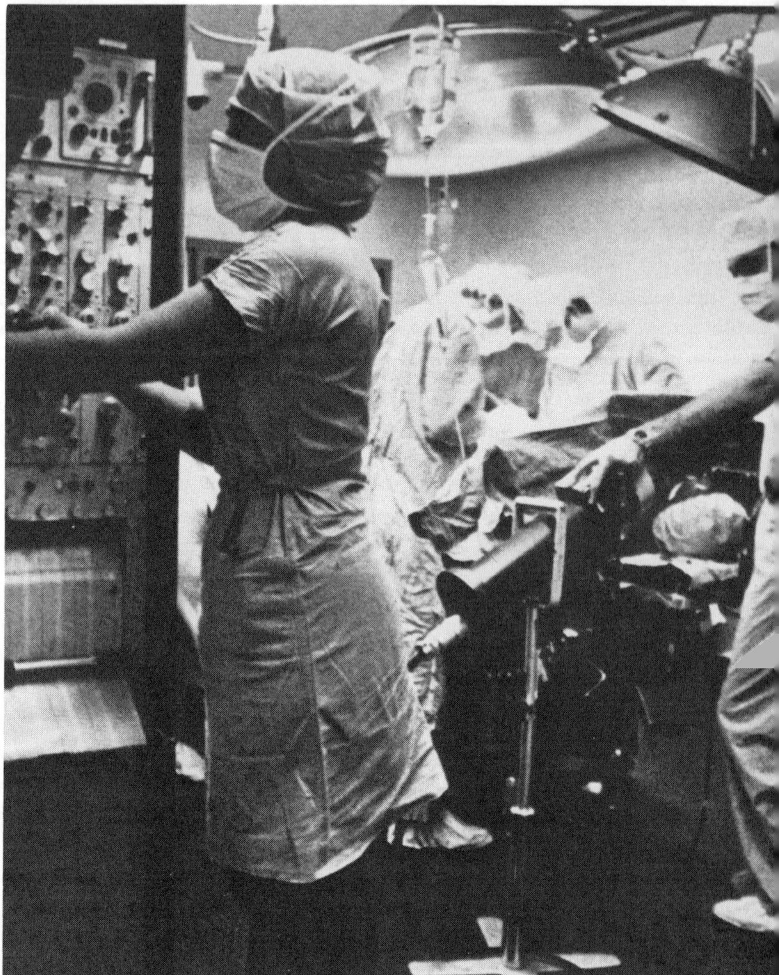

■ Chapter 7

Chronic and Degenerative Diseases

Major Concepts

1. The aging process is accelerated by various acquired diseases.
2. The aging process is accelerated by genetically acquired diseases.
3. Multiple disease syndromes can create secondary degenerative processes.

Throughout history the major cause of death has been communicable disease, i.e., plague, venereal disease, influenza, tuberculosis, pneumonia. In some parts of the world this is still the case, but twentieth-century advances in preventive medicine have vastly altered the pattern of disease in the United States and other western countries. In 1900 the leading causes of death in the United States were tuberculosis and pneumonia, both communicable diseases. Today these diseases are of secondary concern and in their places are cardiovascular disease, the number one cause of death, and cancer, the number two cause of death (see Table 7.1).

The decrease in the number of cases of tuberculosis and pneumonia is credited to improvements in diagnosis, treatment, sanitation, nutrition, housing, and working conditions. More specific measures, such as immunizations, have played the most important roles in the conquest of communicable diseases. Antibiotics and sulfa drugs have greatly reduced the number of cases of communicable diseases as public health hazards.

The significant increase in chronic diseases has been attributed in large to the increased average life span. Chronic diseases are defined as persistent and degenerative diseases. In a period of 100 years, from 1860 to 1960, the proportion of the population in the United States over 45 years of age has climbed from 13% to 29%. This increase in older age groups is currently changing

Table 7.1 Leading Causes of Death in U.S., 1900–1978

1900 Life Expectancy: Male: 46.1 Female: 49.5	1977 Life Expectancy: Male: 69.8 Female: 75.7
1. Tuberculosis	1. Cardiovascular disease
2. Pneumonia	2. Cancer
3. Intestinal disorders	3. Accidents
4. Heart diseases	4. Respiratory disease
5. Infant diseases	5. Diabetes

Source: HEW—1977: Records and Statistics.

Table 7.2

Cause of Death 45–64		Cause of Death 65+
Cardiovascular disease	1	Cardiovascular disease
Cancer	2	Cancer
Cerebrovascular incidents	3	Cerebrovascular incidents
Accidents	4	Influenza
Cirrhosis	5	Arteriosclerosis
Influenza	6	Accidents
Diabetes	7	Diabetes
Respiratory diseases	8	Respiratory diseases
Suicide	9	Cirrhosis
Homicide	10	Kidney failure

Source: National Center for Health Statistics: HEW, 1976.

the whole field of preventive medicine. Early efforts were directed toward the control of communicable diseases of early life. Efforts are now being directed toward the chronic diseases, those thought to be most common in the middle decades of life or later life.

Of the nearly 30 million people over the age of 65 in the United States today, 85% report the presence of at least one chronic condition, with approximately one-half of these individuals encountering limitations in their daily activity because of poor health.

The statistics in Table 7.2 do not tell the whole story. In the early decades of life 6 out of 1000 individuals are afflicted with chronic conditions. Between the ages of 18 and 25 years the rate triples. By the seventh decade 200 out of 1000 are afflicted. This rate doubles again by the eighth decade of life. Inevitably 90% of all individuals over the age of 90 years will be afflicted with chronic diseases.

Even though older people do suffer at least one acute episode of illness every year, there has been a drastic decline since the mid-1940s.

■ Acute Illness and Accidents

Acute illness is defined as a rapidly progressive illness that may lead to rapid death. Older individuals who contract an acute illness or who have an accident are disabled longer. Sixty-eight percent of the accidents had by individuals over 65 are household accidents. Four times as many older women as older men suffer disabilities. As a result of health problems, acute and chronic, as well as accidents, individuals in later life have their activities restricted for approximately 35 days per year as compared to 21 days for individuals between 40 and 50 years of age.

Many individuals in later decades find that the aftermath of ill-health poses more of a threat than death does. From the middle decades to the later decades a large percentage of individuals live with at least one chronic health problem and the likelihood of other severe problems occurring in successive years.

Various respiratory illnesses have become the most frequent acute illnesses among individuals in middle years. This accounts for 78 out of 100 episodes of acute distress by the fourth decade.

For centuries diseases affecting the gastrointestinal tract have plagued individuals in later life. However, individuals in their fourth decade are now experiencing these disorders. Despite the many questions concerning diseases in later life, physicians indicate that treatments used for older individuals are exactly the same as for individuals in their third and fourth decades. The difference among the age groups is the presence of chronic conditions that may further complicate illnesses and the recovery from such conditions.

As significant as these acute conditions are, it is even more significant that these conditions impose limitations on individuals in later years. Such limitations may make these individuals socially isolated. During the fourth and fifth decades of life there is a noticeable increase in the number of individuals who are unable to perform daily routines without constraint. Several unpublished research projects indicate that 50% of the people over 65 are able to maintain their daily routines without limitations. The number of individuals exhibiting constraining factors due to chronic illnesses are shown in Figure 7.1. As expected, the proportion of severely limited individuals increases markedly with advancing age. This number is about four times that of individuals not affected. It has been noted by many physicians that after individuals reach their eighth decade they are more

Figure 7.1 Percentage of adults with limitations.

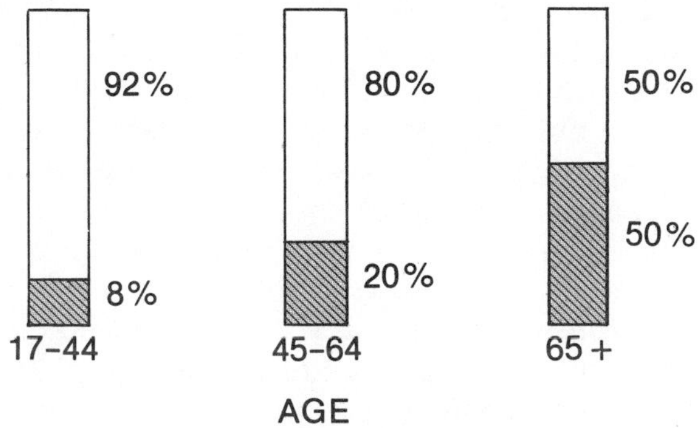

Source: Vital Health Statistics, U.S. Government Pub., May 1978.

inhibited by the effects of chronic conditions and they face greater social barriers. Because of their extensive health problems and diminished resources, many older people become anxious about the possibility of losing their independence. Not all elderly people experience the same health-related problems. It is obvious that factors such as sex, race, and income are very important components of the total health of the society. With very few exceptions, females, nonwhites, and individuals in a low socioeconomic class suffer more from ill-health in the aging process than do others.

The most prevalent chronic conditions among Americans are the various forms of cardiovascular disease, cancer, arthritic conditions, diabetes, and respiratory problems. In Chapter 5 it was emphasized that everyone undergoes certain physiological changes as one ages. These changes are considered unrelated to pathological irregularities. This indicates that medical professionals are able to distinguish between disease and the aging process. However, there is a correlation between degenerative changes and chronic diseases. That is, one does not die from age; one succumbs to a chronic disease.

■ Cardiovascular Disease

Heart disease surpasses all other disorders in terms of both mobility and mortality in western civilizations. According to the American Heart Association, cardiovascular disorders are now afflicting one in five. Prior to the 1960s it was thought that it affected only those individuals past the third decade of life and it was traditionally thought to be part of the aging process. Heart disease among teen-agers has somewhat disproven this. However, various congenital, pathological, and abnormal anatomical changes may contribute to the aging process.

Along with normal intercellular dehydration of body tissue, the aging heart is depicted as having an accumulation of fat, with less efficient valves and markedly widespread atrophy. It has been hypothesized that cardiac output declines approximately 1.3% each year after the age of 31. The most notable changes are the loss of reserve capacities and the loss of rapid response under severe stress. Such degenerative processes are questionable when applied to the general population. However, this disease does produce progressive deposits of fatty tissue with the frequency of increasing inoperable portions of the heart muscle. Such changes are functional as well as structural. The most commonly observed symptoms are visceral pain, loss of breath, irregular heartbeats, and varying blood pressure.

During the twentieth century cardiovascular disease has been responsible for over 50% of the deaths in Western civilized countries. The mortality rate is over three times that of cancer. In the 1970s more males in their twenties were prone to heart disease than were females past menopause. However, the rate of male mortality during the fifth decade and after averages in excess of 1.2 per 1000. The debilitating effect of cardiovascular incidents represents 25% of all disabilities among men in the United States. As chronological age increases, mortality rates double with each decade for males and they triple with each decade for females.

It has been hypothesized that cardiovascular disease is correlated to the high standard of living in Western industrialized countries where overeating, inactivity, and stress are the norm. But, in a 1971 study it was found that nonwhites are more prone to cardiovascular disease than are whites! Public records indicate a 2 to 1 ratio. Offsetting factors are high medical awareness and better quality of medical care among those of higher socioeconomic status. Nonwhite higher incidence is related to high blood pressure, poor diets, high fat consumption, and extrinsic environmental factors.

Cardiovascular disease is radical in onset. Over 30% of the victims die before they can get medical attention. If medical attention is not obtained within 24 hours, additional fatalities may result. Rehabilitation from this disease will be discussed in Chapter 8.

■ Cancer

It is difficult to form an exact definition of cancer, since the many malignant diseases represented by the word "cancer" have few characteristics in common. In general, cancerous or malignant diseases can be described as those conditions in which abnormal cells develop, divide, and grow and are not restrained by the normal controls exerted by the host organism. These cancer cells may resemble the normal cells that make up the tissue in which they originate, but they have the power to grow beyond their normal environment and invade surrounding tissues. A cancer cell somehow corrupts the forces that normally protect the body, invades the well-ordered society of cells surrounding it, colonizes distant areas, and as a finale to this cannibalistic orgy of flesh consuming flesh it commits suicide by destroying its host. In other words, the disease state "cancer" has three qualitative characteristics: (1) the ability to divide and produce abnormal daughter cells, (2) the ability to displace, invade, and destroy normal tissues, and (3) the ability to grow in the presence of control mechanisms that preserve the orderly growth of normal cells.

Of the 100 million million cells in the body, about 500 billion (about one-half kilogram of cells) must be replaced daily. Considering the enormous number of mitotic divisions (cell divisions) that must be completed perfectly for normal development, it is amazing that such a complex organism as a human ever evolved. In fact, not all cell divisions are perfect; the number of abnormal cells formed daily is estimated to be at least 10,000 to 1,000,000. The number probably varies with age and environmental stresses, such as irradiation. A majority of these abnormal cells are probably so defective that they cannot divide into daughter cells or even survive.

The factors that shift the balance of power in favor of the survival of some abnormal cells having the characteristics of cancer are still unknown. It is a biological wonder that a person does not develop cancer early in life. Perhaps a person does, but usually the many abnormal cells are effectively destroyed by the

Figure 7.2 Cancer by site and sex.

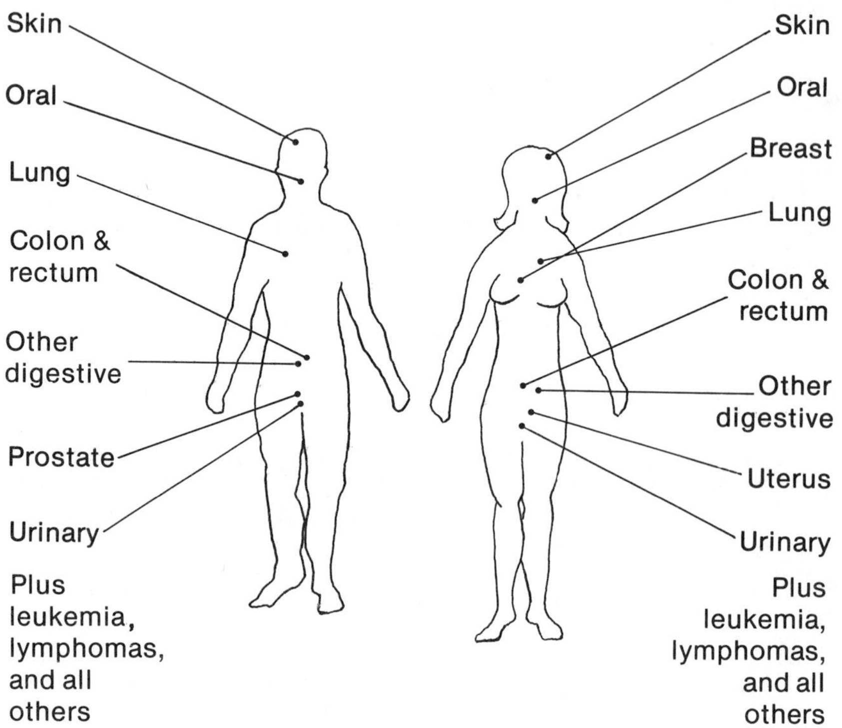

body's natural defenses. If the natural defense against abnormal cells were not so efficient, a person would have a great deal more to fear from the malignant diseases.

The exact nature of these natural defenses is not known (15). One assumption is that some abnormal cells provoke the formation of antibodies against themselves; that is, the abnormal cells perform as antigens and are rejected in the same way that foreign biological material is routinely rejected. A second suggestion is that normal lymphocytes (cells found in the blood) and perhaps other cells recognize that the abnormal cells are foreign and then destroy them.

It is easy to think of cells either as cancer cells or as normal cells, but a good many "normal" cells have some characteristics of malignancy. For example, they may have one or more partially defective enzyme systems among the thousands of malignancies occurring in normal cells, they may sluggishly produce a few noncritical peptides or proteins, or they may even have a group of such defects. Some normal cells have the ability to spread to distant sites and establish secondary colonies; moreover, during the repair of injuries or the replacement of cells—for example, after a loss of blood—the normal cells may divide very rapidly. Other cells, such as the leukocytes, or white blood corpuscles, can, like malignant cells, invade normal tissues.

Many cancer cells are not totally devoid of normal cell characteristics. For example, some cancer cells divide very slowly and some thyroid cancer cells continue to form alveolar structures (compartment-like structures) and produce an enzyme and other normal end products. Moreover, under the microscope, many individual cancer cells look identical to the normal cells from which they were derived. Since this kind of cancer cell is not rare, pathologists prefer to make a diagnosis from sheets of cancer cells and from the patterns of both normal and abnormal cells rather than from a single isolated cell.

Rapid growth and proliferation of the cells are very important factors in determining the relative malignancy of a cancer, but they are not qualitative features unique to cancer cells. Many kinds of normal cells, such as those in the bone marrow and those lining the intestinal tract, may multiply just as quickly as some highly malignant cancer cells. Other normal cells which usually grow very slowly can be temporarily activated to rapid growth when repairs are needed to heal cuts and fractures and other tissue damage. These normal cells stop their rapid growth once the injury is repaired; in other words, they are still under the control of the body and therefore are not cancerous cells. In contrast, cancerous cells do not know when to cease reproducing themselves. Cancerous cells of the thyroid gland or breast may spread into other organs, the bones, and the brain and continue to produce abnormal cells that disrupt the normal tissues.

There are many agents which may cause cancer, but no one knows precisely what happens to a normal cell to transform it into a cancerous one. Probably several factors must be arranged in certain patterns before a cell will become cancerous. At least one important factor must affect DNA (deoxyribonucleic acid), the large molecule in the chromosomes that carries genetic information from one generation to the next. DNA must be affected because cancer cells transmit the characteristics of malignant growth to their daughter cells. Normal cells have 22 chromosomes arranged in pairs, plus 2 sex chromosomes, giving a total of 46. Almost all cancer cells have abnormalities in either the number or configuration of one or more chromosomes. Probably more genetic abnormalities than can actually be observed exist in the chromosomes of cancer cells; since each chromosome may contain from 10,000 to 40,000 genes consisting of sequentially coded DNA components, it would not be surprising to find that an apparently normal chromosome is lacking a significant number of genes.

If it could be established that specific chromosome abnormalities are always observed in patients with certain cancers, then chromosome analysis might become a very useful diagnostic tool in detecting malignant disease. Unfortunately, only one such relationship has been found so far in cases of chronic myelogenous leukemia, in which most of the malignant blood cells of most patients are observed to lack part of a specific chromosome (66). From the time this abnormality was discovered, much research has been devoted to finding other cancers having consistent chromosomal abnormalities.

Some cancer researchers continue to hope that there is an additional fragment of the genetic code that carries the characteristics of malignancy. Others have suggested that the cancerous cells have had a portion of the genetic code deleted and that the absence of this portion frees the cancer cells from normal controls. Still others think that both of these conditions are necessary. Very recent experiments involving the fusion or hybridization of a normal cell with a cancer cell produced a conglomerate cell which always acted like a malignant cell, a result which may favor the addition theory.

In most cancers the malignant cells escape from the tissue of origin and enter the bloodstream, lymphatic vessels, and other tissue spaces. The cancer cells must then migrate through the lymphatic and blood vessels in order to be carried as colonists to distant parts of the body, where they may form additional tumor masses (36). Probably many hundreds of thousands of cancer cells escape from the "mother tumor," but they must be very vigorous to be able to penetrate the walls of the blood vessels, survive the antagonistic defenses of the host, and eventually settle and colonize new areas. Although most cancers grow by spreading throughout the body, some radiate out from a central point, choking off blood vessels and destroying organ functions in

Table 7.3 Death Rate for Cancer, 1976 (per 100,000)

Male 45–54	Male 55–64
1. Respiratory (72.1)	1. Respiratory (202.3)
2. Digestive organs (45.9)	2. Digestive organs (139.0)
3. Lymphatic tissue (12.8) [1]	3. Lymphatic tissue (27.1) [1]
4. Mouth, throat, pharynx (7.9)	4. Urinary organs (26.4)
5. Urinary organs (8.0)	5. Genitals (22.8)
Female 45–54	**Female 55–64**
1. Breast (51.1)	1. Digestive organs (82.5)
2. Respiratory (29.7)	2. Breast (82.2)
3. Digestive organs (29.4)	3. Respiratory (62.2)
4. Genitals (28.5)	4. Genitals (54.1)
5. Lymphatic tissue (7.5) [1]	5. Lymphatic tissue (18.2)

Source: Statistical Abstract of U.S., 1978, p. 77.

[1] Excludes leukemia.

a fairly local area. But no matter how they grow, as the invading cancer cells parasitize more and more tissues, vital functions are progressively weakened until finally the host is destroyed.

Types of Cancer Because cancer is really a large group of diseases, it takes many forms. Most cancers manifest themselves in the form of tumors, but this is not to say that all tumors are cancerous. Many tumors are relatively harmless, for example, the lipomas that are sometimes found in ex-newspaper boys. These benign growths develop over the shoulder blade where the strap of the heavy bag irritated the tissues beneath the skin. Most goiters are also benign tumors. These growths, usually found in women, are enlargements of the thyroid gland in the neck. They are often observed in areas where there is an iodine deficiency.

Benign tumors as well as cancers may occur in any tissue. The medical practice names them according to the tissue of the origin. The suffix oma, meaning tumor, is added to the name of the tissue. For example, fibroma, neuroma, and fibrolipoma are all benign diseases. Malignant diseases are named by using the name of the tissue and the suffix, for example, sarcoma and carcinoma. The suffix refers to the type of cells represented by the tumor; sarcomas, for example, are derived from connective tissue (bone, cartilage, muscle, fat, and fibrous tissue).

Cancers, like the infectious diseases, are caused by many different agents and their effects on the victims range from minor illnesses to life-threatening processes. There are over 100 basic recognized forms of cancer, and there are probably as many different kinds of cancer as there are kinds of normal cells in the body. The uniqueness of each cancer is almost guaranteed, since the behavior of a cancer is the result of the genetic properties of the cancer cells themselves and those of the host, as modified by nongenetic properties of the cells. The malignant diseases, therefore, are represented by a broad spectrum of biological manifestations.

The benign end of the spectrum is characterized by basal cell cancers of the skin. These cancers of the cells in the deep layers of the skin usually occur on areas habitually exposed to sunlight. The cells of these malignant tumors may grow more slowly than many normal cells, but they eventually pile up and form a small tumor mass. Because these particular cancer cells grow slowly, adhere tightly to each other, and do not invade the blood vessels or lymph channels, basal cell skin cancer can be easily treated and cured by surgical excision, X-ray treatment, the application of chemicals or intense cold, and even laser-beam treatment. Of course, if these tumors are not treated, they will grow and gradually destroy the surrounding tissues and even cause death. On the other end of the spectrum are the acute leukemias, which are cancerous diseases of the white blood cells. These diseases are incurable, even when diagnosed very early, because the malignant cells spread rapidly through the body.

Cancer cells are not as stable as normal cells. Normal cells do an excellent job of dividing into daughter cells which are exact replications of themselves. Cancer cells are much less reliable, and the daughter cells may not be exactly like the parent cell. Thus, a cancerous mass may consist of a mosaic of different but related cancer cells, some of which grow slowly and resemble normal cells and others which have the appearance of embryonic cells and grow very rapidly. In general, selective factors will favor the most rapidly growing cells. An understanding of this characteristic of cancers is important to the physician. When the

Figure 7.3 Cancer needs future examination by our society

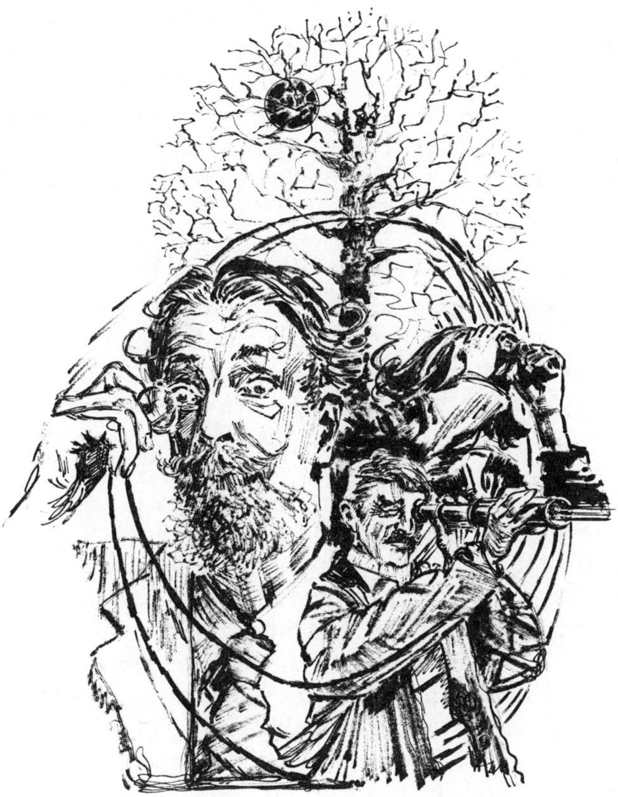

physician treats a patient with an anticancer drug, the treatment may affect only those masses or secondary growths of tumor tissue that were started by a more normal cancer cell; other new growths, which started from one of the wilder cancer cells, may not respond.

Population The devastating effects of the cancerous diseases are not limited to human beings. In every species of multicellular life there are victims of cancerous growth. Some investigators even believe that some one-celled organisms, the protozoa, show peculiar alterations of structure and functions that resemble malignancy. One may observe various kinds of cancerous and tumorous growths on trees and plants, in fish and fowl, and in wild and domestic animals. Even the bones of prehistoric reptiles have defects that probably were caused by cancerous growths.

But few species are more heavily attacked by cancer than the human. Part of the reason for this is that cancer seems to strike most frequently among aging organisms, and human beings live relatively longer than most animals. A yet unproven theory related to cancer is that because many populations exist at a higher trophic level, they may recieve higher than desirable doses of carcinogenic substances. This same observation accounts for the comparative rarity of cancer among primitive people, both in early times and in our own day. Wherever modern medical and sanitary techniques have increased the life span of a population, the rate of death from malignancy has rapidly increased. Also, of course, the keeping of adequate medical records may show the apparent incidence of cancer in a population, since the number of disease victims recognized as having cancer may increase. When we hear of a primitive tribe somewhere in which cancer is almost unknown, we may be sure that the members of the tribe do not live much beyond the age of 30 and that they do not keep medical records.

In our society the malignant diseases develop mostly in people over the age of forty, although children and young people are susceptible to certain kinds of cancer, for example, the leukemias and lymphomas, tumors of the brain and kidneys, and sarcomas of bone. In fact, cancer kills more children between the ages of 1 and 15 than does any other group of diseases; and in rare cases, cancer has occurred even before birth. Teenagers and college students are most frequently afflicted by leukemia and the lymphomas, Hodgkin's disease (a neoplasm of the lymphatic tissues), sarcomas of bone and connective tissue (52), and brain tumors.

Causes The cancerous diseases are so numerous and so different that scientists have been unable to find any one specific and universal event that occurs in the body and causes cells to become malignant. Perhaps there is no single and ultimate cause since there is probably no clearcut distinction between normal cells and cancerous ones. Perhaps only one factor is needed to transform one kind of benign cell into a malignant one whereas several factors may be needed to transform another normal cell into a cancer cell. The degree of malignancy in a cell is related to a series of changes that influence the differentiation (maturation into its specialized function) of a normal cell. Whatever the changes are, they are incorporated into the inheritable part of the cell, which is then able to divide into numerous cancerous offspring.

But even though it is not known exactly what the molecular events are that cause a normal cell to turn cancerous, a great deal has been learned about the circumstances surrounding the development of some cancers. Enough is known about some cancers (such as skin cancer) to prevent them now and others in the future. Thus, the causes of some cancers are known, and the causes of others are suspected. Still, the causes of many remain unknown.

Heredity When cancer strikes more than one member of a family, it is tempting to say that the malignancy was "caught" or inherited. There have been a few rare cases of epidemic-like outbreaks of leukemia among children living in a small area, but there is no conclusive proof that these are attributable to an infectious agent such as a virus; they might be due simply to chance.

A few cancers and a few "precancerous conditions" are inheritable. For example, retinoblastoma, a rare tumor of the eye, is inherited through a dominant gene; and intestinal polyposis, a benign condition which may become malignant, is definitely inheritable. But these cases are exceptional.

Although most cancers are not hereditary, there is good evidence that a predisposition or susceptibility to specific kinds of malignancy may be inherited. For example, individuals whose genes provide them with insufficient pigment-cell protection against the ultraviolet rays of the sun have a predisposition to skin cancer. Albinos and all persons with blue eyes and fair skin, and especially those with red hair, are much more susceptible to damage of those areas of the skin excessively exposed to sunlight. There is a similar, less understood relation between skin pigmentation and malignant melanoma, a cancer of special pigment-containing cells; people who have red hair develop malignant melanoma more often than the rest of the general population.

Environment Other kinds of cancer seem to run in families because family groups are exposed to the same environmental conditions. For example, if a family lived in an area that had a very high background radiation, it might not be surprising that more than one member developed radiation-induced leukemia. On the other hand, cancer is so common that the occurrence of malignant disease in several members of a family usually cannot be attributed to anything other than the statistical fact that the cancerous diseases attack one out of every four persons.

One of the most puzzling things about cancer is its distribution among different countries and among different "racial" groups. These differences can be due to cultural habits. For example, cancers of the mouth and throat are common in countries such as India and Ceylon, where mixtures of tobacco, betel nut, and lime or other ingredients are habitually chewed (58). Cancers of the liver are frequent in tropical Africa but extremely rare in the United States. Cancer of the female breast is much less frequent in Japan than in the United States. Cancer of the uterine cervix is a striking example of low incidence in a special group; it is relatively infrequent in Jewish women. A particular kind of cancer of the hypopharnyx is found among Swedish women who have chronic anemia. Gastric cancer has been most frequent in countries with colder climates, especially those having access to the sea, such as Iceland, Chile, Norway, Japan, and Finland (15). Gastric cancer also used to be the most common kind of fatal cancer among American men, but in the last 10 years the incidence has dropped off rapidly. It is also becoming less frequent in Europe and seems to be decreasing in Japan, where it is the most important fatal cancer. There is no idea why gastric cancer is decreasing. Some think that the preventive factor has been an improvement in our diet; but exactly what dietary improvement has decreased the incidence of stomach cancer no one is able to say.

The cancers whose etiology, or causes, have been easiest to trace are those connected with the hazards of a particular occupation. The first so-called "occupational cancer" was recognized in 1775 when Sir Percival Pott suggested that the "lodgment of soot" on unwashed young chimney sweeps probably caused the scrotum cancer so frequent among them. This clinical observation of the correlation between soot and cancer of the scrotum stimulated the formation of safety regulations, i.e., bathing requirements. As a result, the incidence of this cancer decreased sharply, even though the carcinogenic or cancer-causing ingredient in soot was not identified until more than 150 years later, when in 1916 Yamagiwa and Itchikawa painted coal

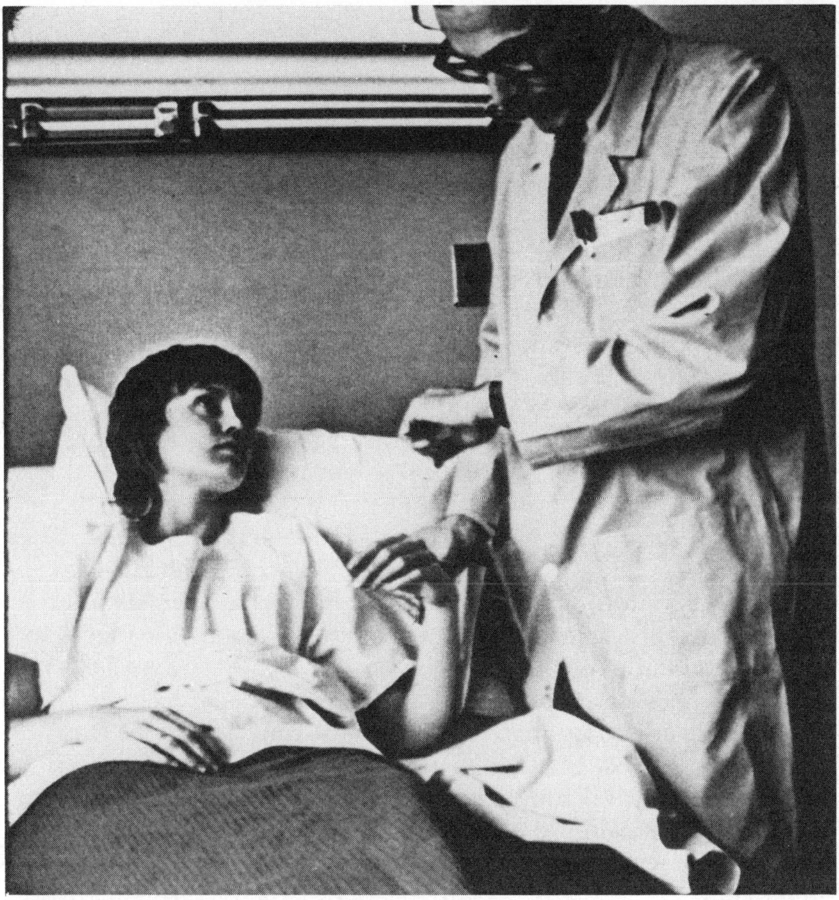

Figure 7.4 Immediate diagnosis is a must.

tar on the ears of rabbits for many months and proved it to be the carcinogenic agent. In 1932 Kennaway and his associates isolated a specific carcinogenic compound, benzopyrene, in coal tar. Subsequently, a very large group of hydrocarbons have been synthesized or isolated and shown to be carcinogenic for one or another species of experimental animal.

Recently many chemical compounds have been identified as carcinogens; for example, arsenic is known to cause skin cancer; compounds related to aniline dyes produce bladder cancer; metallic compounds like the chromates and nickel can cause cancer of the lung and nasal cavity; asbestos may be the cause of unique cancers of the cells lining the chest and abdominal cavities (66). Benzol, anthracene oil, petroleum fuel oil, and diesel oil have all been reported to cause skin cancers. Additional chemical carcinogens will undoubtedly be found among the new and more powerful chemicals that are constantly being developed.

Carcinogens There is a real necessity for continuous vigilance in checking new industrial techniques in order to prevent the inadvertent introduction of a carcinogen which may affect not only a specific group but also the general population. To protect the public and those workers engaged in processing these potentially dangerous chemicals, the public health departments of the federal and state governments, together with private industries, have devised screening tests for carcinogens.

More perfect methods are required, however. One problem is that testing is generally done on experimental animals and a chemical that is harmless to one species may cause cancer in another. For example, men who use arsenic sprays in orchards year after year or who were exposed to arsenic during the "roasting" of crude copper ores developed characteristic skin lesions. Naturally, scientists wished to study arsenical cancers in experimental animals, but after many years of testing no susceptible species besides the human has been found.

Another disadvantage of animal-testing programs for carcinogenic agents is the long period of observation required. For example, several hundred mice must be kept for nearly one and one-half years in order to ensure that a single compound at a single dosage level and with a single method of application is not carcinogenic. It probably would be better to use primates for some studies, but the expense would be prohibitive and the animals might have to be studied for more than 10 years. It is evident that a newly marketed chemical or a food additive might cause a great deal of damage before its carcinogenicity is detected. It took years of intensive effort by research groups in several countries to trace the cause of liver damage and liver cancers in domestic fowl and hatchery trout to aflatoxin, a compound from a mold that contaminated the peanuts that were part of the feed mixture for the animals. Hopefully, more effective carcinogen-detection systems will be made available through the use of cultured human cells and tissue fragments instead of test animals and through the development of even better techniques of predicting carcinogenicity from chemical structure.

Another problem in identifying carcinogenicity is that relatively little is known about the principles of the cancer-producing activity of multiple carcinogens in subcarcinogenic doses. Nor are the effects of combinations of carcinogens and cocarcinogens fully understood. These are substances which in themselves are not cancer-producing but which heighten the reaction to true carcinogens. We clearly recognize that the human is exposed to small doses of a wide variety of carcinogenic stimuli and carcinogens, including chemical, physical, and microbiological agents. But individual susceptibility to carcinogens varies greatly, and not everyone exposed to a carcinogen develops cancer. Just as a very few persons exposed to a virus may develop a virus disease, so some persons may be susceptible to one carcinogen but not to another.

An important environmental source of carcinogenic activity is radiation in all of its various forms. It has already been mentioned that the ultraviolet rays of sunlight are carcinogenic for humans. People who are exposed to intense sunlight, such as sailors, farmers, and high-altitude dwellers, are most likely to develop skin cancer of the face, especially on the nose, forehead, and ears. Mail carriers sometimes develop a characteristic skin cancer on the left hand, the hand most frequently exposed to the sun year after year.

Radiations that have very much shorter wavelengths are even more dangerous. Radiations from radium and other natural radioactive sources, such as X-ray machines, nuclear fission, and artificial radioisotopes, are potent carcinogens for many species of animals and for humans. Radiation damage may result in various kinds of precancerous lesions and malignancies, depending upon the body site, the tissue exposed, and the particular susceptibility of the individual.

Perhaps the most tragic case of occupational carcinogenic radiation involved a group of young women who were employed by watch manufacturers in the early part of this century. These women painted the luminous dials of wristwatches with a mixture of radium, mesothorium, and zinc sulfide. They used fine-pointed brushes for this purpose, and to preserve the fine tips, they rotated the bristles between their lips. The radioactive "paint" coated their lips and mouths, and some of the mixture was unavoidably swallowed. After a few years many of the young women became chronically ill from a combination of heavy metal poisoning and radiation damage. Some of them developed cancers where the radioactive metals had selectively deposited in their bones, thus both damaging the bone marrow and causing bone sarcomas.

In retrospect, it seems unbelievable that the causal link between "the sisters of death" and their experience as dial painters was not immediately accepted. But, in fact, lawyers, ill-informed physicians, and representatives of the watch manufacturers avoided taking immediate responsibility for the watch dials painted with radium. They insisted that the causal relationship between the workers' illness and their exposure to radium was not proven and that a controversy over the relationship existed between scientists and physicians.

There was indeed a controversy, but no one bothered to notice that the experts in cancer research and radiation biology were on one side and a miscellaneous group of poorly informed men whose good intentions were obscured by their poor judgment or financial interests were on the other side. (The parallels between this episode and the present "controversy" about the health hazards of cigarette smoking are amazing!) Several books were written in support of the thesis that the radioactive materials were not at fault, even though radiation had been known to be associated with tissue injury since 1907. The books negated the observed fact of clinical disease in humans exposed to radiation on the grounds that similar diseases could be caused in only a few experimental animals.

This objection, of course, did not take into account the great variation in susceptibility to radiation injury that exists among species. One species may react very strongly to radiation, while another may react hardly at all. Even individuals of the same species react differently to similar stimuli. Among the watch-dial painters examined in one study, all were found to have considerable amounts of radioactivity in their bones. But while two-thirds of them had developed severe bone diseases, depression of the blood-forming organs, and multiple cancers, the remaining one-third showed little or no evidence of disease. This great individual variation is one of the factors which makes it very difficult to establish meaningful standards for the amount of radiation a "normal" person can tolerate without harm.

By obscuring the relevance of this tragic clinical "experiment" with confusing claims and counterclaims, the radium-dial defenders did society a great disservice. They indirectly prevented the public from protecting itself against the dangers of excessive radiation. For many years parents continued to expose their children's feet to unnecessary radiation for shoe fitting. Shoe fitting by fluoroscopy was a dangerous procedure even when carried out properly, but salesmen often allowed children to look at their feet repeatedly. The salesmen even removed the protective filters over the X-ray tube in order to provide a brighter image, and thus they greatly increased the radiation dosage.

Even trained people made mistakes in the use of X-rays and fluoroscopes. Dentists and physicians paid too little attention to the need for protecting themselves and their patients. The results of this carelessness are now being seen as an increased incidence of cancer and leukemia among early practitioners using radium and radiation equipment. Some doctors erred by treating newborn infants for "enlarged thymus" by X-ray therapy. These children later had an unusually high incidence of thyroid cancer and leukemia (36).

The increased susceptibility of youngsters and unborn infants to radiation effects has now been recognized; most dentists protect their young patients and pregnant women by using lead bibs, and most medically accredited radiologists are careful to expose a minimal amount of tissue to the X-ray and protect the rest of the body with lead shields. Unfortunately, some practitioners are still advertising "spinal X-rays" as a part of the routine examinations, a procedure which is usually both unnecessary and dangerous.

Among untrained people, the errors in judgment were even more widespread. Some "skin specialists" used Z-rays for removing unwanted hair and for treating acne. From 10 to 40 years later the victims of these treatments developed many deforming skin lesions and multiple cancers (16). And people still continued to buy watches with radium dials and to demonstrate industrial fluoroscopes to their friends by exposing their hands to the X-ray beam. The atomic bomb made the dangers of radiation terrifyingly clear. Ever since Hiroshima and Nagasaki, there has been increasing concern about protecting people against radiation. Today, there is almost universal legislation limiting the use of radiation and X-ray machines and requiring licenses for those administering radiation and radioactive isotopes. There is still additional need for protective devices and techniques for monitoring and regulating the new industrial uses of fission. Danger is faced from radioactive sources in every part of living, from radioactive fallout as well as from industrial, medical, and natural sources.

Regretfully, educational programs about the dangers of radiation have caused some people to fear all X-ray examinations. This overreaction is not justified because properly administered

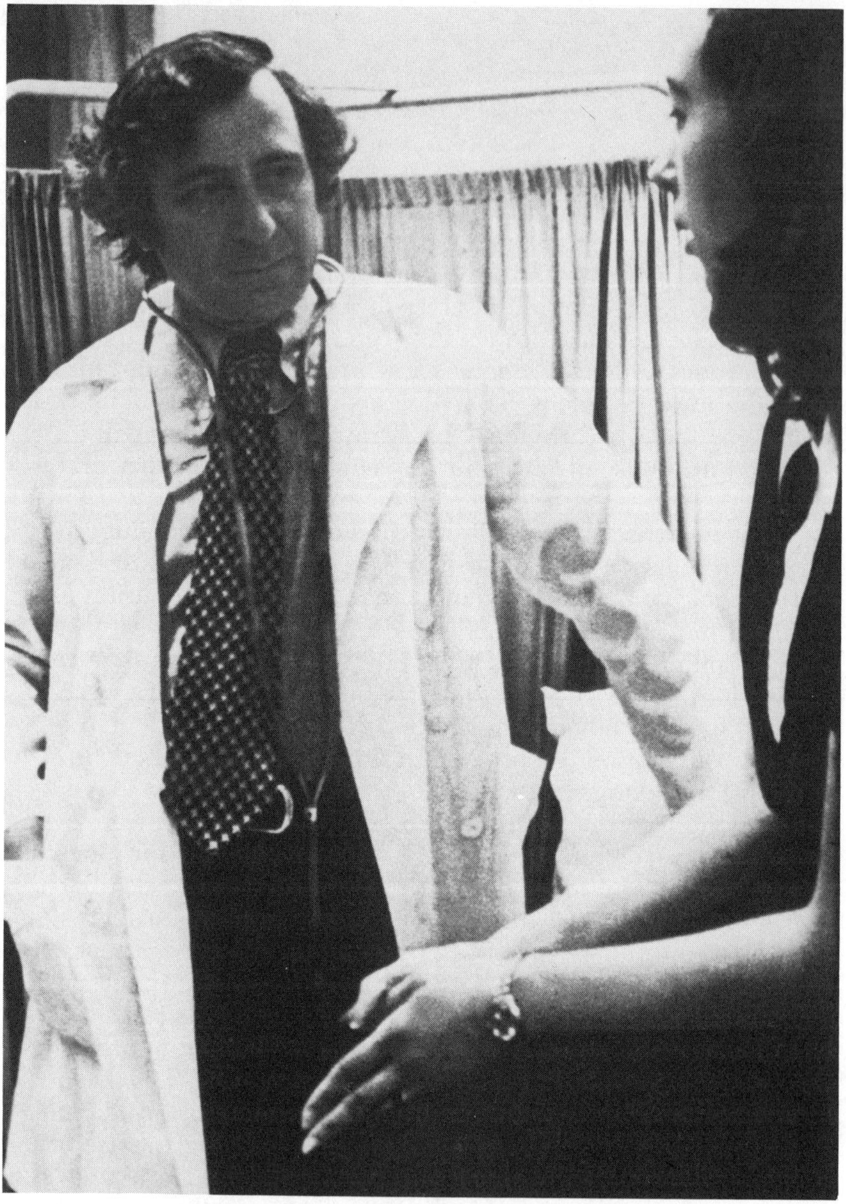

Figure 7.5 Careful follow-up for any medical problem is preventive medicine.

X-ray examinations for diagnosis of the teeth or the chest expose one to less radiation than does the normal background radiation from the earth and from outer space.

Although many factors may cause cancer, there are many more things which do not cause cancer but which have been implicated erroneously because of rumors, old wives' tales, and unjustified extrapolation of animal data to humans. It is truly amazing that so many common foods and additives are shunned because of an unwarranted fear of cancer. Periodically cancer research centers are asked if it is true that aluminum cooking utensils, or asparagus, or hair sprays, or cranberries, or vegetable colorings cause cancer. They are also asked for information about carcinogenic hydrocarbons and the possible dangers of charcoal-broiled steaks or the use of hickory-smoke extracts. So far there is very little information about the carcinogenic effects of barbecued foods, but preliminary animal studies have not revealed any dangers.

A much-maligned "cause" of cancer is a previous fracture or other injury. Although it is possible in extremely rare instances that an injury might affect the growth rate of a preexisting cancer, there is no proof that the usual kind of injury is a cause of cancer. When malignant lesions are discovered after a bone has fractured, it almost always is found that instead of the fracture causing the lesion, the fracture was caused by the damaging effects of the preexisting cancer. Similarly, a fall followed by a persistent bruise and lump usually results from a hemorrhage into a preexisting tumor. It is noteworthy that many attempts have been made to induce cancers in experimental animals by single and repeated injury but all attempts have failed.

There are, however, several kinds of tissue injury that may result in cancer. Wounds or old burns which remain infected or inflamed for many years must be observed closely for malignant changes. Fortunately, these conditions are not frequently encountered in the United States. A somewhat related and more common condition is ulcerative colitis, a disease in young people that causes chronic and acute inflammation of the colon. This condition may also present the threat of malignancy.

There is a need to find and identify more of the factors that cause cancer and somehow to prevent people from coming into contact with them once their carcinogenic activity is established. We are only now beginning to identify carcinogens that actually initiated carcinogenic processes 5 to 20 years ago. In the future an increase in the use of atomic fuels will also increase carcinogenic activity. The possibility of mutations in infectious organisms that will give fuels the capacity to cause cancer will be present, as will the ever-increasing exposure to air and water pollutants. Trained biologists, chemists, and microbiologists who can screen substances and microorganisms for carcinogenic activity are needed.

In addition, the public should be promptly informed about any dangerous carcinogens.

■ Diabetes Mellitus

Diabetes mellitus is one of the oldest diseases known to the human. More than two thousand years ago Hippocrates described it as excessive amounts of sugar in the urine (74). Ever since that time it has been studied, but so far the cause and the cure have not been discovered. Diabetes mellitus is the third leading cause of death in the United States, with about 300,000 deaths annually. Ten million Americans have diabetes, and 600,000 new cases are diagnosed each year. This is an annual 6% incidence rate. The cost for treatment is reaching $5.3 billion per year.

In 1921 Banting and Best, from Canada, discovered the use of insulin in controlling diabetes and allowing diabetics to function almost normally (24). Diabetes is a dynamic disease that

Figure 7.6 Death rate for diabetes by age and sex, 1976.

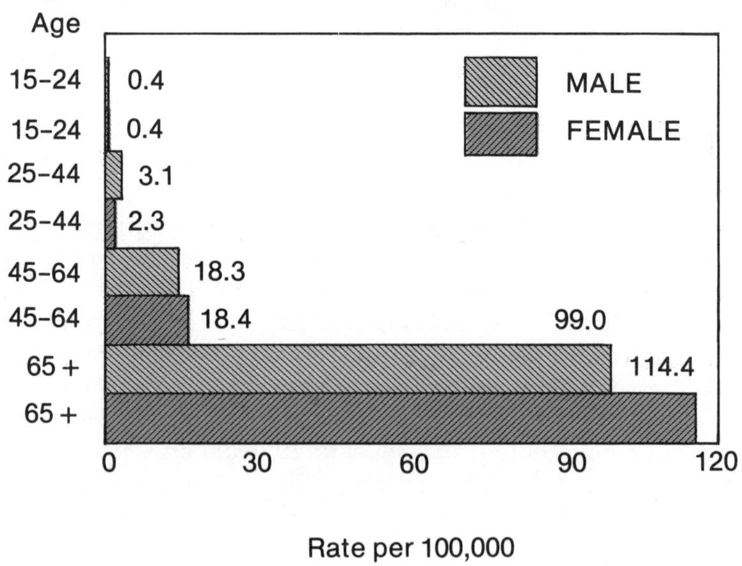

Source: Statistical Abstract of U.S., 1975, p. 76.

is undergoing dramatic changes as well as fundamental advances. These advances have not only prolonged the life span of the diabetic but have also created new problems associated with the chronic nature of the disease.

Diabetes is physiologically defined as a chronic systemic disease which is characterized as a malfunction in the metabolism of insulin and of carbohydrates, fats, and protein. The main disorder is associated with glucose, which the body needs for energy. Insulin is the hormone secreted by the beta cells of the pancreas and it does the following:

1. Enables glucose (the product of carbohydrate metabolism) to be transported across cell membranes into muscle.
2. Converts glucose in the cells into energy.
3. Converts glucose into glycogen in the liver to be stored as reserve energy (74).

Types of Diabetes There are three different types of diabetes mellitus. Each type is categorized according to the amount of insulin secreted by the pancreas. In *insulinopenic,* or juvenile-onset, diabetes there is a complete absence of insulin production by the pancreas. This type represents 10% of the diabetic population. Because insulin is no longer produced by the pancreas, daily insulin injections are required for the rest of the diabetic's life. *Insulinotardic,* or adult-onset, diabetes, is characterized by a delayed response in insulin secretion. These adults are usually of normal weight but may require insulin or pills for control rather than just diet. They represent about 15% of the diabetic population. *Insulinoplethoric,* or adult-onset, diabetes, occurs in those who are obese. These diabetics, which represent about 75% of all diabetics, can be controlled mainly with weight reduction diets. The loss of even from 7 to 10 pounds may frequently result in a dramatic lowering of the fasting blood sugar.

Saul Kent has asked whether or not diabetes is a form of accelerated aging (42). The decreasing glucose tolerance with age has been demonstrated repeatedly with the normals for a fasting blood sugar increasing 10 milligrams per 100 milliliters for each decade after the sixth. Overt diabetes mellitus is observed in 20% of the population over 65 years of age in Western society (80). It has been speculated that the decreased glucose tolerance is the result of the loss of the normal insulin sensitivity and the increasing prevalence of obesity in middle and late years (62).

Symptoms The symptoms of diabetes (hyperglycemia), include extreme thirst, large amount of and frequent urination, and extreme hunger. Other symptoms are blurred vision, fatigue, and slow healing of cuts (74). These symptoms disappear when blood sugar levels return to normal. The causes for the symptoms are associated with the elevation of blood sugar. The high levels of sugar in the blood cause the viscosity of the blood to increase which causes a large amount of fluid to enter the bloodstream and urine in an attempt to dilute both the blood and the urine. This process causes increased urination and thirst.

Diagnostic Procedures The diagnostic procedures for diabetes include testing the urine for glucose and serum blood sugar levels, testing after fasting and 2 hours after eating, 24-hour urine tests for glucose, and 3- or 5-hour glucose tolerance tests. Glucose tolerance is affected by many variables, for example, certain medications, previous carbohydrate restriction, liver disease, alcoholism, and prolonged rest. These variables are likely to alter the results and may result in a wrong diagnosis (65). The glucose tolerance test indicates the person's ability to burn glucose and is given to a person whose fasting blood sugars are normal.

Genetics The role of genetics in diabetes has been studied infrequently and with little predictability because it has been impossible to identify genetic markers. There is a controversy over shared environmental factors and genotypes. Heredity is seen more readily as a factor in juvenile-onset diabetics, with 70% to 81% having a positive family history for diabetes. In adult-onset diabetes in people over 55 years of age, a positive family history is found in only 30% to 40% of the cases. Since more juvenile-onset diabetics are growing to adulthood, studies have shown that one-third of the fertile marriages of two diabetic parents do not produce any diabetic offspring (32).

Juvenile-Onset Diabetes Juvenile-onset diabetes manifests itself at any age from infancy to the mid-twenties. Such diabetics require special considerations, especially as children go through the various stages of growth and development. Good control of diabetes exhibits normal growth, but fair and poor control exhibits poor growth. Because an adolescent has rapidly fluctuating needs for insulin, the adolescent must have a good understanding of the disease (6). An acceptance of the disease and the adjustment to their needs by all those associated with the disease will help the adolescent adjust to the condition (11). Although juvenile diabetics are living into adulthood now, their life span is still shortened by one-third. The juvenile-onset diabetic is prone to ketoacidosis, which is a result of poor control. It is demonstrated by three major symptoms of diabetes: abdominal pain, rapid breathing, and fruitlike odor to the breath. If ketoacidosis is not recognized, it could lead to death. Ketoacidosis is an extreme elevation of serum glucose concentration, increased fat oxidation, and increased ketones (67). Because diabetes is a chronic disease, it manifests certain complications about 20 years after the onset of the disease. The complications, which accelerate the aging process, lead to the final demise of the juvenile-onset diabetic.

Treatment The goals for the treatment of diabetes include prevention of acute diabetes, retardation of chronic manifestations, and modification of the biochemical composition of the blood (65). Methods of treatment for diabetes include diet, medication, monitoring blood sugars, exercise, and education. Since 70% of adult-onset diabetics are obese, diet plays a very important role in the control of the disease. The diet, which is calorie controlled, is divided into 25% fats, 20% protein, 45% carbohydrates, excluding simple sugars, and 10% dietary supplements. Since it is known that elevated blood lipids have an effect on vascular disease, the fat and carbohydrate content of the diet may be altered to improve blood lipid levels (43). The only restrictions placed on juvenile-onset diabetics are that simple sugars must be eliminated from the diet and that they must eat three meals every day.

Insulin and oral hypoglycemic agents are the two types of medication used in controlling diabetes. Insulin is a hormone given by injection to replace the endogenous insulin that is not being produced by the pancreas. There are several kinds of insulin and their action times vary from 3 hours to 48 hours. Insulin is necessary in the juvenile-onset diabetic but in the adult-onset diabetic it must be used with care. Some adults are very susceptible to hypoglycemic reactions and others are insulin resistant. The complications resulting from insulin therapy include hypogylcemic reactions, or low blood sugars, local infection, and local atrophy of the tissue (67). Oral medication includes various types of pills which have a variety of action times. The sulfonureas are the main oral medications and stimulate the pancreas to produce more insulin. Those who should start oral medication are the nonketosis-prone adult-onset diabetic and the mild to moderate diabetic who has failed on the diet. Those who should not take oral medication are the insulin-dependent, those suffering from acute complications, pregnant women, and those who have renal insufficiency. There may be times when control is not maintained on oral medication and insulin is initiated as treatment (65). There has been much reluctance to start oral hypoglycemic agents because of the results of the University Group Diabetes Program study. These results were concerned with the development of vascular complications and the number of cardiovascular deaths in the oral hypoglycemic agents. Recently, the validity of the study has been questioned. Some variables questioned include improper patient selection, inadequate follow-up, frequent drug changes, and fixed amounts of oral drugs.

The monitoring of urine glucose levels at home with test tape or Clinetest tablets is important to detect any change in the course of the disease (44).

Exercise is an important aspect of the management of the diabetic. Exercise acts like "insulin" because it reduces blood sugar. Extra calories may be required if the blood sugar drops to too low a level during the exercise. Establishing a regular daily exercise program for both adult and juvenile-onset diabetics is essential for control of their disease. For example, the result of walking one-half hour a day will be a 20-pound weight loss over the period of one year (44).

Aging and Degeneration The degenerative complications related to diabetes have become an ever-increasing concern because there is a prolonged life span in the diabetic, both adult and juvenile. Diabetics are 17 times more prone to kidney disease, 25 times more prone to blindness, 5 times more prone to gangrene, and 2 times more prone to heart attack and stroke. It is the third leading cause of death. The complications may manifest themselves prior to the diagnosis of diabetes in the adult-onset diabetic. In the juvenile-onset diabetic the complications do not begin to appear for more than a decade after the onset of the disease.

The degenerative complications are classified as *macrovascular* disease, *diabetic microangiopathy*, and *diabetic neuropathy* (24).

Macroangiopathy. Macroangiopathy is related to the large blood vessels in the brain, heart, and extremities. Vascular disease accounts for most of the morbidity and mortality associated with diabetes. It is unknown whether the diabetic structural changes are complications or manifestations of the disease. The large vessel disease is related to the abnormalities of both blood sugar and lipid levels which leads to plaque formation followed by calcification of the large blood vessels. Three-fourths of the cerebral vascular accidents are associated with diabetes. The coronary artery disease in the diabetic is more diffuse, especially in the adult-onset diabetic. It is related to more than one-half of the diabetic deaths (20). Silent myocardial infarctions are related to a nerve disorder in the heart as well as the macroangiopathy. This vascular disease is characterized by decreased circulation in the arms or legs. The decreased circulation is caused by an occlusion of the blood vessels in the extremities due to plaque formation. Vascular insufficiency can cause cramping in the legs when the diabetic exercises. An increased incidence of infection is a result of the combination of neuropathy and macroangiopathy. This infection can lead to gangrene. The large vessel disease in the poorly controlled diabetic is demonstrated by increasing frequency, earlier onset, accelerated progression, and more severe and diffuse involvement.

Visual Problems. Microangiopathy, or small blood vessel disease, is the cause of diabetic retinopathy and diabetic nephropathy. Diabetes, the leading cause of blindness in the United States, causes diabetic retinopathy, glaucoma, and cataracts. Cataracts are not related to microangiopathy, but they should be considered in any discussion of visual problems and diabetes. It has been speculated that cataracts are caused by an increased accumulation of sugar in the lens since insulin is not required for sugar to pass into the lens (27).

Diabetic retinopathy is characterized by the abnormalities of the blood vessels in the retina of the eye. These abnormalities can be new blood vessel formation, blood leakage into vitreous, and formation of scar tissue that leads to traction on the underlying retina. It is commonly found in patients who have had diabetes for 20 or more years. Background retinopathy, the milder form of the disease, may cause only minor visual changes.

Background retinopathy is diagnosed when the vascular lesions are contained within the retina. Proliferative retinopathy can cause absolute blindness as the new blood vessels begin to form. These blood vessels can easily hemorrhage. Following hemorrhages, more scarring results and retinal detachment is common in this process. Blurred vision can be caused by fluctuations in blood sugars, but if it persists for several days, it should be evaluated by an ophthalmologist. The treatment for background retinopathy is frequent monitoring to observe the progression of the disease (57). Proliferative retinopathy is treated aggressively because there is an increasing incidence of blindness. The treatment utilized mostly is *photocoagulation.* The heat caused by the lazer destroys the abnormal blood vessels which readily bleed and secrete exudate. The treatment results in a small scarring of the retina (67). The blindness caused by these hemorrhages is known to improve slowly as the blood is reabsorbed.

Kidney Problems. In the kidney the vascular disease caused by diabetes is related to a thickening in the cellular basement membrane of the blood vessels. This aspect of vascular disease has been discovered only recently through the use of the electron microscope, which examines the tissue from a renal biopsy. A thickening in the cellular basement membrane has also been identified in the prediabetic. The thickening is diffused throughout the kidney which, as a result, decreases the filtration of the blood. The treatment of vascular kidney disease has been diuretics, antibiotics to prevent infection, hemodialysis, and renal transplant when the kidney has failed completely (46).

Diabetic *neuropathy* is the most common manifestation of chronic kidney complications. Diabetic neuropathy appears in every *visceral* and *somatic* system of the body. The somatic involvement is bilateral and is characterized by pain and *paresthesia* with nocturnal intensification. Paresthesia is the sensation of burning, tingling, numbness, or coldness of the involved area. The pain may be so intense that narcotics are necessary. The diabetic *amyotropathy* is a progressive weakness and wasting of the pelvic girdle which improves slowly over a period of several months. It requires special care of the feet because there is the possibility of infection and trauma, which may lead to amputation. A sensory deficiency in the upper extremities can cause an impairment in reading braille (24). Diabetic neuropathy may occur independently and can mimic other disease states. The systems involved are:

Eyes: The main disorder is extraocular muscle palsy.

Gastrointestinal Tract: The disorders are characterized by delayed emptying of the stomach, irregular and unpredictable absorption, and diabetic diarrhea.

Genitourinary Tract: The disorders include paralytic bladder, retrograde ejaculation, and impotency.

Research and the Future A study of 4400 diabetic patients was made between 1947 and 1973 in France. Jean Pirart reported the following on degenerative complications:

1. Incidence and prevalence of neuropathy, microangiopathy, and much less macroangiopathy are functions of the known duration of diabetes.
2. There is an interrelationship between retinopathy and neuropathy.
3. Sex doesn't appear to make a difference in the incidence of degenerative complications.
4. Family history has no role in the development of degenerative complications.
5. Age has yet an unproven effect on specific complications.
6. Obesity has no influence.
7. Unrecognized diabetes mellitus demonstrates an earlier onset of degenerative complications.
8. Severity of diabetes has no role in the incidence of degenerative complications.
9. Poor control is related to increased incidence and prevalence.
10. Atherosclerosis is unrelated to poor control (59).

Statistics show an increasing probability that the number of diabetics will double in the next 15 years. It is probable that researchers should look for methods of diabetic control that will prevent the onset and progression of the degenerative complications. It has been felt that although *exogenous insulin* stimulates the *endogenous insulin* in control of diabetes, it doesn't prevent the onset of organ damage. Patients who have experimentally received pancreatic islet cell transplants have experienced an improvement in end organ damage (50). The islet cell transplants have been done rarely and only in patients with severe kidney

Figure 7.7 Activity limitation for arthritis by age and sex, 1976.

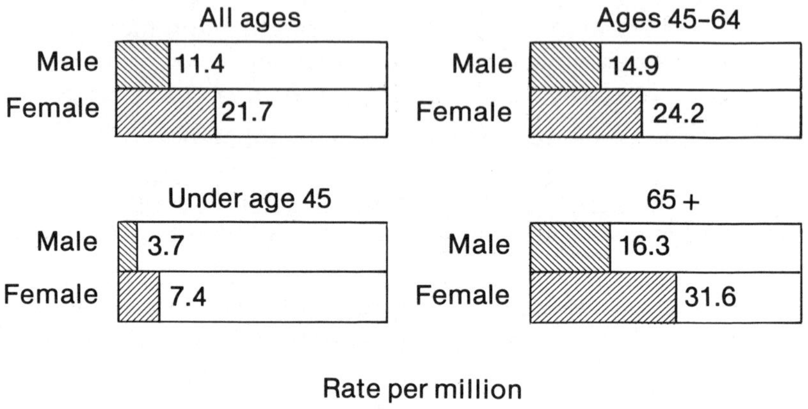

Source: Statistical Abstract of U.S., 1978, p. 120.

disease as a result of diabetes. Other studies include the use of *vitrectomy* in the patients with proliferative retinopathy. The vitrectomy is a surgical procedure in which the vitreous of the posterior chamber of the eye is removed. It is done as a last resort with the hope of improving the vision of the blind diabetic (53).

■ Arthritis

Most adults will at some time suffer from some form of arthritis. The word "arthritis" is a general term used to describe many different conditions that induce aches and pains throughout the body. The joints and surrounding connective tissue are the most frequent sites of attack, although not all involve inflammation.

Arthritis is one of the oldest diseases known to humans and evidence of arthritis is seen in the bones of prehistoric humans and Egyptian mummies dating as far back as 8000 B.C. The most common forms of arthritis are rheumatoid arthritis, osteoarthritis, and gout. Rheumatism is also a general term used to describe stiffness and aching pain. This group of diseases afflicts more people than do cancer, diabetes, heart trouble, and tuberculosis combined. Yet, little was being done to help these sufferers until the Arthritis and Rheumatism Foundation was founded in 1948. This and other organizations have been able to point out the magnitude of this health problem. As a result, there is much more new knowledge about the forms of the disease and new treatments of them are available.

Rheumatoid Arthritis Rheumatoid arthritis is a severe chronic inflammation of the joints, especially in the knees and fingers. It was once considered a specific joint disease, but now it is recognized as a chronic systemic disorder in which inflammation is the dominant factor. Rheumatoid arthritis is the most severe and the most painful form of arthritis; and it exerts the most potential to cripple its victims.

Rheumatoid arthritis attacks more women than men. Because arthritis symptoms seem to increase during menses and decrease during pregnancy, specialists hold to the theory that there is a link between rheumatoid arthritis and the endocrine glands. It would seem that it is a disorder of metabolism which is the sum of the physical and chemical processes of the body. Attacks cause pain and swelling of the joints, weakness, fatigue, and stiffness, especially in the morning. These manifestations may last for weeks or months and may vary in intensity. Arthritis frequently hits after an illness and in young mothers after the first child. Fatigue from work is a contributing factor. Fear and worry can trigger the onset. The signs and symptoms should be considered warning signals and a physician should be consulted. If neglected, they may recur and progress to fusion of the joints.

Statistics. Arthritis is the number one crippling disease in the United States and is ranked second only to heart disease as the leading cause of limitation of activity for persons who suffer from a chronic disability. In 1966 it was estimated that 1 in every 20 persons suffered from some form of rheumatism. According to the National Center for Health Statistics' latest report, in 1976 there were 31½ million people who fell victim to some form of arthritis in the United States. This means that 1 out of every 7 people or 1 in 3 families were affected. Of the 31½ million arthritics, 6½ million were diagnosed rheumatoid arthritics. The center estimated 1 million new cases each year. As of May, 1978, the statistics grew to nearly 1 in 4 people adding up to 50 million affected Americans, 40% of whom required some form of medical attention. The incidence of arthritis more than doubled in the 10 years from 1966 to 1976 and from 1976 to 1978 it doubled again. This increasing incidence of arthritis may be the result of the growing numbers of people advancing into their later decades of life, the growing number of people seeking medical attention, and a better diagnostic procedure which enables quicker diagnosis.

Rheumatoid arthritis affects women three to five times more often than men. Three-fourths of the cases begin between the ages of 20 and 50. Whites are victims more often than blacks and the occurrence of the disease is greatest in the temperate climates. There is a diminishing effect as the Arctic and equator are reached, and the disease is almost unheard of in the tropics.

In the United States the annual cost of all forms of arthritis from medical bills, lost wages, and quackery is a whopping $13 billion.

Treatment. Rheumatoid arthritis is an incurable, crippling, chronic disease and must be diagnosed and treated by a physician. Presently, no "miracle cures" or self-treatment programs have proven effective. Even with medical assistance there is no simple method for long-lasting control of the disease over its natural course, but it can be controlled and joint destruction can be avoided with proper care.

A major problem in controlling rheumatoid arthritis is diagnosing it correctly because it may be confused with several diseases that produce joint pain. Diseases mistaken for rheumatoid arthritis are listed in Table 7.4

The best treatment of the disease includes different methods and techniques. Drugs and a balance of exercise, activity, and rest prescribed by a physician can prevent progress of the disease. Rest reduces the joint inflammation and exercise retains muscle and joint function and prevents the onset of deformity. Drugs prescribed by the physician may include aspirin, gold salts, corticosteroids, and quinoline derivatives (73). There is no single drug or other method of treatment that will cure or relieve this form of arthritis. The advice of a physician is absolutely essential.

A physician has a variety of programs available to choose from in order to combat inflammation and its destructive process. The most popular treatment involves chemotherapy with salicylic acid (aspirin). It is the safest and offers minimal side effects. Aspirin is administered in amounts much greater than normally used for non-arthritic patients. As a result, gastric distress, bleeding, and peptic ulcerations may occur. Nevertheless, when compared to other chemotherapeutic treatments, these results are

Table 7.4 Diseases Mistaken for Rheumatoid Arthritis

Periarticular fibrositis	Angina pectoris
Rheumatoid fever	Lipomas
Syphilis	Osteochondritis dissecans
Subdeltoid bursitis	Osteomyelitis
Gout	Herpes zoster
Weak, painful, pronated feet	Polycythemia
Peripheral neuritis (associated with alcoholism, diabetes mellitus, primary anemia, chronic arsenic poisoning)	Intermittent claudication
Serum sickness	Drug intoxication
Hypertrophic pulmonary osteoarthropathy	Deficiency diseases: scurvy, beriberi, rickets
Tuberculosis (pulmonary)	Hyperparathyroidism
Psoriatic arthritis	Paget's disease
Myxedema	Trichiniasis
Hyperthyroidism	Erythralgia
Malingering	Infantile paralysis
Hemophilia	Periarteritis nodosa
Arthritic purpura	Malignant disease of joints
Leukemia	Leprosy
Hysteria	Lupus erythematosus
Cervical rib and scalenus anticus syndrome	Acromegaly
Raynaud's syndrome	Ochronosis
Scleroderma	Subacute bacterial endocarditis
Acrosclerosis	Coronary thrombosis
Calcinosis	Boeck's sarcoid (Lupus Pernio)
Parkinsonism	Dermatomyositis
	Milkman's disease
	Archachnodactyly (76)

minimal. The majority of individuals respond positively to aspirin, but some cases may require additional quick relief action. At this point gold salts or corticosteroids may be initiated.

Gold salts effects are gradual. Often it is several weeks and even months before the effects are apparent. Reactions involve the kidney and bone marrow, are potentially serious, and may even be fatal (68).

Corticosteroids, such as prednisone and cortisone, offer an individual quick relief of joint symptoms by suppressing pain and increasing joint mobility. Masked remissions are temporary and continued treatment results in undesirable side effects. These side effects include skin conditions, abnormal fat deposits around the face, and emotional imbalances which range from insomnia to depression.

Antimalaria drugs are yet another option. These include chloroquine and hydroxychloroquine which are derivatives of quinoline. Like gold salts, these drugs act slowly and the benefit is rarely evident before 3 months. Maximum improvement is not evident before 6 to 12 months. The side effects are high. To date, research has focused on irreversible retinal vasculitis as a side effect. As a precaution, ophthalmological examinations are recommended every 3 months for patients taking antimalarial drugs.

Myths About Arthritis. The media constantly reaffirms that arthritis sufferers are the most exploited victims of disease in the United States. It is estimated that more than $400,000,000 a year is spent on worthless and even harmful devices, treatment, and so-called cures. Some of the treatments include filtered sea water, so-called "immune" milk, honey and apple vinegar combinations, and alfalfa tablets. Not only are they usually worthless, they are also expensive. Athritis sufferers are especially vulnerable because there is no known cure and because the pain can often cause great discomfort, victims are willing to try anything for relief.

Arthritics have been said to suffer the greatest from the psychological implications of the pain and disfigurement. This is especially true among people who were socially active in their earlier years. The trauma may cause depression and withdrawal.

Osteoarthritis Osteoarthritis is a progressive degenerative joint disease that involves the breakdown of the cartilage and other tissues that make a movable joint operate properly (5). It has been estimated that some 40½ million Americans are affected with some degree of osteoarthritis. In addition, 97% of all people over 60 show signs of this disease. The rate of occurrence increases with advancing chronological years, as does the degree of severity.

Synonyms. Osteoarthritis has several synonyms by which it is known. These include "degenerative joint disease," arthrosis, osteoarthrosis, and hypertrophic arthritis. The suffix "itis" usually indicates an inflammation. However, in the term osteoarthritis this is usually unjustified since inflammation is not generally a characteristic of this disease (45).

Joint Tissue and Joint Motion. To comprehend what takes place when degeneration occurs, it is necessary to understand how the normal skeletal system functions with regard to the joints and joint tissue. Every bone in the body, with the exception of the hyoid bone in the neck, connects to at least one other bone. Every bone except the hyoid bone forms a joint with some other bone. Joints perform two functions: they hold our bones together securely and they simultaneously make it possible for movement to occur between the bones. Freely movable joints are constructed in a similar manner. These joints have a *joint capsule,* a joint cavity lined with smooth, slippery *synovial membrane,* and a layer of cartilage over the ends of the two joining bones (2).

Joint Tissue Degeneration. Osteoarthritis, said to be the most common of all joint diseases, is also related to the "wearing out" of the articular structures. One of the first changes that takes place is a slight roughening of the cartilagenous surfaces. The joint cartilages degenerate and atrophy; the smooth surfaces soften and fray. Elasticity is lost and stress causes further damage. As these irregularities become more prominent, the cartilage wears away and the underlying bones become exposed to each other. With the absence of the cartilage cushion, the joint becomes painful to move (12). Cysts form in the bone near the joint and fragments of bone or cartilage become loose within the joint (5).

Affected Joints. Osteoarthritis may occur in any joint, but certain joints are more involved than others. These are the weight-bearing joints of the knees, hips, and spine, as well as the distal interphalangeal joints and the cervical and lumbar spinal articulations. The proximal interphalangeal joints usually do not show changes until notable pathology has appeared in the distal interphalangeal joints. Joints which undergo injury or trauma or those subjected to repeated stress and strain may also be affected (5).

The knee is a most commonly affected site of osteoarthritis. Early changes are characterized by damage of the articular cartilage. Cartilage cells show various stages of degeneration. Injuries in early years may accelerate the process. Osteoarthritis of the hip is usually the most disabling form of the disease. Managing hip involvement includes measures to reduce stress and repairing weight-bearing progressive joint damage and irreversible joint damage (14).

Primary and Secondary Osteoarthritis. Osteoarthritis is often separated into "primary" and "secondary" arthritis. Primary osteoarthritis has been described as occurring, for the most part, in middle-aged women and as being more generalized. Heberden's nodes and involvement of the proximal interphalangeal joints, knees, and spine are common. The metacarpophalangeal joints other than the first and wrist joints are seldom affected (5). Although pain may be severe at first, after a period of several months pain and inflammation subside. Primary arthritis appears to be genetically linked and there is a strong tendency for this form of arthritis to run in families. Secondary arthritis is usually the result of a traumatic injury or overexposure to excessive stress and strain. It has a tendency to affect the larger joints or the small joints that are exposed to severe use or trauma. Characteristically, secondary osteoarthritis occurs later in life, but it may show earlier if the joint suffers excessive abuse (21).

Heberden's Nodes. The development of *Heberden's nodes,* like other forms of osteoarthritis, is slow and usually causes little inconvenience; often it does not interfere with the normal movements of the joints. Many times joints are free from tenderness and pain. However, in the early stages one may experience great pain and some limitation of movement. At this stage the nodes do become swollen and tender. Usually several or all of the distal phalangeal joints are involved (12). These nodes usually begin to appear in middle life, particularly in females. They manifest themselves as bony outgrowths at the base of the terminal phalanges of the fingers. The nodes are found to develop in those individuals whose hands undergo excessive strain or hard work. Those who have large "well-defined" Heberden's nodes may not have osteoarthritis anywhere else in the body (14).

Cause of Osteoarthritis. The cause of osteoarthritis is unknown, but there are several possible contributing factors that should be considered. As previously mentioned, heredity may predispose an individual to "primary" osteoarthritis. The genetic linkage theory is one of the most widely accepted theories, but there is also the theory that if an individual were to live long

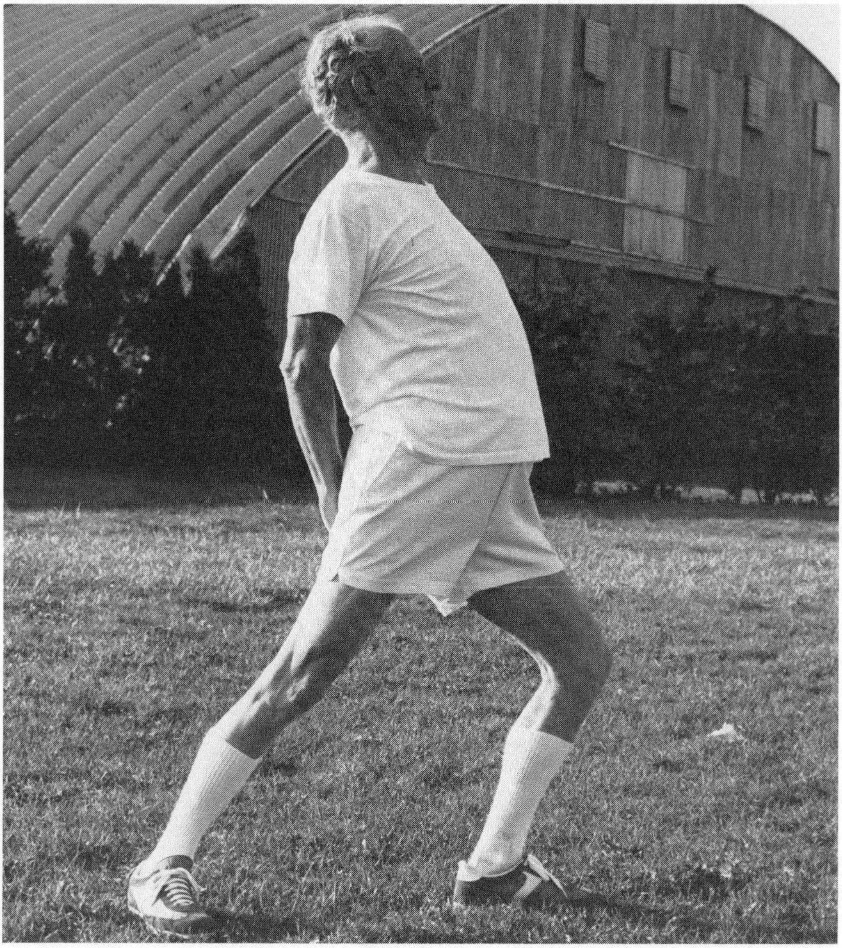

Figure 7.8 Stretching can be important to the maintenance of healthy joints.

enough, he or she would eventually develop osteoarthritis (21). Joint injuries related to sports, occupation, and so on, give credence to the "wear and tear" theory. Mild, long-continued irritation or an acute violent attack, such as from an accident or fracture, may also result in the onset of this disease.

Obesity is also a predisposing factor. The strain of too much weight adds unnatural and unequal pressure on joint surfaces, causing poor posture and deterioration. This may lead to a strain on the lumbar spine and the knees, thus resulting in osteoarthritis (5).

Some researchers believe that some individuals have better cartilage than others and those individuals who get osteoarthritis have chemical abnormalities. Another theory maintains that some individuals inherit mechanical imperfections in their joints which predispose the joints to "wear out."

Symptoms. The onset of *hypertrophic arthritis* (osteoarthritis) is insidious. The individual often first notices a slight stiffness in the affected joint which may gradually become more uncomfortable, especially during use. As time progresses, the symptoms become more marked and there may be constant pain in the involved joint. The affected joints rarely swell. Loss of mobility and an inability to perform normal movements and activities are unusual, but they do sometimes occur. Subsequently, posture and coordination are often affected as muscles become weakened (14). Pain is usually caused by irritation and pressure on nerve endings at bone endings. Affected joints are painful following use or following a period of inactivity.

Treatment. Osteoarthritis cannot be cured. Symptoms can be alleviated and joint function may be improved. A successful treatment of osteoarthritis depends upon a correct and accurate evaluation of the diagnosis.

No particular drug is "the" answer. Analgesics, especially aspirin, are thought to be most useful. Aspirin is widely used, and it is used for so many reasons that its effectiveness is often downgraded. Perhaps one of the most important features of the treatment of osteoarthritis is rest for the affected joint (12). For the obese person, weight reduction is of prime importance. However, diet does not play any part in the treatment except in relation to obesity. Progressive moderate exercises repeated several times daily can be helpful. One long period of exercise is not recommended.

Occasionally surgery is indicated in severe cases. If hip joint motion is seriously restricted, a hip *arthroplasty* may be needed. Years ago surgery was considered only as a last resort. Orthopedic surgeons now consider surgery sooner if they feel that it will benefit the afflicted individual. Sometimes a total hip replacement is made. Splints, crutches, and braces reduce pressure and relieve the weight and strain on the affected joints. Canes and crutches protect as well as assist in weight bearing.

Heat is another traditional and effective means of relieving pain in morning hours. A hot bath early in the morning lessens the stiffness. Heated wax, heat lamp treatments, and electric pads have also been considered helpful (5).

Drugs. Many drugs are prescribed in the treatment of osteoarthritis. A drug is prescribed because a physician has a specific reason for it. Some people think that because a friend is taking a medication this medication is also the answer for them. Conversely, they may have an adverse reaction or sensitivity to the drug. Drugs of choice include the following:

Aspirin: Aspirin is the single most widely used medication prescribed for the treatment of osteoarthritis. Aspirin is one of the most effective and safest drugs available without prescription. It is prescribed in larger doses when it is used in the treatment of osteoarthritis, and it is repeated several times daily.

Phenylbutazone: Phenylbutazone is a recently developed drug that does not alter the course of osteoarthritis. Although is does relieve pain and stiffness, it is not without side effects (5).

Indomethacin: Indomethacin is an anti-inflammatory drug. Many people cannot tolerate its short-term effects, but the side effects do not seem to be intense in long-term usage and the drug is beneficial in long-term treatment. It has been especially successful in treating osteoarthritis of the hip.

Corticoids: Some cases dictate relief of pain with a cortisone compound injection. This, however, is a very painful process. It does not affect the disease process, and apparently it is only helpful if injury to a joint, knee, hip, or elbow has caused inflammation of the surrounding tissues (5).

Gout Gout is an ancient but by no means rare disease. Of the 20 million persons in the United States who have arthritis in one form or another, more than 1 million are victims of gout. The disease has had an unusual appeal to medical historians. Recordings of it are found in earliest medical literature. Its ancestry is a most distinguished one and no disease has enjoyed a more royal patronage. Descriptions of its dramatic appearance, the ensuing pathos, and the whimsical aspects of the disease have been documented in both fiction and biography. The excellent clinical accounts of gout ascribed to Hippocrates and others testify to the Greek and Roman physicians' intimate knowledge of its varied characteristics. The term "gout," derived from the Latin word *gutta*, meaning a drop, was introduced in the thirteenth century and refers to the belief that the disease is caused by a poison of some sort falling into the joint.

The relationship of *uric acid* to gout was not discovered

until chemicals needed for analytical methods were developed. In 1848 Garrod's discovery of the "thread test" for increased amounts of uric acid in blood of gouty patients finally established the relationship between uric acid and gout. A series of independent investigators provided evidence that uric acid is the end product of human purine metabolism. Giant steps forward in modern scientific research have made it possible to control for life (7).

Symptoms. Gout affects the entire body, but it manifests itself chiefly by recurring attacks of acute painful swelling in various joints, the large toe being the most commonly affected. Gout is a *metabolic* disease in which something has gone wrong with the body's chemical mechanism. The metabolic defect in gout is the buildup of too much uric acid in the tissues and blood. In some cases, too much uric acid is produced, and in other cases, too little uric acid is eliminated. Uric acid is formed as the body uses certain chemical compounds present in many foods and in body cells (17).

Uric acid, which circulates in the blood and is eliminated through the urine, comes from two sources. The first is from the purines from foods as they are broken down. Purine-rich foods include organ meats (kidneys, sweetbreads, liver, brains), wild game (venison, rabbit, duck, bear), shellfish, anchovies, and sardines. Red meats and herring are considered moderately high in purines and legumes, asparagus, cauliflower, mushrooms, spinach, oatmeal, and whole wheat are slight. The second source is from the purines in tissues of the patient's own body which are constantly being broken down as new tissues are being built up. Biologists speak of this as normal cell turnover. But in certain blood conditions, such as polycythemia, which produces too many red cells, and in skin conditions, such as psoriasis, the cell turnover is greatly increased. Thus, people having these conditions are particularly susceptible to gout (9).

Uric acid is carried by the blood to the kidneys where it is filtered through the kidneys into liquid which becomes urine. However, only a small portion of it passes out with the urine. In fact, almost 90% is reabsorbed into the bloodstream. The average person excretes about ½ gram of uric acid a day. The main problem with gout centers around the formation and removal of this uric acid. If one produces too much uric acid or fails to get rid of it, then the waste accumulates in the body and sooner or later gout results.

Most gouty patients form uric acid in greater quantities than do normal individuals and since the kidneys eliminate approximately the same percentage of that which is brought to them, there is constantly an increased amount of uric acid circulation in the bloodstream. Other gouty patients seem to form uric acid in normal quantities, but their "uric acid clearance" is reduced. Thus, they too will have an increased amount of uric acid circulating in the blood. In an attempt to get rid of excessive amounts of uric acid, the blood deposits these fine needlelike crystals in and around various joints, in certain cartilages like the ear, and in other organs, especially the kidneys (17).

These crystals are very small and can only be seen under the highest-powered light microscope. In the joint, these tiny crystals are engulfed by white blood cells. Unfortunately, these cells find the crystals indigestible. The lysomes and enzymes within the cell are burst by the crystals and the enzymes are liberated within the cell and then into the joint where they produce severe inflammation and pain. The inducing agent is crystals of uric acid, a relatively insoluble chemical that is deposited from the blood (41).

Heredity. Although gout is not always hereditary, it tends to run in families. The defect in body chemistry that leads to an overabundance of uric acid in the blood and body tissues is hereditary and is passed through either the mother or father. It does not mean that offspring of a gouty parent are sure to get the disease, but it does mean that they have a greater than average chance (1).

Gout is most prevalent among middle-aged and overweight men. It is rare in women (no more than 5% of those who have gout are female) and the symptoms in women are most likely to occur after menopause. It is also rare in young children, but when it does occur, it can be rapidly crippling if not properly treated. Gout is not contagious. Gouty patients are found in all areas of the world and in all climates. Gout appears in all races.

Phases. True uric acid gout passes through two phases. Initially, there is an acute stage in which the subject suffers from recurrent attacks of acute painful swelling in various joints which may be moderate or severe. The first attack is usually sudden, severe, and dramatic. After each succeeding attack the joint seems to return to normal until the next bout. Strangely, attacks come on early in the morning between 2 and 4 A.M. and awaken the patient. Any joint may be involved, but the toe joint is the most common. The joint swells rapidly and takes on a reddish-purple hue which turns white on pressure. The joint is usually warm and extremely painful and tender. Exactly what governs the severity of an attack is not known. Under modern treatment, painful swelling can be relieved in several hours, but if it is untreated, painful swelling will last several days before subsiding. After this attack the patient may be free for many months or years but not forever.

There has been much speculation on why gout usually starts in the joint of the big toe, but there seem to be two main reasons. (1) The big toe joint often shows osteoarthritis due to wear and tear before any of the other joints do. (2) Since the big toe joint is the farthest joint from the heart, it is the coldest joint in the body. These two factors both enhance the crystallization of uric acid from its solution in blood (9).

In the second phase, attacks become more frequent and do not subside as rapidly. Also, more than one joint may be involved and the patient may experience symptoms of weakness, malaise, and fever. Eventually, some joints will not clear completely and though acute symptoms subside, low-grade pain remains because uric acid crystals sooner or later destroy joint surfaces. The joint becomes filled with large masses of crystals that look like chalk. The joint appears to be swollen and movements are limited. Gout mainly tends to damage the big toe joint, but joints in the fingers, elbows, and elsewhere can also be damaged. Uric acid may be deposited in other tissues. It is often found in the skin on the backs of the elbows, on margins of the ears, and in the hands. Usually the spine, shoulders, and hips do not give symptoms (17).

Excess uric acid that is converted into crystals of sodium biurate accumulate in certain areas as nodular deposits or *tophi* of varying size. The most frequent site is along the free edge of the ear and behind the elbow. They also form in the cartilage and capsules of joints. They are not usually found with the first attack of gouty arthritis and may not show up for 10 to 12 years, if at all. Only about 30% to 40% of gouty patients develop tophi (17).

The kidneys are the only internal organ of the body which is commonly damaged by urate crystals. Collections of crystals of uric acid accumulate in the kidneys and in time can gradually destroy the kidney. Damaged kidneys threaten life itself, either directly because they fail to get rid of waste products or indirectly because they lead to high blood pressure which in turn may lead to heart disease and stroke. Even when kidney damage is not too severe, the results are unfortunate since uric acid itself is one of the waste products of the body and is normally eliminated by the kidneys into the urine, hence its name. If the kidney damaged by gout becomes even less efficient at getting rid of uric acid, the condition becomes worse (41).

Uric acid crystals may form kidney stones of varying sizes. The amount of pain depends upon the size and location. The stone may or may not pass of its own accord or it may cause blockage and necessitate surgery.

Purine-Rich Food. Specific precipitating factors are thought to bring on an attack of gout. The belief that certain purine rich foods and high living promote the onset of gout has persisted since ancient times and is still accepted today. It is important to remember that it is not only the type of food that matters but also the amount consumed. However, it has been found that most gouty patients do not show an adverse response to occasional excess purine feedings and the frequency of attacks does not vary in alternating intervals of high and low purine intake. The natural course of the disease is characterized by very sudden changes in an erratic, unpredictable pattern (7).

Alcohol. Overindulgence in alcohol is a predisposing factor in gouty arthritis. People who drink alcohol burn it. In the body the alcohol passes through the stage of transformation to lactic acid. So people who drink excessively have lots of lactic acid in their blood and this can affect the kidneys and stop them from getting rid of uric acid. The greater the alcohol intake, the less uric acid is eliminated. It is easy to see that people who eat well, producing more uric acid, and who drink well, disposing of less uric acid, are candidates for gout (41).

Injury. Probably the most frequent cause of a gout flare-up is an injury or trauma to a joint. The injury need not be severe; a minor twist of an ankle or knee may touch off a very severe attack. The frequent involvement of the joints of the large toes has been attributed to chronic strain sustained in walking or from the pressure of ill-fitting shoes.

Surgery. Patients with gout are particularly prone to suffer acute attacks during the week after an operation unless certain precautions are taken. This means a purine-free diet for 5 days before and after an operation and the taking of small doses of colchicine regularly during that time.

Medicine. A number of medicines may start attacks of gout and therefore they must be taken with caution. These include liver extract, penicillin, vitamin B^{12}, insulin, and diuretics. In addition, the sudden withdrawal of ACTH or cortisone may precipitate an attack (17).

Prognosis. The key to understanding the role of uric acid in gout lies in the solubility of uric acid. Uric acid circulates in the blood in the form of poorly soluble salt, sodium biurate. Blood is thicker than water and the thickness is due to plasma proteins which are able to keep uric acid in solution at levels far above the natural solubility. Because of this, all persons with gout who are not on treatment have two or three times more uric acid in blood than is desirable. In chemical terms, the blood is a supersaturated solution of uric acid and therefore can be made to deposit crystals. So persons with gout have a strong tendency to form crystals and the tendency is strongest in joints and kidneys.

For gout patients, the prognosis depends largely upon the patient and how closely he is willing to follow the prescribed regimen. Since the actual cause of gout is not known, it is not surprising that there is no cure. It is not yet known how to alter the basic underlying metabolic defect. But the clue to the cure of gout is the *solubility* of uric acid. If the amount of uric acid dissolved in the blood can be kept below 6 milligrams in 100 cubic centimeters, then crystals of uric acid will steadily dissolve back again into the blood. At least at this point, thanks to modern scientific research, the disease can be controlled during the lifetime of the patient (41).

The drug treatment of gout is now so effective that it is hardly necessary to impose severe dietary restrictions on patients, other than using common sense in not overeating purine-rich foods and not overdrinking alcoholic beverages. It is helpful to drink plenty of nonalcoholic fluids; up to 5 or 6 pints a day will increase the flow of urine considerably and will help prevent kidney damage or the appearance of stones.

Treatment. The treatment of gout is divided into two distinct phases. The first phase is that of the *acute attack* during which one or more joints are painful and swollen. The second phase might be called the *quiescent* or *interval* phase during which the patient is apparently normal but during which time excessive uric acid is building up in his body and depositing in tissues. The treatment therefore is divided into two separate regimens. In the acute attack the purpose of the treatment is to relieve the patient of the acute pain and disability. The purpose of the treatment in the second phase is to prevent the excess accumulation of uric acid. Treatment during this time is by far the more important so far as the eventual outcome of the disease is concerned (17).

Until recent years the only known remedy was a drug called colchicine. Even the Egyptians and other ancient peoples who suffered from gout knew about this drug. It was gout sufferer Benjamin Franklin who is credited with the introduction of colchicine in America. Colchicine is a poisonous crystalline alkaloid extracted from the saffron crocus and it has been responsible for providing relief to gout sufferers for many years. But colchicine, while it alleviates acute attacks, can produce unpleasant side effects. It is extremely powerful and the amount needed to control an attack of gout is about the same as the amount that will cause abdominal cramps and diarrhea.

The most common program is to start with 2 tablets and then to take 1 additional tablet every hour through the day until the pain is relieved or intestinal symptoms develop. After the first day, 1 tablet three times a day for a week is usually enough to prevent recurrence. The value of colchicine is that it stops the production of lactic acid and consequently reduces the inflammation.

Other common drugs used are *ACTH*, *indomethacin,* and *phenylbutazone*. When taken in correct amounts, they relieve the severe pain and swelling in an acute attack, but they do nothing to reduce the uric acid in the body. It is important that gout patients use these drugs under the close supervision of their doctor in order to keep the side effects under control (17).

It is interesting to note that gout and *aspirin* do not mix. Aspirin affects the complicated pathways by which uric acid is lost from the body through the kidneys. Instead of helping the situation, it may do the opposite by actually reducing the loss of uric acid from the body.

Telling a man who is having a severe attack of gout to rest is like telling a man without legs not to walk. The joint is so painful that the patient is not capable of anything but resting. However, people with milder attacks should be instructed not to walk because walking will usually make them worse (41).

In recent years, a better understanding of the complicated pathway by which uric acid is formed and removed has led to the development of effective drugs designed to reduce the amount of uric acid in the body. These drugs are of two types: those that reduce the formation of uric acid such as *allopurinol* and those that increase the loss of uric acid through the kidneys such as *probenecid.*

Allopurinol interrupts the "metabolic breakdown" of purines before they reach the stage of uric acid. Probenecid, which has been available long enough to have had adequate time to prove its usefulness, does not lose its beneficial effects over a long period of time and serious side reactions are rare. When the drug is started, there may be a tendency for mild gouty flare-up; for this reason, some colchicine is often prescribed during the first few weeks. The gouty patient taking probenecid excretes about twice as much uric acid in a day as he does without the drug but there is no deleterious effect on the kidney (17).

Once it is necessary to start taking these drugs, it is essential to continue treatment throughout life. To put it bluntly, treatment for gout is treatment for life. Fresh attacks of gout will be prevented and the joint swellings and visible deposits of uric acid in the skin will heal. Unfortunately, during the first few weeks of treatment, these drugs will actually stir up the gout because they exert such a profound influence in moving the uric acid from the deposits that free uric acid gets into the new sensitive areas. This problem should not dismay those who want a long-term cure for gout because these initial painful attacks can be prevented by taking small doses of the acute attack drugs during the first few months of treatment with the chronic gout drugs (41).

Today gout can be completely controlled with drugs designed to correct the abnormal chemistry. If the gout patient receives adequate medical care and follows his physician's advice, he can be spared the agonizing pain and crippling and can lead a normal, symptom-free life.

Pseudo-gout. Uric acid is not the only crystalline substance that can produce acute joint inflammation. For years doctors have recognized a specific form of arthritis caused by chalklike substances other than uric acid being deposited in joints. It is a crystalline form of calcium pyrophosphate. The similarities of the inflammation induced by calcium pyrophosphate to that induced by uric acid are reflected in one of its names: *pseudo-gout.* It is also called *calcium gout* and *chondrocalcinosis.* (Condro means cartilage and calcinosis means calcium.)

Pseudo-gout can affect adults at almost any age. Its major distinction is that it sometimes runs in families. It is generally the knee joint that is affected, but the wrist, elbow, hip, shoulder, or spine can also be affected. The trouble usually starts as a result of repeated attacks of severe arthritis. Sometimes the condition produces chronic wear and tear or osteoarthritis. Here the symptoms take the form of aches and pains and grating in the joints.

It is the X-ray that produces the clue to the diagnosis of pseudo-gout. The X-ray shows abnormal chalky material which leads the doctor to examine the joint fluid. The particular crystals of calcium pyrophosphate will then be discovered. The treatment for pseudo-gout is similar to that for gout with the exception of the use of aspirin. Indomethacin and phenylbutazone are usually effective and the severe pain subsides within a day or two (41).

As with gout, the picture has improved dramatically in recent years. In both diseases the joint disability and deformity that were once inevitable can be prevented with proper treatment. The classic middle-aged, self-indulgent gentleman with the aching toe has been the butt of slapstick humor for years, but now with effective drugs available, he may have the last laugh.

■ Allergies

An allergy is an abnormal reaction of the body to a harmless foreign substance, usually a protein. Instead of building a resistance to the allergen, as the body would to a harmful bacteria or virus, it builds a sensitivity. The sensitivity is established when the tissues of the nose or bronchi, for example, develop antibodies to pollens, grasses, weeds, molds, dust, dander, drugs, feathers, various foods, plants, insect stings, and others. Once the antibodies have been developed, the tissue reacts to that specific allergen. Also at this time histamine may be released. Histamine causes dilation of the blood vessels, increased flow of secretions, and local irritation (35, 75, 78).

Allergies plague some 19 million people, two-thirds of whom suffer from hay fever or asthma. Prolonged and repeated sneezing, red, swollen, teary eyes and itchy nose and eyes are characteristics of hay fever. Actual fever is not. The pollens of trees, grasses and weeds, and molds are easily air-borne. The hay fever victim suffers only when his or her specific allergen is in the air. Those who are sensitive to tree pollen suffer in the spring; those sensitive to grasses suffer in the early summer; those sensitive to ragweed may suffer from spring to late fall. People who are allergic to house dust, dog or cat dander, or other inescapable airborne material may suffer all year long. The degree of suffering depends upon the amount of pollen in the air and the sensitivity of the person. Some people may develop complications such as chronic sinusitis, nasal polyps (growths), and asthma (35).

Asthma develops because of the sensitivity of the bronchial tissues. When the allergen is airborne, the lining of the bronchial tubes swells and the secretions thicken. The muscles, particularly in the branchlike extension of the bronchial tree, fail to release or dilate, thus making it most difficult for the victim to expell air. The characteristic wheezing, coughing, and gasping ensue. Children get asthma; so do adults in every age, race, and occupation. In asthma, as with most all allergies, there is usually a family history of sensitivity and usually the victim has suffered from skin rashes, hives, or hay fever before getting the first asthma attack. The attacks occur most often at night and the squeezing of the chest and throat bring a fear of choking. Attacks of asthma, though distressing, are rarely fatal. Children, when under care, often recover permanently when they reach their teens. Effective medicines can be prescribed to relieve the distress and to end long-lasting attacks. The causes are the same as in hay fever. Recent research has dispelled the myth that asthma may be a psychosomatic disease (22).

Hay fever and asthma are controlled by removing the cause so far as is practical and by building up the patient's resistance. Avoiding the specific substance is the best way to control the allergy, but it is not always easy for the patient or the doctor to discover the offending substance. A careful history of when the attacks occur may reveal the agent. If this method gives no clue, the doctor may have to perform as many as 30 or 40 skin tests. The doctor does this by scratching a powder or solution made up of the allergen into the patient's skin; if a red welt or wheal appears, the test is positive. Some people may be allergic to several different substances. Once the causative agent is identified, it may be possible to avoid it. Seasonal vacations and air conditioning may help, but they have their limitations. If the agent is dander, the family pet may have to go (22, 35).

In many cases, it is impossible to avoid the substance. The doctor may then suggest that the patient build an immunity to it by taking a series of graded injections. The solution to be injected contains a minute amount of the allergen; this amount is increased in each injection until the body can tolerate larger doses without reaction. The injections have to be repeated annually even though after several years desensitization to the specific substance may occur. The availability of testing and desensitization is limited because there are few specialists in the field.

The sticky sap of poison ivy, poison oak, and poison sumac contains an active ingredient known as urushiol which causes allergic skin reactions. Seven out of ten persons may become sensitized to any of the three plants. The rash may be mild or severe, and it may appear a few hours or several days after contact. The skin may turn red and itch or large blisters and swelling may appear depending upon the sensitivity of the person and the degree of exposure. Avoiding the plants is the best preventive measure because urushiol must make contact with the skin for a reaction. Smoke may carry drops of the chemical and pets may rub up against the plants and pass the sap to a person indirectly. It is well to wear long sleeves and trousers in the woods and pastures and maybe in the backyard, for poison ivy and poison oak grow almost everywhere. There is little risk of developing scars unless there is a secondary infection. Spreading is not due to the discharge from the blisters but from the original or a new contact. The best treatment is sudsing the skin and washing clothes that may be contaminated. Most cases disappear by themselves. Calamine lotion is a good drying agent and relieves itching.

Skin conditions may be of special concern to individuals in later life who have developed high sensitivity levels. Such levels may be attributed to high incidences of anaphylactic shock among the elder population afflicted with organic poisons. Medical advice is a must in such cases (60).

Hives is an allergy most often caused by drugs and food. It starts below the skin surface and manifests itself in red surface swellings not unlike large mosquito bites. Common foods that are involved are cows milk in children, eggs, wheat, nuts, strawberries, and shellfish. Once a food, and it can be any food, is identified, it can be avoided. The American Dietetic Association has suggested allergy recipes for people sensitive to foods.

Drugs, particularly antibiotics, such as penicillin, are being used more frequently than in the past. Therefore, it is not surprising to find more people sensitive to them. A person who has had a reaction to a specific drug or antitoxin should be aware of the greater danger that may arise if the drug is used again, especially if it is injected. Such a person should wear a medical identification tag or carry a warning card for the allergy risks with medicines.

Summary

Few time periods in life are totally free from illness or disability. In life's early decades and during the middle decades acute conditions are the most prevalent. Chronic conditions occur in later life. Throughout life social and economic factors influence an individual's health. These factors become more significant when examined in conjunction with various degenerative physiological conditions. Twentieth-century industrialized societies no longer fear infectious diseases. Instead, degenerative diseases are claiming lives and remaining with the afflicted for decades of life in later years. The single factor that makes these health problems in later decades baffling is their multiple etiology and gradual alterations. Mortality from some diseases, cardiovascular and cancer among these, is more common than from others, showing evidence among males and females and among whites and nonwhites at differing rates. Many nonfatal diseases may be found among almost all elderly individuals. A prime example is hardening of the arteries. However, nonfatal diseases are by no means found totally among the elderly. Individuals in their first two decades of life may be subject to such diseases as diabetes, gout, and arthritis. Assuming that some portion of the population may not face the aforementioned illnesses, then it can be assumed that management and treatment are the answers in providing a homogenous quality of life for those affected.

References

1. "Allergies Plague 19 Million." *Science Newsletter* 88 (1965): 42.
2. Anthony, Catherine Parker. *Textbook of Anatomy and Physiology.* St. Louis: C. V. Mosby, 1971.
3. Arky, Ronald. "Current Principles of Dietary Therapy of Diabetes Mellitus." *Medical Clinics of North America* 62 (1978): 655–62.

4. Arthritis Foundation. *About Gout.* Atlanta, Ga., 1978.

5. ——. *Osteoarthritis.* Atlanta, Ga. 1977.

6. Ashburn, Shirley Smith. "The Health Care System—How Do Teenagers Use It?" In *Approaches to the Care of Adolescents,* edited by Audrey J. Kalafatich. pp. 13–30. New York: Appleton-Century-Crofts, 1975.

7. Bauer, Walter, and Krane, Stephan. "Gout." In *Diseases of Metabolism,* Philadelphia: Saunders, 1977.

8. Blau, Sheldon, Paul, and Schultz, D. *Arthritis, Complete Up to Date Facts for Patients and their Families.* Garden City, New York: Doubleday, 1974.

9. Bluhm, Gilbert, McCarty, Daniel, Jr., and Wallace, Stanley. "'Live with It' Is Out for Gout." *Patient Care* 7 (1977): 131.

10. Boyland, Brian, and Weller, Charles. *The New Way to Live with Diabetes.* Garden City, New York: Doubleday, 1976.

11. Bruce, Nancy, and Dawson, Alice E. "The School—Its Relationship to Health Services." In *Approaches to the Care of Adolescents,* edited by Audrey Kalafatich, pp. 56–60. New York: Appleton-Century-Crofts, 1975.

12. Brunner, Lillian Sholtis, Emerson, Charles Philips, Ferguson, L. Kraeir, Suddarth, and Smith, Doris. *Textbook of Medical Surgical Nursing.* Philadelphia: Lippincott, 1970.

13. Coleman, Lester. *All Your Medical Questions Answered.* San Francisco, Calif.: The Hearst Corporation, 1977.

14. Conn, Howard F. and Conn, Rex, B. *Current Diagnosis.* Philadelphia: Saunders, 1968.

15. Conway, H., and Hugo, N. E. "Radiation Dermatitis and Malignancy." *Plastic and Reconstructive Surgery* 38 (1976): 255–68.

16. Cowdry, E. V. "Malignant Neoplasms of the Stomach." *Etiology and Prevention of Cancer in Man.* New York: Appleton-Century-Crofts, 1970.

17. Crain, Darrell. *Arthritis Handbook.* New York; Arco, 1972.

18. Davis, Paul J. "Endocrines and Aging." *Hospital Practice* 12 (1977): 113–28.

19. Dong, Collin H., and Banks, Jane. *New Hope for the Arthritic.* New York: Thomas Y. Crowell, 1975.

20. Dortimer, Anthony C., Shenoy, Prokashi N., Shiroff, Robert

A., Leaman, David M., Babb, Joseph D., Liedke, A. James, and Zelis, Robert. "Diffuse Coronary Artery Disease, Fact or Fiction." *Circulation* 57 (1978): 133–36.

21. Driscoll, Pamela Webb. "Rheumatoid Arthritis: Understanding It More Fully." *Nursing* 1 (1975):19–21

22. Ducas, Dorothy. "Winning the Battle Against Asthma." *Today's Health* 45 (1967): 28–32.

23. Ehrlich, G., ed. *Total Management of the Arthritic Patient.* Philadelphia: Lippincott, 1973.

24. Ellenberg, Max. "Managing Diabetic Neuropathy." In *Diabetic Rounds,* pp. 68–79. New York: MEDCOM Learning Systems, 1973.

25. ———. "Diabetes: Our Leading Health Problem." In *Diabetes in Theory and Practice,* pp. 1–8. New York: Pfizer Laboratories, 1978.

26. Foreman, Issac, Faccio, Enrique, and Milei, Jose. "Autonomic Neuropathy and Painless Myocardial Infarction in Diabetic Patients." *Diabetes* 26 (1977): 1147–58.

27. Forsham, Peter H. "Diabetes: Back to Basics." In *Diabetic Rounds,* pp. 8–17. New York: MEDCOM Learning Systems, 1973.

28. ———. "Hyperglycemia and Vascular Complications of Maturity—Onset Diabetes Mellitus." In *Diabetes in Theory and in Practice,* pp. 28–38. New York: Pfizer Laboratories, 1978.

29. Fraser, Marianne. *Balancing the Scale: Diabetic Patient Education.* Salt Lake City, Utah: University of Utah Medical Center, 1974.

30. Freinkel, Norbert. "Nature of Research." *Diabetic Forecast* 31 (1978): 22–23, 31.

31. Gangong, W. F. *Review of Medical Physiology,* 8th ed. London: Lange Medical Publications, 1976.

32. Goldstein, Samuel, and Podolsky, Stephen. "The Genetics of Diabetes Mellitus." *Medical Clinics of North America* 62 (1978): 639–54.

33. Good, Robert A. "Diabetes: Relentless Progress Against a Relentless Disease." *Hospital Practice* 12 (1977): 15–16.

34. Gorich, John. "Diabetic Control and the Late Complications of Diabetes." *American Family Physician* 16 (1977): 84–91.

35. *Hay Fever, The Facts.* New York: National Tuberculosis and Respiratory Disease Association, 1979.

36. Hempelmann, L. H., Pifer, J. W., Burke, G. J., Terry, R., and Ames, W. R. "Neoplasms in Persons Treated with X-rays in Infancy for Thymic Enlargement: Report of Third Follow-up Survey." *Journal of the National Cancer Institute* 48 (1977): 317–41.

37. Hernandez, Luis A. "Gout." *Nursing Times* (1976):47–48.

38. Hoover, Joan. "What Exactly Is a DRTC?" *Diabetic Forecast.* 31 (1978): 24–27.

39. *It's Women 3 to 1.* New York: The Arthritis and Rheumatism Foundation, 1978.

40. Jackson, Robert L., Holland, Edward, Chapman, Ira D., and Guthrie, Diana. "Growth and Maturation of Children with Insulin Dependent Diabetes Mellitus." *Diabetes Care* 1 (1978): 96–107.

41. Jayson, Malcom, and Dixon, Allan. *Understanding Arthritis and Rheumatism.* New York: Pantheon, 1974.

42. Kent, Saul. "Is Diabetes a Form of Accelerated Aging?" *Geriatrics* 31 (1976): 140–50.

43. ———. "Re-evaluating the Dietary Treatment of Diabetes." *Geriatrics* 33 (1978): 99–107.

44. Kilo, Charles. "Controlling Diabetes: Should You Believe UGDP?" *Modern Medicine* 46 (1978): 49–53.

42. Kent, Saul. "Is Diabetes a Form of Accelerated Aging?" Jovanovich, Inc., 1976.

46. Lange, Kurt. "Managing Diabetic Neuropathy." *Diabetic Rounds,* pp. 50–55. New York: MEDCOM Learning Systems, 1973.

47. Lee, Elizabeth. *Diabetes.* Bowie, Md.: Robert C. Brady, 1972.

48. Litch, Sidney, ed. *Arthritis and Physical Medicine.* New Haven, Conn.: Elizabeth Litch, Publisher, 1969.

49. Littler, T. R. *Understanding Rheumatism.* London: Tavistock Publications, 1966.

50. Marjarian, John S. "Islet Cell Transplantation in Treatment of Diabetes." *Hospital Practice* 13 (1977): 63–69.

51. McFadden, Maureen. "Ravages of Rheumatoid Arthritis." *Nursing* 4 (1975):239–41.

52. McKenna, R. J., Schwinn, C. P., and Higginbotham, N. L., "Osteogenic Sarcoma in Children." *California Medicine* 103 (1965): 165–70.

53. Michels, Ronald G. "What Role for Vitrectomy in Managing Diabetic Retinopathy." *Hospital Practice* 13 (1977): 73–78.

54. Mihich, E. *Immunity, Cancer and Chemotherapy.* New York: Academic Press, 1975.

55. Nowell, P. C., and Hungerford, D. A. "Chromosome Studies in Human Leukemia." *Journal of the National Cancer Institute* 27 (1961): 1013.

56. Palumbo, P. J. "How to Treat Maturity-Onset Diabetes Mellitus." *Geriatrics* 32 (1977): 57–63.

57. Patz, Arnall. "Managing Diabetic Retinopathy." In *Diabetic Rounds,* pp. 44–49. New York: MEDCOM Learning Systems, 1973.

58. Paymaster, J. C., and Gangadharan, P. "Oral and Pharyngeal Cancer in India." *Cancer* 13 (1973): 71.

59. Pirat, Jean. "Diabetes Mellitus and Its Degenerative Complication: A Prospective Study of 4,400 Patients Observed Between 1947–1973." *Diabetes Care* 1 (1978): 168–88.

60. *Poison Ivy, Oak, and Sumac.* Public Health Service Bulletin No. 1723. Washington, D.C.: U.S. Government Printing Office, 1967.

61. Prevention Magazine Staff. "Gout." In *The Encyclopedia of Common Diseases.* Emmaus: Pa.: Rodale Press, 1976.

62. Reaven, Gerald. "Does Age Affect Glucose Tolerance?" *Geriatrics* 32 (1977): 51–54.

63. Rodman, Ferald, ed. *Primer on the Rheumatic Disease,* 7th ed. New York: Arthritis Foundation, 1973.

64. Schuman, Charles. "Managing Maturity-Onset Diabetes." In *Diabetic Rounds,* pp. 30–37. New York: MEDCOM Learning Systems, 1973.

65. Schuman, Delores. "Assessing the Diabetic." *Nursing* 76 (1976): 62–67.

66. Selikoff, I. J., Churg, J., and Hammon, E. C. "Relation Between Exposure to Asbestos and Mesothelioma." *New England Journal of Medicine* 272 (1965): 560.

67. Skillman, Thomas, G., and Tzagournis, Manuel. *Diabetes Mellitus.* Columbus, Ohio: Upjohn, 1977.

68. Smyth, Charley J. "Therapy of Rheumatoid Arthritis." In *Management of Arthritis Patients and Patience,* Arthritis Foundation Series No. 16, pp. 24–39. New York: McGraw-Hill, 1972.

69. Spirtz, Norton. "Nerve Disease in Diabetes Mellitus." *Medicinal Clinics of North America* 62 (1978): 787–98.

70. Taylor, T. G., and Irwin, J. "Some Audiological Aspects of Diabetes." *Journal of Laryngology and Otology* 92 (1978): 99–112.

71. Thornton, George F. "Infections and Diabetes." *Medical Clinics of North America* 55 (1971): 931–38.

72. Timiras, P. S. *Developmental Physiology and Aging.* New York: Macmillan, 1972.

73. *Today's Health Guide.* Chicago: American Medical Association, 1965.

74. *Understanding Your Diabetes.* New York: Pfizer Laboratories, 1977.

75. Unger, Donald L. "The Sneezin' Season Is Here." *Today's Health* 45 (1967): 3.

76. Warmbrand, Max. *Overcoming Arthritis and Other Rheumatic Diseases.* Old Greenwich, Conn.: Devin-Adair, 1976.

77. Weiss, L. *The Cell Periphery, Metastasis, and Other Contact Phenomena.* New York: North-Holland Publishing, 1967.

78. "What Is an Allergy" *Science Digest* 64 (1968): 87–88.

79. Whitehouse, Fred. "Get Wise Exercise." *Diabetic Forecast* 31 (1978): 20–22, 51.

80. Williams, T. Franklin. "Diabetes Mellitus in Older People." In *Clinical Aspects of Aging,* edited by William Reichel, pp. 327–30. Baltimore: William & Wilkins, 1978.

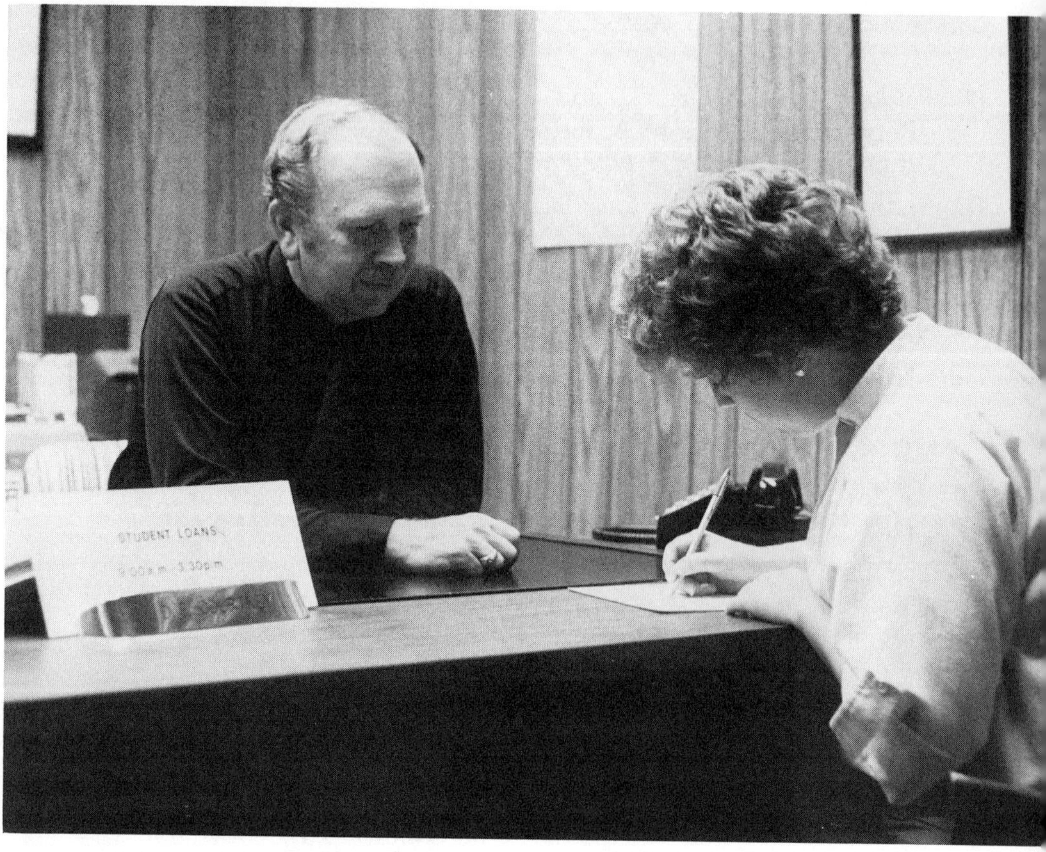
STUDENT LOANS
9:00 a.m. 3:30 p.m.

■ Chapter 8

Cardiovascular Disease

Major Concepts

1. Heart disease is inevitable if one lives long enough.
2. Hypertension, often called high blood pressure, potentially is the most destructive cardiovascular disease afflicting Americans.
3. Cardiovascular risk factors are elements of twentieth-century American life.

Cardiovascular disease is a disease of the vascular system that causes narrowing, hardening, or loss of strength in the vasculature of the heart and its immediate arterial system. Included in this system are the coronary arterial vasculature, the ascending and beginning segment of the descending aorta, and the carotid arteries. The remainder of the arterial tree containing such sections as the subclavian, renal, and femoral arteries is not part of this discussion. The pathological changes that can lead to a blocking that decreases resilience or rupture of the vessels are included in this definition. The disease manifests itself in such forms as hypertension, angina pectoris, myocardial infarction, and cerebrovascular accident (stroke). Generally, the diseases of the heart proper are referred to as arterio-atherosclerotic coronary heart disease (41).

Heart disease in the aged is seldom, if ever, distinct and it usually consists of changes due to aging and one or more of the conventional types of heart disease. This chapter will discuss these changes and their effects on the development, manifestations, and treatment of heart disease during one's life. The primary objectives are to identify that subject material relevant to the aging process and heart disease which may facilitate the diagnosis and management of the heart patient and to stimulate greater interest and curiosity about heart disease in the aging process. The natural processes of aging cannot be counteracted, but longevity may be extended and disability may be reduced by better total medical care of the aged cardiac patient. The aging process and the special features of heart disease in elderly patients are a major concern for life extension.

This focus on heart disease in the aging process is important because heart disease is the most common cause of death in the population aged 65 and over. The death rate from heart disease in this age group is twice as high as that of stroke, the next most common cause of death. Together, these two diseases account for a death rate of 9319.8 per 100,000 persons, almost 10 times the rate of cancer, the next most common cause of death (993.4 per 100,000 persons). Furthermore, the social, psychological, and economic toll of these diseases in terms of disability, disruption of family life, and money constitutes an enormous drain on the resources of the patient, the family, and the nation.

Although the aging heart can function adequately in most old people as long as the coronary system is not damaged, the following physiologic alterations may occur with age:

1. The cardiac reserve diminishes and the heart reacts poorly to sudden stress.
2. The cardiac output drops about 1% per year below the normal value of 5 liters per minute found in younger persons. The reduction in cardiac output results from a decreased stroke volume due to aging and a slower heart rate (11).
3. The estimated left ventricular work declines at rest (25).
4. The maximum blood flow through the coronary artery tree at the age of 60 is about 35% lower than in youth (13, 14).
5. The aged myocardium shows a delay in the recovery of contractility and irritability. Despite its slow rate of recovery, it functions well when there is an adequate period of rest between beats, but it reacts poorly to rapid heart beat (tachycardia). Simple tachycardia (120 to 150 beats per minute), caused by fever, emotional upset, or other conditions can precipitate heart failure in older people, even without a rise in blood pressure.
6. Normal vasomotor tone decreases while vagus nerve influences increase.
7. Peripheral vascular resistance rises 1% per year, about the same as the decrease in cardiac output per year (25, 40).
8. The heart is less sensitive to the effect of atropine (a drug used to relieve spasms) and more sensitive to carotid sinus stimulation.
9. The aged heart has a decreased ability to utilize oxygen.
10. An increased pulse wave velocity found in older persons whose blood pressure is normal reflects the increased rigidity of the larger and medium arteries with age (19, 22, 44, 45).

Blood pressure in the aging human depends upon:

1. The loss of elasticity in the walls of the larger arteries, which tends to raise systolic and depress diastolic pressures.
2. The increased ability of vasopressor control to change, which tends to raise both systolic and diastolic pressures.

The first is a structural, vascular factor; the second is a functional, neurogenic factor. Since their effects on systolic blood pressure are additive, systolic blood pressure rises with advancing years. The diastolic pressure, however, may rise or fall with age (20). The variability of the vascular and neurogenic factors with aging accounts for the controversy over normal blood pressures in elderly people. In the literature the range is from a very conservative upper limit of 120 millimeters of mercury systolic and 80 millimeters of mercury diastolic, regardless of age and sex, to more liberal values (26, 27, 28). In extreme old age, normal blood pressures generally range between 100 and 140 millimeters of mercury systolic and between 70 and 90 millimeters of mercury diastolic.

■ Statistics

Cardiovascular disease kills three times as many people as do various forms of cancer. Younger males are susceptible targets, but women prior to menopause apparently have some hormonal protection but after menopause there is a greater likelihood of their experiencing coronary problems. The rate of male mortality from heart attacks during the second half of life ranges from a low of only 719 per 100,000 in the countries of southwestern Europe to a high of over 1225 in the United States and 1400 in Finland. Incidences among females are comparably broad, with a low of 376 in a few Scandinavian countries to over 520 in the United States. Even when not fatal, heart diseases take their toll; about 22% of all the disabilities found in men and 15% of those found in women during the middle years are attributed to heart problems. With advancing age, mortality increases dramatically, doubling every decade or so for men and tripling for women. In some of the Scandinavian countries the rate among women climbs even more rapidly, approaching a fourfold increase per decade. Still, female deaths average only about half those of their male counterparts (37).

■ Artherosclerosis

Atherosclerosis is a general label for all arterial diseases; however, the form most prevalent in the elderly is called atherosclerosis. It is characterized primarily as a hardening of the *intima* or interior walls of major vessels and it is considered the leading precursor of other retrogressive coronary changes. In a recent report on the worldwide distribution of heart diseases, the World

Health Organization noted that atherosclerosis is almost a universal health problem that singularly stands in the way of any appreciable prolongation of life. The same report also predicted that in those countries where the incidence of atherosclerosis is not yet a widespread cause of death, rapidly changing social and technological conditions may indicate future increases (46). Indeed, evidence indicates that this was clearly the case historically both in industrialized countries and in countries currently undergoing rapid industrialization. The disease is not a modern malady, for it was described in explicit detail in ancient Greek medical literature. Examination of mummies also suggests that it was known in Egypt and probably throughout the ancient world (42). The extent to which heart diseases alone claim lives is overwhelming. In the United States over 600,000 die yearly from the various forms of cardiovascular disease, and more than 28 million exhibit some form of the disease. Add in atherothrombotic diseases (such as cerebral hemorrhage) not involving the heart and the number of fatalities increases by another one-third. Despite a recent slight decline, middle-aged American men stand about one chance in five of developing clinically significant cardiovascular problems before they reach retirement age. Aside from Finnish men, Americans have the highest cardiac mortality rates in the world. Like so many other generic cardiovascular diseases, atherosclerotic conditions discriminate on the basis of sex; they occur among American males at a rate of three times the incidence among similarly aged females. And like other chronic illnesses, atherosclerosis need not prove fatal and it need not disrupt normal routines; its prevalence approches 100% among the very old in certain populations, seriously impairing their way of life.

Only among sufferers of diabetes or other high-risk illnesses does atherosclerosis make much of an impact before late in the fourth decade, although its inception usully dates from early adolescence. Individuals having a family history of heart disease seem particularly prone to cardiovascular disorders, although the mechanism by which susceptibility is transmitted is still a puzzle to medical science. The most important factors that have been linked to heightened probabilities of arterial diseases are diets high in saturated fats, sedentary activities, obesity, cigarette smoking, and psychological stress.

Over the past century there have been numerous attempts to trace the pathogenesis of atherosclerotic conditions, but to date no theory has won uncontested acceptance. The appearance of fatty streaks in the inner wall of the arteries has prompted many investigators to conclude that the blood deposits fatty substances that are absorbed through the *endothelial lining* separating the actual blood flow from the intima of the artery. These in turn are trapped inside the artery wall rather than passing through with the nutritive substances. Ultimately, a roughening and swelling occur and promote the formation of fibrous plaques in the *lumen,* or artery channel. Once the irregularity has taken shape, further buildup follows and constricts the space through which blood may flow. The actual fibrous plaque buildup is called a *thrombosis* and may eventually bring about a complete *occlusion* or closing of the artery. Under stress, thromboses may break loose and float through the artery until they become lodged in one of the smaller branches. Since the artery is a living form of connective tissue, damage begins immediately after any individual cell dies, no matter what the cause. With tissue death comes calcification, loss of elasticity, and lowered permeability. Which factors actually initiate the damage is hotly debated among physiologists, and while it is agreed that certain preventive steps may inhibit the development of plaques, nothing can be done about reversing their effects until the process is more fully understood (43).

■ Hypertension

Hypertension, what many people call high blood pressure, affects roughly the same percentage of older people as does heart disease, and like other coronary problems, it is much more prevalent among blacks. Essentially, hypertension is the rise in blood pressure causing an accelerated heart rate. Part of the difficulty with diagnosing hypertension in older people is the general tendency for blood pressure to elevate throughout most of life, especially among women. Also, the tissue of appropriate levels for a given individual poses questions that are not easily answered. In addition, blood pressure is affected by the presence of other illnesses, fever, obesity, and even air temperature. In turn, hypertension may cause other bodily homeostatic functions to become unbalanced, thus indirectly contributing to death. Cerebral hemorrhage and cardiac failure appear to be the most frequent terminal conditions associated with high blood pressure, but renal insufficiency and bronchopneumonia are not unusual. Among the clinically significant symptoms are fluctuations in systolic and diastolic pressure, changes in the structure of certain parts of the eye, and mental confusion, especially late in the day. Again, personal history and family background are important factors that must be taken into account (23). Hypertension factors will be discussed later in the chapter.

■ Cerebrovascular Accidents

Cerebrovascular accidents, or strokes, rank as the third most common cause of death in the second half of life. Each year strokes claim over 200,000 lives in the United States and leave many times that number impaired. Although quite a number of traumatic events may cause brain damage, most of them stem from other circulatory difficulties. In referring to strokes, most practitioners mean either cerebral hemorrhages caused by embolisms that have traveled to the brain and leave occluded one of the cerebral arteries or a thrombosis that develops in the brain's own ventricular system. In either event, the result is a cutting off of oxygen-rich blood supplies to some part of the brain, with a subsequent degeneration of the affected sections. Part of the insidious aftermath of a stroke is a loss of memory, aphasia, emotional problems, partial paralysis, loss of bowel control, and so on. Epidemiological studies of stroke suggest that strokes occur more frequently in industrialized countries than they do in underdeveloped nations and they are more likely to strike nonwhites than whites, with both sexes equally prone, under comparable occupational conditions and activity levels. Almost all researchers agree that cigarette smokers impose a greater survival risk on themselves in terms of both strokes and other coronary difficulties than do nonsmokers. Immediate medical attention may alleviate many complications and rehabilitation can help stroke patients overcome physiological malfunctions, but the neural injury can never be undone. Recent investigations of the toxic effects of the chemical components present in neurotransmitters, but released in unusually large doses during and after infarction, may provide new avenues for minimizing stroke damage (47).

Various degenerative diseases of the brain are yet another form of pathology affecting the elderly. Because of their diffuse character, cerebral atrophy, senile plaques, Parkinson's disease, and numerous other disorders are generally lumped together under the label organic brain damage. Brain damage is difficult to diagnose, and many symptoms of functional disorders are incorrectly labeled organic disorders. Many of the related cerebral conditions are long standing and only manifest themselves during stressful episodes in later life or when cardiovascular accidents trigger them.

■ Risk Factors

The risk factors discussed below are associated with or are generally considered to be the causitive agents involved in the development of cardiovascular disease. There is an extensive amount of documented data that generally agree that the same factors involved in the pathological consequences affect the cardiovascular system.

Two aspects of diseases involving the peripheral vascular system are important. These involve circulatory problems of the extremities such as *Raynaud's disease* (hands) and *Buerger's disease* (legs). In the later decades there are symptoms seen in the legs (e.g., brown colorization changes and scaling) that are related to decreased circulation, which can be the result of decreased cardiac output caused by cardiovascular changes. In addition, there are valvular problems, which include papillary muscle dysfunction, papillary muscle rupture, and rupture of the chordae tendenae. These are not caused by atherosclerotic processes, but they are dysfunctions that can cause sufficient restriction of blood flow to the point of necrosis (dead tissue) (10).

Process of Atherosclerotic Development There are differences of opinion on the concept of atherogenesis, but the discussion here will concern itself with only one of those opinions, the opinion that it is progressive and developmental.

Blood contains fat molecules and low-density lipids. These low-density lipids carry fat molecules into the tunica intima (the innermost layer of an artery) cells between most other cells and the elastic layer. As the fat molecules crowd into this region, their eventual overcrowding causes the elastic layer to begin to disintegrate because there is a lack of normal nutrition. Note that early diagnosis is possible and trends develop through exercise, diet, and monitoring of high-density lipids! With the continued invasion of fats and lipids, the cells of the intima fill with these materials, causing them to appear "foamy." Again, with this invasive action continuing, the foam cells build up in quantity until with additional lipids, the fat becomes visible to the naked eye as yellow spots or streaks on the surface of the intima. This condition has been observed and noted in children and young adults. This observable change and its vascular involvement are in the intima of the aorta. In arteries smaller than the aorta these early lesions involve not only the intima and elastic layer but also some of the nearby myocardium muscle cells. These cells are also foamy in appearance.

There is more information available on people in their later decades and the process of degeneration is more traceable in them. Additional fats and lipids accumulate into the fatty streaks. The foam cells increase in number because more cells are dying. The lipids released from the dying cells assemble into large "pools" as cholesterol crystals and a mixture of triglycerides, phospholipids, and sterols. The entire mixture appears as a soft paste or gruel. "Ather," the first part of the word atherosclerosis, is a Greek word meaning gruel.

An aorta riddled with these streaks and pools may contain up to 100 times its normal content of lipids. This extracellular mass of lipids, etc., irritates the arterial wall and brings about an inflammatory response. A scar develops in the shape of a sac that encloses the gruel. It is thicker on the lumen side where it is forming a thick barrier between the bloodstream and the gruel. This cushionlike formation, which is called a *raised or fibrous plaque,* protrudes into the lumen. Characteristically, it is pearly in color and is called *pearly plaque.*

As the plaque continues to grow it consumes more of the arterial wall, forming more foam cells and damaging more of the elastic layer. With time, the intima media is involved and is destroyed. Finally the intima adventitia (the outer layer of the artery wall) is invaded. The inflammation is now causing excess blood to congregate at the site and lymphocytic infiltration.

The capsule of the atheroma thickens, possibly as a compensatory effort, and builds a "new" arteriole wall. The new wall does not contain muscle fiber or elastic fiber. Instead, it contains only scar (connective) tissue, and thus it is a much less efficient wall section.

Figure 8.1 Anatomy of a heart attack.

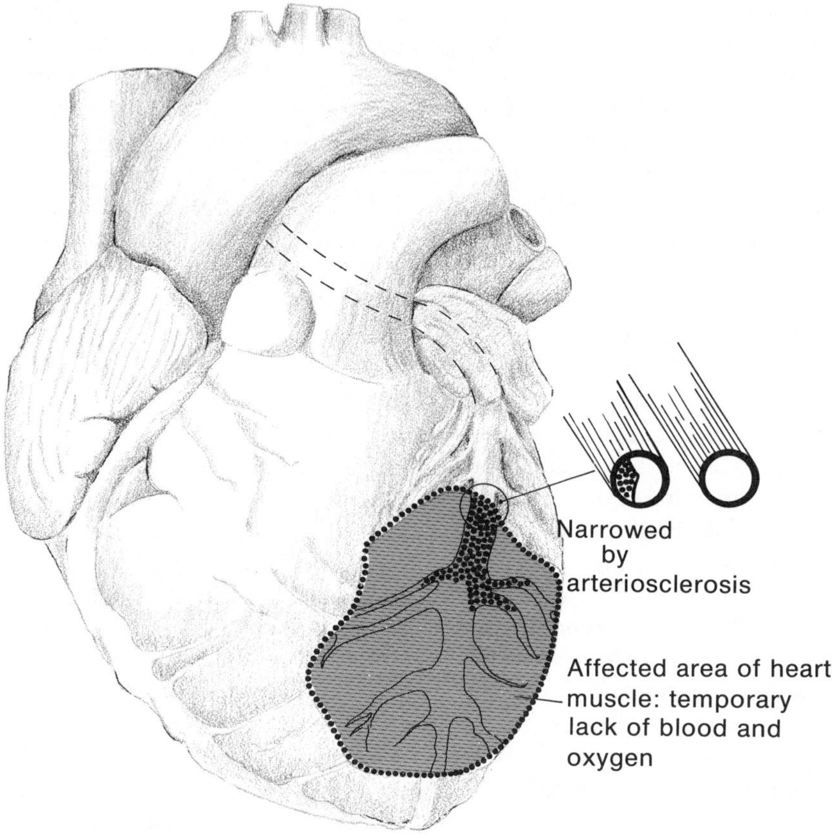

Deposits of calcium form on the gruel, on the capsule, or on both. These deposits may be in the form of fine granules, thin strips, or huge masses. When they are in large amounts, the artery hardens. Up to now, the repair processes have essentially been a form of protective scarring. The vessel is not too impaired although the wall is thickened. There still remains a smooth intimal surface and the lumen remains open, allowing blood to flow to the tissues. If no further involvement occurs, the scar may remain in this form indefinitely.

There are two possible directions of degeneration. The first vessel may begin breaking down, making atherosclerosis a deadly disease. With continuing degeneration, the capsule next breaks away. Then an ulcer forms from the plaque and some of gruel is carried away. The remainder forms an uneven, abnormal surface over which the blood clots. Alternatively, a hemorrhage may occur within the ulcer or under the edge of it. Before the wall size increases by atherosclerosis, the ulceration may break through the remainder of the wall and cause the artery to rupture.

The narrowing process, generally, is common for coronary arteries imbedded in the unyielding environment of the *myocardium*. Since the occlusion is usually a slow process, *collateral circulation* may develop. If this does not occur, the result is a bulge because the vessel is unable to widen. In the aorta, the bulge occurs along with a lengthening and twisting of the vessel.

Where the blood clotted over the exposed plaque as a result of the sac breaking away, the rough surface is covered by a clot. This clot may break away and this thrombus, if it is large or if it has developed in a smaller artery, may occlude the artery and cause an infarction or area of myocardial tissue death.

Atherosclerotic lesions prefer certain locations. This suggests that hemodynamic forces (blood pressure or turbulence) may play a role in where the atherosclerosis develops. Some evidence supporting this is suggested by the fact that the lesions are not found in veins where pressures are much lower. There are cases in which venous hypertension can occur and lesions have been found. The lesions are found most frequently in the aorta rather than in the small arterioles and they are generally prevalent at a point of declining size of large vessels or at the origin of small branches or where there are bends against a bony surface (descending aorta). How the process actually occurs is still a question (42). The effects of the risk factors do appear to correlate with this overall procedure and will become apparent later in the chapter.

Risk Factor Statistics In 1900 the fourth largest cause of death in the United States was reported to be diseases of the heart. These accounted for 8.3% of deaths from all causes. Pneumonia, tuberculosis, diarrhea, and enteritis were the first four causes, but advances in medicine and technology have been able to diminish these as major causative factors.

In 1959 diseases of the heart were reported to be the major cause of death in the United States. They accounted for 38.6%

of all causes of death, an increase of over 400% in the 59 years between these two reports. Pneumonia, one of the leading three causes of death in 1900, remained in the list of the first ten causative factors, but its 11% standing had been reduced to 3½% (42).

In 1975 statistics indicated that cardiovascular disease accounted for 52% of the major causes of deaths. Over 994,000 people died from cardiovascular diseases. The report also stated that more than 29 million people have some form of this disease and that more than 24 million have hypertension, 7 million of which are unaware of the condition.

Below are listed additional statistics on cardiovascular disease:

1. Twice as many blacks as whites have hypertension.
2. Generally, more white males than females are affected.
3. Strokes killed 194,000 individuals in the year 1975.
4. In 1978 there were 643,000 people who died of "heart attacks."
5. There are an estimated 4,120,000 individuals with histories of heart attacks or angina symptoms.
6. With relation to age, the percentages of deaths from heart attack are: ages 25 to 34, 11%; ages 35 to 44, 27%. As age increases, the percentage continues to rise, but there is no other range change in which any figure near such a 16% jump occurs (2).

A comparison of male and female incidences revealed the following:

1. Atherosclerosis begins earlier in males than in females.
2. The incidence of cardiovascular disease increases in males until it reaches a maximum during the seventh decade of life.
3. Decade by decade the incidences are greater for males through the seventh decade of life.
4. After the seventh decade the female incidences increase.
5. The female incidence peaks in the eighth decade and then declines in the ninth (18).

In 1978 more than 1 million people died from cardiovascular disease. The most prevalent cardiovascular disease is atherosclerosis (24).

Figure 8.2 Heart disease is our leading killer.

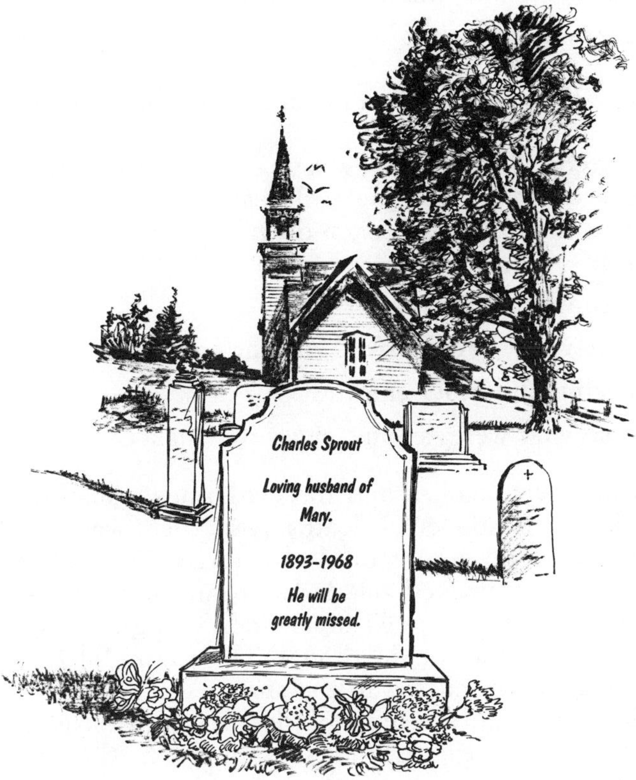
Charles Sprout
Loving husband of
Mary.
1893-1968
He will be
greatly missed.

Elements of Risk Below are listed the elements of twentieth-century living that have been identified or assumed to be causative factors in the degenerative processes leading to cardiovascular disease:

- Cigarette smoking
- Hypertension
- High levels of cholesterol or other fatty substances in the blood
- Stress and tension
- Heredity
- Diabetes

Lack of exercise

High intakes of animal fat (diet)

Obesity (17)

These are affected by factors including age, sex, and geographical location.

Cigarette Smoking. The Lung Association made a study comparing cigarette smoking and deaths (per thousands each year). The variable was broken down into the following four categories:

Those who never smoked

Those who never smoked regularly

Smoking and other causes

Those who were regular cigarette smokers

Those who never smoked and those who never smoked regularly had the lowest incidence of deaths. Also, there was no difference between these two groups until about ages 55 to 59 at which those who never smoked regularly began to show a slightly higher death rate. At age 65 to 69 these two groups again were found to be equal in the death rate. The reason for this return to equality was not discussed in the study.

The next highest cause of death was associated with smoking and other causes (not identified). In the 65 to 69 age range the death rate for individuals in this group consistently ran higher than the death rate for those who never smoked and for those who never smoked regularly. Those who smoked regularly had the highest death rate for all the age groups studied. The increase over the third category was approximately two to five more deaths per thousand (18).

An individual who doesn't smoke has a higher risk of having a heart attack than of having a stroke but is below the average risk of having either. An individual who smokes one pack or less of cigarettes per day has an above average risk of having a heart attack or a stroke. The risk of stroke for this person now also exceeds the risk of heart attack, which is just the opposite for the nonsmoker. When a person smokes more than one pack a day, the risk of heart attack is almost twice that for the nonsmoker and the risk of stroke is five times greater (2).

The following are the consequences of smoking.

1. There is a 70% increase in heart attacks.
2. Coronary artery disease is accelerated.
3. Emphysema is aggravated and it further compromises the heart.
4. The heart rate increases.
5. The blood pressure increases.
6. The peripheral vasculature constricts and if the cardiac output is reduced, the extremities are further compromised.
7. Stopping may, after some years, allow a return to the group in the low-risk category.
8. Risk increases with the number of cigarettes smoked.
9. Physical fitness and endurance are impaired.
10. Smoking cigars or a pipe does not exclude an individual from the risk group (4).

There is evidence that there is an allergic reaction to tobacco. For example, an individual suffering from hypertension (a nonsmoker) goes for a ride in an auto with a friend who smokes. At the beginning of the trip the individual's diastolic pressure measures 74 millimeters of mercury, which is lower than normal. An hour later, at the end of the trip during which the friend smokes, the individual now has a diastolic pressure of 96 millimeters of mercury. At the end of 4 hours, the individual's pressure is just over 100 millimeters of mercury diastolic (30).

Carbon monoxide poisoning is linked to increased permeability of the vascular walls. In turn, these may facilitate precipitation of penetrated lipoproteins and the accumulation of lipids. Epidemiological data indicate that smokers who have a carboxyhemoglobin (a compound formed when hemoglobin is exposed to carbon monoxide in the blood) content of 5% or more have an incidence of atherosclerotic coronary disease 21 times higher than nonsmokers do. Less than usual exercise after smoking may lead to angina because the nicotine increases the demand for myocardial oxygen and there is decreased myocardial oxygen delivery because of the carboxyhemoglobin (10).

Hypertension. The second of the three elements of risk that lead all others in their relationship to cardiovascular disease is hypertension (29). The American Heart Association refers to hypertension as an unstable or persistent elevation of pressure above the normal range. Along with the organs affected, such as the brain and eyes, is the heart. Hypertension is classified as either essential or secondary. *Essential hypertension* is the result of increased peripheral resistance caused by degenerative constriction of the arterioles. This produces visual problems in later life. From 80% to 90% of all cases of hypertension are in this category. The remaining cases are classified as being secondary hypertensive, which is the result of renal vascular stenosis or occlusion (visual acuity problems).

There are many statistics available that indicate that an adverse diastolic blood pressure level is related to causing pathological changes in humans. There is also controversy over systolic levels being a factor. When the systolic level exceeds 130, an individual is considered to be above the average risk point for having a heart attack or other cardiovascular degenerative problems (2).

With increasing age, the blood pressure seems to rise as a result of not only degenerative processes but also tension, smoking, lack of exercise, obesity, kidney disease, and arterio-sclerosis. The diastolic pressure changes from typical values of from 60 to 70 during the teen years to from 80 to 90 at age 65. Systolic pressures of 110 during the teens rise to from 140 to 150 or more at age 65. Interestingly, the pressures of females rise higher than the pressures of males after age 35. The most marked increase is that of the female systolic pressure (42).

Hypertension, and usually the diastolic pressure level, is believed to be a factor in heart attack. The increased work load places a high (over 90) diastolic pressure on the left ventrical. This elevated pressure is the resistance the heart must pump against, which in turn can cause fatigue in the heart muscle.

High blood pressure is attributed to the narrowing of blood vessels or their "hardening." These vessel changes are caused by the several factors described in the atherosclerotic degenerative process. If the heart has to pump against an elevated pressure, other hemodynamic factors which accelerate the atherosclerotic process (e.g., turbulence), must be considered.

The Health Insurance Institute has noted that the salt intake in the United States is too high. This excessive intake is thought to contribute to hypertension (6). Other sources say that if people eliminate additional salt intake, they may not have to take medications all their lives to combat the resulting hypertension. Hypertension is related to the weight problem caused by the salt intake (8). Obesity may aggravate preexisting hypertension or it may possibly hasten the development of the problem in individuals who are genetically predisposed to hypertension (36).

Hypertension is now seen as one cause of cardiovascular diseases. Primarily, it causes the blood to move through vessels at higher than normal pressures to maintain a higher resting pressure. There appears to be a relationship between a hypertensive state and the development of atherosclerosis during the aging process. Both increase at an accelerated rate.

Cholesterol. Cholesterol is one of the main serum lipids. Premature arteriosclerotic vascular disease has been noted to be a major clinical manifestation of increased cholesterol buildup. In addition, studies have indicated that elevated levels of cholesterol are associated with increased risks in the development of coronary heart disease (21).

A number of foods contain high amounts of cholesterol, for example, eggs, liver, shrimp, and other shellfish. These foods cause the blood level of cholesterol to increase above the usually accepted normal levels produced by the body of from 200 to 250 milligrams per 100 milliliters (21).

Recent studies have indicated that lipoproteins are available in two forms: high-density lipoproteins (HDL) and low-density lipoproteins (LDL). The LDLs are responsible for causing deposits of cholesterol onto and within the arterial walls. The HDLs prevent the LDLs from causing this deposition. It is recommended that the intake of foods containing LDLs be reduced and that the intake of foods containing HDL's be increased.

Cholesterol is always found in plaque. How it gets there is the subject of intensive research. It may be an attendant substance carried along into the plaque formation and other factors may really be the responsible agents for the development of atherosclerotic lesions. In individuals who suffer from hypothyroidism the cholesterol and fat-related atherosclerotic evidence have been found to display a consistent correlation. It has also been found that medically removing the hypothyroid condition has almost removed the accelerated atherosclerotic process from both test humans and animals. Four hundred ninety patients over 60 years of age were put on a regimen designed to alleviate hypothyroidism. At the completion of a 20-year effort none of these individuals experienced any heart damage symptoms. Additionally, 172 patients under 60 years of age with either hypertension and/or high serum cholesterol levels also experienced no heart failures while treated for hypothyroidism. Over the past 25 years the patients kept on thyroid therapy programs have rarely had heart attacks (33). Could it be that more studies should be made on the causes of the degenerative processes of the cardiovascular system? Obviously, the American Heart Association believes there should be because it continues to give grants for studies in this area.

Smoking and hypertension can be a deadly combination. But when excessive amounts of cholesterol are found in an individual who smokes excessively and who has hypertension, the risk of a heart attack occurring is more than tripled. The risk that such an individual will suffer from a stroke is seven times higher than the risk taken by one who smokes but does not have hypertension and does not have excessive amounts of cholesterol. And the risk is three and one-half times higher than the risk taken by one who does not have hypertension but does have excessive amounts of cholesterol and smokes (2).

Stress. Many individuals who would not have survived in the days before the discovery of antibiotics are now remaining alive. Within this new population one may find that many individuals are suffering from "premature" heart attacks and other cardiovascular problems. One of these causative agents producing early death is stress.

Stress, broadly speaking, is difficult to define. It should be looked upon as any condition from within an individual, or in the environment, that causes a response in the defense mechanisms of greater value than would be expected for normal existence. Because of this increased defensive action, stress has been considered an important factor in the process termed *atherogenesis*.

Stress caused, or was considered responsible for, advanced degrees of damage to the cardiovascular systems of the soldiers who fought in the Franco-German War of 1871, World War I, World War II, the Korean War, and the Vietnam War.

In Graz, Germany, a German physician during World War I found many civilians who were cardiac cripples. These individuals were functioning under great stress because of their involvement in the war's activities at home. Increases in civilian atherosclerosis were four times greater during wartime.

Stress is believed to cause the adrenal gland to secrete

large quantities of adrenalin. The hyperactivity thus produced puts increased pressure and flow conditions into a state in which the hemodynamic effects accelerate the process of atherosclerosis. It appears that if stress persists for an extended period of time, this chronic oversecretion of adrenaline, etc., is responsible for the cardiovascular degenerative diseases (34).

The National Institute for Occupational Health and Safety (NIOHS) reported the following: Twenty-two thousand workers in 130 occupations were evaluated in 1977 in reference to their jobs versus stress-related cardiovascular damage. The top 12 stress occupations are listed below:

1. Unskilled laborer
2. Secretary
3. Assembly line inspector
4. Clinical Lab Technician
5. Mid-level office manager
6. Manager-administrator
7. Foreman
8. Waitress/waiter
9. Machine operator
10. Farm owner
11. Mine worker
12. House painter

The stress ratio for nonskilled, nonmachinist laborers was far off the normal curve, making it impossible to compare this category of worker with the next category of worker. Stress, according to NIOHS, as do dairy products, produces high levels of cholesterol and triglycerides, but stress increases these cholesterol and trigylceride levels four times as much as dairy products do. In other words, diet can be managed, but death from a heart disease can still take its toll (9).

Heredity. Studies have been conducted in which mechanical stress (changes in either blood turbulence or pressure) has been implicated as a causative agent in the localization of atherosclerotic lesions. It appears that in some of these areas where lesions occur the degenerative process is the result of genetically induced differences in the anatomical makeup of arterial systems such as the coronary arteries. Changes in the structural development have occurred during the embryonic development state. The atherosclerotic lesions may have begun very early and can be traced back to embryonic development. The lesions show a uniform relationship to various ethnic groups in terms of where they specifically develop. The differences between ethnic groups in the degree and the extent of the lesions may be assumed to involve tissue differences in the arterial wall.

Combinations of autosomal chromosomes (any chromosome other than the sex chromosomes) have been identified and related to (over 1200) *Marfans syndrome*. Individuals with this syndrome are generally tall and have long legs and spidery fingers. Two degenerative conditions were discovered in these individuals. They have a predisposition to suffering from aortic rupture and they invariably have hypercholesteremia. In addition, there are multifactoral disorders resulting from the interaction of one or several predisposing genes with environmental factors. When examined thoroughly it was found that other traits were localized. In an adult population ranging from middle age to later years, there has been a predisposition to hypertension and coronary artery disease.

The risks in adults who may have inherited factors related to ischemic heart disease depend upon age, sex, diet, smoking, blood pressure, lipids, family history, and glucose tolerance. It is thought that this predisposition to atherosclerosis, possibly caused by hypertension, could be managed by controlling environmental factors (16).

Diabetes. Seventy percent of those who have diabetes die from complications resulting from vascular disease. Athero-sclerotic lesions have been found in the large arteries, the smaller arteries, and the arterioles. The primary site is the larger arteries where the lesions tend to be both diffuse and progressive. These lesions have been found in the cerebral and coronary arteries. The length of time that individuals have diabetes is related to the incidences of vascular disease. In juvenile-onset diabetics, 92% of those who have had diabetes for over 20 years display the vascular degenerative process. It is important that diabetes be controlled since it has been found that hypoglycemic episodes may precipitate vascular accidents (21).

Three types of vascular disease are found in individuals suffering from diabetes mellitus: diabetic microangiopathy, arteriolar disease, and atherosclerosis. In *diabetic microangio-*

pathy diffuse capillary basement thickening is evident. *Arteriolar disease* displays lesions in these vessels and it is frequently associated with hypertension. In *atherosclerosis* the lesions are located in the larger vessels of the arterial tree. These three types of vascular disease are classified under diabetes arteriosclerotic disease. No pathologic differences can be found between the diabetic and the nondiabetic atherosclerotic lesions. In general, the incidence of atherosclerotic lesions is higher in diabetics, and atherosclerosis develops at an earlier age in those who have diabetes.

Among women diabetics the appearance of coronary artery disease is greater than in men and the life expectancy of these women is shorter than that of nondiabetic women. Gangrene is about 50 times more prevalent in diabetic men over age 40 than it is in nondiabetic men over age 40. Gangrene is 70 times more prevalent in diabetic women over age 40 than it is in nondiabetic women.

Unexplained geographic differences have been found in the incidence rates of vascular involvement in diabetics. Diabetics in Israel, North Africa, and the Middle East have a low incidence of coronary artery disease as compared to other areas of the world.

Lack of Exercise. Lack of proper exercise may be the reason for a higher than normal resting heart rate. The higher the resting rate, the less fit (cardiovascularly) the person. This "unfit" individual has been found to have a small heart and a small stroke volume capacity. In addition, the blood volume is small, and when this individual stands up, the heart rate increases.

Among bedridden individuals the number of arteries and the interconnections between them are significantly reduced. The importance of these interconnections in relation to preventing myocardial infarction cannot be understated (35).

There is no doubt that exercise is beneficial, but the simple truth is that exercise may not prevent coronary atherosclerosis. There are people who have regularly engaged in high levels of vigorous exercise and have maintained the endurance of an athlete. These same people have extensive coronary artery disease and some have died from heart disease while exercising.

It has been suggested that before beginning an exercise program, one should try walking two miles. If chest pains develop during this test or if the individual experiences dizziness, gastrointestinal upset, breathing difficulty or flulike symptoms, the individual should consult with a physician before continuing with such an activity (38). Obviously, an individual in any of the other risk factor categories should consult with a physician before starting any exercise program.

Exercise is not a singular cure, just as it probably isn't a singular cause of cardiovascular disease. Regular, vigorous exercise is not necessarily going to prevent coronary artery disease. Similarly, coronary artery disease may not prevent exercise (29). Individuals suffering from this disease may be encouraged to exercise in order to alleviate any additional problems brought about by obesity and poor diet. Exercise might improve the psychological outlook of the person prone to coronaries. It may increase the effects of a diet used to control obesity and hyperlipemia. And, again, with proper supervision, exercise may improve the prognosis following a heart attack (35). Exercise will be discussed in greater detail in Chapter 10.

Diet. It has been shown that the amounts of calories, fats, cholesterol, and salt that are ingested are related to cardiovascular disease. These amounts are considered to be in excess of the amounts usually recommended by nutritionists. There appears to be a correlation between atherosclerosis and diet, particularly with regard to the amount of fat consumed. Excessive amounts of saturated fats and cholesterol appear to raise serum cholesterol levels. The total number of calories is also important. The people in eastern Finland obtain 22% of their calories from saturated fats. It has been documented that they had the highest 5-year incidence of coronary artery disease of any population in the world. The people in western Finland, Holland, Crete, southern Italy, and Yugoslavia and railroad workers in the United States have lower percentages of calories from fats and lower incidences of coronary artery disease. The correlation persists, but what actually aggravates atherosclerosis has not been positively identified (29).

Studies of the effect of vitamin C on cholesterol levels have shown that for some reason the inclusion of therapeutic amounts of vitamin C in the diet produced the following changes: a lowering of cholesterol levels in the young individuals studied (those under 25) and an increase in cholesterol levels in people of later decades of life. When this second change was explored, it was found that the increase in serum levels was the result of plaque being dislodged from the arterial walls. Further investigation revealed that the walls became more impervious to invasion by lipids and cholesterol. The recommended levels of vitamin C intake have been theoretically set at 55 milligrams per day. Vitamin C is one of the vitamins the body does not store. The body excretes excess amounts not used (5).

A summary of additional studies of the degenerative heart diseases in humans revealed the following:

1. In the United States men between 45 and 49 years of age whose fat calories were 40% of their total intake had the highest death rate of the nations examined.
2. In the United States for men between the ages of 55 and 59 whose fat calories were 40% of their total intake, the death rate was almost triple that of the norm (12).
3. If there is a genetic tendency to overeat and if the family environment encourages overeating, the rates of atherosclerotic problems are accelerated (16).

Obesity. Obesity directly influences the risk factors related to cardiovascular disease. These factors are *hypertension* and *hyperlipemia.* Diabetes, stress, exercise, smoking, and personality types also may be related. If a child is obese in the first year of life, it will be difficult to eliminate this fat cell development in the later years of development and in the adult stage. Most people become obese in their middle years. Fifty percent of black women have become obese by the age of 50.

Obesity increases the left ventricular work load because of the increased vascular lengths required to supply nutrition to the excess tissue mass. A higher pumping rate and pressure are suspected as accelerating the development of atherosclerosis.

Obesity is related to hyperlipemia in which low-density lipids are prone to invading the arterial walls and carrying cholesterol, another suspected risk factor, along with them. It is essential that obesity be eliminated. This requires modifying the behavior of an obese-prone individual. Poor eating habits must be exchanged for approved good eating habits because it is believed that good eating habits will result in maintaining the recommended weight reduction (29). Behavior modification and nutritional control will be discussed in Chapter 9. Statistics from various life insurance companies show that there is a far greater evidence of coronary artery disease in those individuals who are considered overweight (12).

Aging and Risks Every age group has its risks. The following paragraphs describe the risks for each of the various age groups.

Ages 1 to 4. Whole milk, butter, ice cream, desserts high in fats, egg yolks, and salt supposedly start the artherosclerosis processes. These pathological changes in the vasculature have been documented. Accidents account for the greatest number of deaths in this age group.

Ages 5 to 14. Accidents are responsible for the greatest percentage of deaths in this age group, which is odd in that this is generally considered the safest age range. It is now important to encourage all forms of exercise. The total fat load must be reduced. Strangely, the human is the only animal that continues to drink milk after being weaned. "Fat" foods should be avoided. Obesity from the 1 to 4 year range could persist and there could be an increase in atherosclerotic development.

Ages 15 to 24. The greatest percentage of deaths in this group are caused by accidents and suicides. Alcohol use and smoking increase with this age group and there is a significant increase in the development of atherosclerotic plaque. Generally, there are fewer heart attacks in this age group than there are in the 5 to 14 age group. Cardiorenal disease has increased by a factor of three. During college years students are preoccupied with matters that may later lead to cardiovascular disease (see chapter opening illustration).

Ages 25 to 34. Accidents account for the greatest number of deaths in this age group. Major cardiovascular and renal diseases show that they have increased in the total degenerative processes of the body.

Ages 35 to 44. The major cardiovascular and renal diseases claim the most victims now. In deaths per 100,000:

Rheumatic heart disease has a value of 6.0.

Atherosclerotic, degenerative, and coronary disease has a value of 55.5.

Hypertensive heart disease has a value of 5.0.

Ages 45 to 54 and Ages 55 to 64. The death rates from cardiovascular diseases show great increases. Cerebrovascular accidents trail only heart disease and cancer as causes of death.

A man at age 60, in the United States has no greater life expectancy than did a man living during the days of the Roman Empire.

Ages 65 to 74 and Ages 75 to 84. In the 65 to 74 age group 55% die of heart attacks. In the 75 to 84 age group, 67% die of heart attacks. Generally, exercise is limited to walking. People in their "golden years" should keep active, both physically and mentally. It is said that more people "rust out" than wear out (32).

The Individual and Risk How close is anyone to having a heart attack? It is thought that if conditions were to remain normal, an individual's heart would start out prepared to continue pulsing life-giving substances through the body approximately 3½ billion times (heart beats) in a lifetime. The average heart beat rate was taken to be 70 beats per minute. If the individual were to use these beats on fear, anger, stress, and overexertion or if the individual were to attempt to force the heart to send blood through a fat-overburdened body, the heart beats would be wasted. Evidence shows that the processes causing heart disease are reversible (31).

The signals of impending fatal heart attack often go unheeded. Signals are chest pains, indigestion symptoms, and pain in the left arm. In addition, there may be dizziness, difficulty in breathing, or flulike symptoms. The time lapse between the signal(s) and the attack varies. It may be only one to two hours or it may be as long as eight weeks. Americans tend to dismiss chest pains and these other symptoms even though they know they are part of the generally accepted risk factors for cardiovascular disease (39).

What causes sudden cardiac death? Because of the apparent relationship between atherosclerotic development and cardiovascular changes, it isn't surprising that sudden cardiac death should be found 70% of the time when *intraluminal reduction* is present. The incidence of *thrombosis* involvement is there. In addition, the longer the site of stenosis has existed, the higher the incidence of thrombosis (15). Atherosclerosis has the characteristics of *not* being in evidence or of developing into a possible disaster as time progresses. Thus, the general appearance of atherosclerosis is sudden stenosis, thrombosis, aneurysm, or embolus. The sign is dramatic and all too often fatal (36).

Summary

People in the United States must be doing something about the risk factors of heart disease, or at least they must be doing something right. The heart disease death rates began to decline about 30 years ago, but two-thirds of the entire reduction has occurred in the last 10 years. The death rate has reduced by from 18% to 20% for middle-aged white males. Statistically, this is a significant change. Cardiovascular problems are still the number one killer, but the rate is decreasing and no explanation is yet available. Research is just beginning to determine why there has been this improvement. People may be taking the advice to cut down on fats, to stop smoking, and to reduce high blood pressure. The United States is now doing better than any other industrial country at reducing the death rate due to cardiovascular incidents (7).

References

1. American Heart Association. *Cigarette Smoking and Cardiovascular Disease.* New York: American Heart Association, 1971.
2. American Heart Association. *Heart Facts.* New York: American Heart Association, 1977.
3. American Heart Association. *Risk Factors and Coronary Disease.* New York: American Heart Association, 1968.
4. American Heart Association. *Smoking and Heart Disease.* New York: American Heart Association, 1973.
5. Atherosclerosis Research Fund. "Vitamin C for Cleaner Arteries." A reprint from *Prevention Magazine,* Emmaus, Pa.: Rodale Press, 1977.
6. Baltimore Evening Sun. "Curtail Intake of Table Salt, Authorities Urge." *The Evening Sun,* 30 October, 1978.
7. Baltimore Evening Sun. "Heart Disease: Americans Are Doing Something Right." *The Evening Sun,* 25 October, 1978.
8. Baltimore Evening Sun. "Hypertension." *The Evening Sun,* November 6, 1978.

9. Baltimore Evening Sun. "Stress Study Results Amazing." *The Evening Sun,* 27 October, 1978.

10. Baroldi, John B., and Scomazzoni, Anthony. *Coronary Circulation in the Normal and the Pathologic Heart.* Washington, D.C.: U.S. Government Printing Office, 1967.

11. Brandfonbrener, M., Landowne, M., and Shock, N. W. "Changes in Cardiac Output with Age." *Circulation* 12 (1965):557.

12. Cooper, W., Barber, J., Mitchell, A., Runbergen, R., and Green K. *Nutrition in Health and Disease* 14th ed. Philadelphia: Lippincott, 1963.

13. Dock, W. "The Capacity of the Coronary Bed in Cardiac Hypertrophy." *Journal of Experimental Medicine* 74 (1941):177.

14. ———. "Aging of the Myocardium." *Bulletin of New York Academy of Medicine* 32 (1956):173.

15. "Early Warning Systems for Genetic Risk." *Emergency Medicine,* 10 (1978):417.

16. Eliot, H., Baroldi, Q. J., and Dzindozio, T. "What Causes Sudden Cardiac Death?" *R.N.* 2 (1976):18–20.

17. Georgia Heart Association. *Heart Attack, What Now?*, 12th ed. Atlanta, Ga.: Georgia Heart Association. 1977.

18. Guyton, A. C. *Basic Human Physiology,* 2nd ed. Philadephia: Saunders, 1977.

19. Hallock, P. "Arterial Elasticity in Man in Relation to Age as Evaluated by the Pulse Wave Velocity Method." *Archives of Internal Medicine* 54 (1934):770.

20. Harris, R. "Clinical Use of Reserpine (Serpasil) in Geriatrics." *Annals of the New York Academy of Science,* 59 (1954):95.

21. Harvey, C., Johns, H., Owens, T., and Ross, T. *The Principles and Practices of Medicine,* 18th ed. New York: Appleton-Century-Crofts, 1972.

22. Haynes, F. W., Ellis, L. B., and Weiss, S. "Pulse Wave Velocity and Arterial Elasticity in Arterial Hypertension, Arteriosclerosis, and Related Conditions." *American Heart Journal* 11 (1936):385.

23. Howell, T. H. *Geriatrics.* Springfield, Ill.: Charles C Thomas, 1970.

24. Johnson, G. T., "Health." *Chicago Tribune,* 23 July, 1978.

25. Landowne, M., Brandfonbrener, M., and Shock, N. W. "Relation of Age to Certain Measures of the Performance of the Heart and Circulation." *Circulation* 12 (1974):567.

26. Master, A. M., Garfield, C. I., and Walters, M. B. "Normal Blood Pressure and Hypertension." In *New Definitions.* Philadelphia: Lea & Febiger, 1952.

27. Master, A. M., and Lasser, R. P. "Relationship of the Blood Pressure to Weight, Height and Body Build in Apparently Healthy Subjects 65 to 106 Years of Age." *American Journal of Medical Science* 235 (1958):278.

28. Master, A. M., Lasser, R. P., and Jaffe, H. L. "Blood Pressure In Apparently Healthy Aged 65 to 106 Years." *Procedures in Social and Experimental Biological Medicine* 94 (1957): 463.

29. McIntosh, I., Stamler, C., and Jackson, C. *Introduction to Risk Factors in Coronary Artery Disease. Heart and Lung Journal* 7 (1978).

30. Medical Electronics and Data. *The Heart Watcher,* No. 13. Columbus, Ohio: United Color Press, 1975.

31. ———. *How Close Are You to a Heart Attack?* Columbus, Ohio: United Color Press, 1974.

32. ———. *The Heart Watcher,* Nos. 14, 15, 17. Columbus, Ohio: United Color Press, 1975, 1976.

33. ———. *The Heart Watcher,* No. 22. Columbus, Ohio: United Color Press, 1977.

34. ———. *The Heart Watcher,* No. 23. Columbus, Ohio: United Color Press, 1977.

35. ———. *The Heart Watcher,* No. 25. Columbus, Ohio: United Color Press, 1977.

36. *Merck Manual,* 13th ed. Rahway, N.J.: Merck and Company, 1977.

37. Metropolitan Life Insurance Company. *Statistical Bulletin,* Vol. LII. New York: Metropolitan Life, 1971.

38. Mitchell, J. H. "Exercise Training in the Treatment of

Coronary Heart Disease." *Advances in Internal Medicine,* Vol. 20, edited by G. H. Stollerman. Chicago: Yearbook Medical Publishers, 1975.

39. Shock, N. W. "Age Changes in Some Physiologic Processes." *Geriatrics* 12 (1957):40.

40. Smith, and Gips, *Care of the Adult Patient,* 2nd ed. Philadelphia: Lippincott, 1966.

41. Timiras, P. S. *Developmental Physiology and Aging.* New York: Macmillan, 1972.

42. "Unheeded Signals of Fatal Coronary Heart Disease." *R.N.* (Aug., 1973):147

43. Walton, K. W. "Atherosclerosis and Aging." In *Textbook of Geriatric Medicine and Gerontology,* edited by J. C. Brocklehurst, pp. 75–112. Edinburgh: Churchill/Livingstone, 1973.

44. Wezler, K. "Arterienelastizitat." *Zeitschrift fur Kreislaufforschung* 27 (1965): 721.

45. Wiggers, C. J. *Physiology in Health and Disease,* 5th ed. Philadelphia: Lea & Febiger, 1959.

46. "The World Health Situation." In *World Health Chronicle.* Geneva: World Health Organization, 1967.

47. Wurtman, R. "A New Look at Stroke." *Men and Molecules,* 701 (1974):87.

PART FIVE

Habits of Enhancement

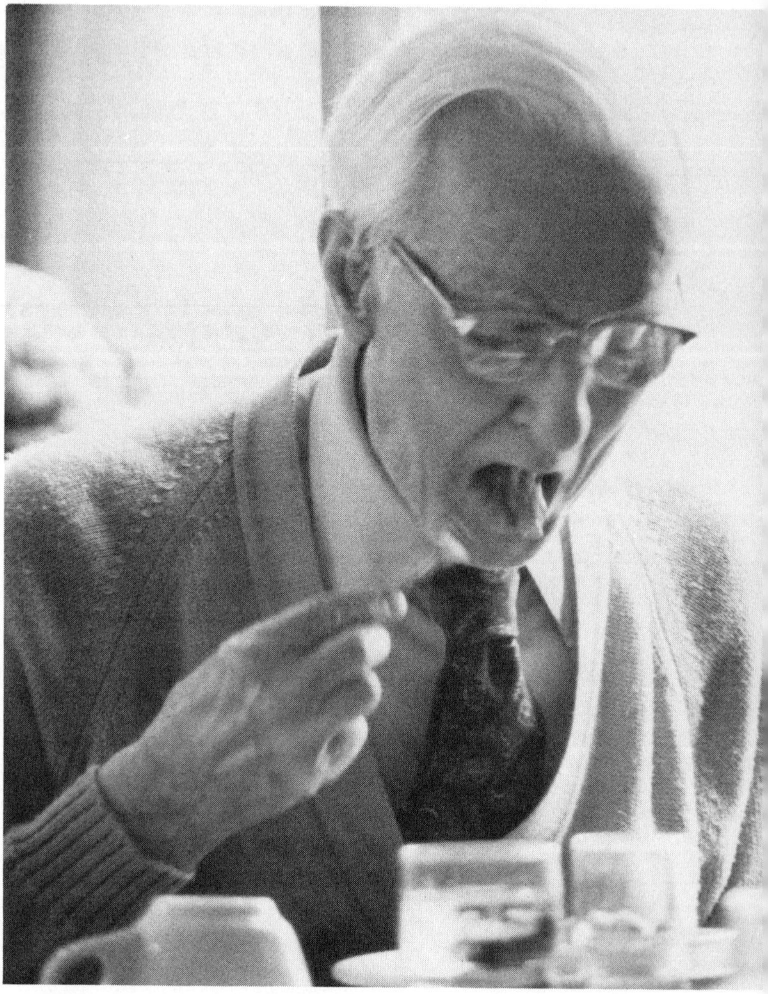

■ **Chapter 9**

Nutritional Practices and Aging

Major Concepts

1. Nutrient requirements for all age groups vary slightly.
2. Physical change, disease and disorders, lack of finances, and reduced mobility influence nutritional status.
3. Psychosocial variables influence nutritional status.

The Role of Nutrients

The nutrients in food provide energy, maintain body functions, and help the body grow and repair itself. These nutrients include protein, fats, carbohydrates, vitamins, and minerals. Water, although not considered a nutrient, is a necessary part of the diet. It enables nutrients to be transported throughout the body, aids in cooling the body, and is important in the elimination of wastes. Nutritional needs remain fairly constant throughout life. The one exception is caloric requirement. As people age, they are usually less active and the body's metabolism gradually declines; therefore, there is less need for calories. The other nutrients (protein, fat, carbohydrates, vitamins and minerals) have the same physiological function and basically the same intake requirement in all people regardless of age. A deficiency in any of the nutrients at any age is harmful to health.

Protein Approximately 15% of the dietary intake should be calories from protein. According to experts, it is recommended that children up to age 10 eat about 45 grams of protein per day, boys and girls between the ages of 10 and 18 from 45 to 60 grams, adult men from 60 to 65 grams and adult women 55 grams per day. These recommendations vary as people are physically active or sick. Young recommends that the older adult have an intake of 1 gram protein per kilogram per day (31).

Proteins are highly complex substances found in all living organisms and are made up of chains of amino acids. There are around 100 amino acids. Eight are called essential amino acids because they cannot be biochemically synthesized in the body and must be obtained through dietary intake. The best sources of the essential amino acids are animal products. Protein is also obtained from plants.

Protein has three basic functions in the diet: (1) It aids tissue growth and maintenance, (2) it aids in the production of enzymes, antibodies, and hormones, and (3) it provides energy. Although protein can be used as a source of energy it is less efficient than fats or carbohydrates. When energy reserves are low, the body can convert stored protein into glucose and utilize it for energy.

Fats Fats provide the most concentrated form of energy and tend to burn up slowly, thus producing a more lasting source of energy. One gram of fat is equivalent to 9 calories.

Approximately 30% of the caloric intake should be comprised of fats.

A fat molecule is made up of atoms of hydrogen, carbon, and oxygen. The atoms are bonded, or chemically attached, to each other. The number and type of molecule and the manner in which the molecules are bonded determine the type of fat molecule. Two types of fats are consumed in the diet: saturated fats and unsaturated fats.

Saturated fats. A fat molecule is considered saturated when the central chain of carbon atoms is double-bonded, or chemically attached, to two hydrogen atoms. Sources of saturated fats are animals, especially beef, and some vegetable plants.

Unsaturated fats. When some of the hydrogen atoms are missing in a fat molecule, the fats are called unsaturated fats. There are two types of unsaturated fats: mono-unsaturated and polyunsaturated. A mono-unsaturated fat, also called oleic acid, has one unsaturated double bond in the molecular structure. Sources of mono-unsaturated fats are plants, poultry, and fish. A polyunsaturated fat, also called linoleic acid, has two or more unsaturated double bonds. Polyunsaturated fats are also known as the essential fatty acids because they are needed for normal cell function. Sources of polyunsaturated fats are plants.

Fats have several functions in the body: They are sources of energy and they transport and assist in the body's utilization of fat-soluble vitamins (A, D, E, and K). Accumulated fats provide insulation for the body and protect vital organs.

Cholesterol is an organic compound belonging to the steroid family. Cholesterol occurs either free or as esters of fatty acids in almost all animal tissue. It is important for the production of bile acids, steroid hormone, and provitamin D_3. The body, especially the liver, produces cholesterol and additional supplies are obtained through the diet. There seems to be a relationship between cholesterol levels of 400 milligrams a day, serum cholesterol, and health. The average American diet exceeds 600 milligrams of cholesterol a day.

Polyunsaturated fats lower serum cholesterol, mono-unsaturated fats have little or no effect on serum cholesterol, and saturated fats tend to elevate serum cholesterol. There is a great deal of controversy in the scientific community over the exact role of these dietary factors and heart disease.

Since 1900 the proportion of saturated fats in the diet have decreased from about 40% of total fats to 38% in 1975. However, the overall quantity of saturated fat has steadily increased. In

1900 each person consumed about 50 grams of saturated fat compared to about 58 grams in 1975. According to unpublished data from the Consumer and Food Economics Institute, 72% of the saturated fats are from animal sources and 28% are from vegetable sources. At the same time, the increased use of salad and cooking oils has caused mono-unsaturated and polyunsaturated fats consumption to grow even more rapidly.

The breakdown on fats consumption for 1976 was as follows:

16% calories from saturated fats

7% calories from mono-unsaturated fats

19% calories from polyunsaturated fats

The United States Senate Select Committee on Nutrition and Human Needs recommended in its 1977 report that less than 10% of the total caloric intake be saturated fats, up to 10% be polyunsaturated fats, and 10% be mono-unsaturated fats (27, pp. 39–40).

Carbohydrates About 55% of the caloric intake should be carbohydrates. This nutrient, in the form of sugars (simple carbohydrates) and starches (complex carbohydrates), is converted by the body into glucose and is rapidly oxidized into energy, heat, water, and carbon dioxide. Unlike fats which provide long-lasting energy, carbohydrates provide the body with quick energy. Other functions of carbohydrates include: (1) regulating fats used for fuel, (2) preventing protein from being used for energy, and (3) maintaining interrelationships with vitamins, particularly the B vitamins. One gram of carbohydrate is equivalent to 4 calories.

Sources of carbohydrates include breads, cereals, noodles, macaroni, spaghetti, fruits, vegetables, milk products, and prepared foods and beverages containing refined sugars.

In the early 1900s, 68% of the carbohydrates intake in the United States was from starch foods and 32% was from sugars. By 1976, 47% of the carbohydrate intake was from starch and 53% was from sugars. In a 30-year period changes have been seen in pounds per capita per year of foods containing complex carbohydrates and "naturally occurring" sugars. In this same 30-year period the consumption of vegetables other than dark green or yellow vegetables decreased 12 pounds per capita per year; flour and cereal products decreased 31 pounds; fruits (other than citrus) decreased 30 pounds; potatoes decreased 21 pounds; citrus fruits (including frozen orange juice) increased 10.5 pounds; and dark green and dark yellow vegetables decreased .3 pound. The consumption of grain products varies by geographical location. For example, the northern states, which include the North, Northeast, and the West, consume greater quantities of bread, breakfast cereals, macaroni, and noodles, while the southern states consume greater quantities of bakery products (other than bread) flour mixes, cornmeal, grits, and rice (27, pp. 12–13, 21).

In recent years the consumption of sugars in the United States has increased from 18% of total caloric intake to about 24%. The largest percentage of sugars, 14%, comes from refined sugars (cane and sugar beets) while processed sugars (corn sugar, syrups, molasses, and honey) account for 4%. The remaining 6% of total calories consumed as sugar are derived from fruits, vegetables, and milk products. In 1971 it was reported that each person was consuming over 70 pounds of refined sugar per year in food products and beverages and only purchasing about 25 pounds per year for household use. The soft drink industry, which uses huge quantities of sugar, reported that the sales of soft drinks more than doubled in a 15-year period. Individuals who consumed cola beverages increased their intake from 13.6 gallons a year in 1960 to 27.6 gallons in 1975. In other words, each person who consumed colas drank 221 sixteen-ounce cans of cola and took in 21.5 pounds of refined and processed sugar a year (27, pp. 30, 33).

Vitamins Vitamins are substances the body needs in order to function, but they are required in very small quantities. Vitamins provide no energy. Water-soluble vitamins are transported and dissolved in water and include the B vitamins, niacin, pantothenic acid, folic acid, and vitamin C. The general physiological roles of these vitamins are many, and as a group they are responsible for stimulating the functioning and/or maintenance of the following body systems or processes: digestion and appetite, metabolic processes, functioning of the central nervous system, lactation following childbirth, functioning of the endrocrine system including the thyroid, adrenal, and anterior pituitary glands, blood cell regeneration,

Table 9.1 Water-Soluble Vitamins

Vitamin	RDA [1]	Result of Deficiency	Food Source
B_1 (thiamine)	1.0–1.4 mg	Beriberi, loss of appetite, indigestion, fatigue, neuritis, irritability	Pork, beef, liver, legumes, whole grains
B_2 (riboflavin)	1.5–1.7 mg	Dermatitis, eye irritation	Milk, liver, enriched cereals
B_6 (pyridoxine)	2.0 mg	Anemia	Wheat, corn, meat, liver
B_{12} (cobalamin)	3.0 mg	Extrinsic factor in pernicious anemia	Liver, milk, eggs, cheese, meat
Niacin	13–18 mg	Pellagra, neuritis, dermatitis, lassitude, weakness	Meat, peanuts, enriched grains
Pantothenic acid	— [2]	Decreased breakdown of glucose to energy	Liver, eggs, skimmed milk
Folic acid	400 mg	Megaloblastic anemia	Liver, green leafy vegetables, asparagus
Biotin	— [2]	Decreased breakdown of glucose to energy	Egg yolk, liver
Ascorbic acid	55–60 mg	Weakened capillary walls	Citrus fruits, tomatoes, cabbage, potatoes, strawberries, broccoli, Brussels sprouts

[1] U.S. Recommended Daily Allowance for females ages 18 to 35 (first number) and males ages 18 to 35 (second number).
[2] No current recommendation for dietary intake.

and functioning of the integumentary and muscular systems. Table 9.1 lists the water-soluble vitamins, their recommended daily allowance for the 18 to 35-year-old male and female, the results of deficiency, and food sources.

The fat-soluble vitamins (A, D, E, and K) are transported and dissolved in fats. These vitamins influence the following body systems or functions: integumentary system, digestive system, calcium equilibrium, mineral metabolism, blood platelets formation, and blood clotting. Table 9.2 lists the fat-soluble vitamins, their recommended daily allowance for the 18 to 35-year-old male and female, the results of deficiency, and food sources.

When a person consumes more vitamins than the body requircs, small amounts are stored in the body and excesses are excreted in the urine or feces. Excesses of vitamin C are not stored in the body; therefore the daily intake of food high in

Table 9.2 Fat-Soluble Vitamins

Vitamin	RDA [1]	Result of Deficiency	Food Source
A	5000 IU	Reduced ability to adapt from bright light to darkness, decreased appetite, physical weakness, retardation of growth and development	Liver, kidney, cream, butter, egg yolk, yellow and green vegetables, fortified foods
D	400 IU	Reduced ability of body to utilize calcium	Sunlight, yeast, fish oil, fortified foods
E	12–15 IU	Less integrity in red blood cell, anemia	Vegetable oil, milk, eggs, muscle meats, fish, cereal, green leafy vegetables
K	— [2]	Reduced blood clotting ability	Green leafy vegetables, cheese, egg yolk, liver

[1] U.S. Recommended Daily Allowance for females ages 18 to 35 (first number) and males ages 18 to 35 (second number).

[2] No current recommendation for dietary intake.

vitamin C is necessary. Large quantities of most vitamins do not have a toxic effect on the body, but there are some exceptions. An intake of 100 milligrams of niacin can produce dilation of blood vessels and in larger amounts can impair liver function. Excessive quantities of vitamin K have no toxic effect on the body, but they may have an effect on the therapeutic use of anticoagulant drugs.

Table 9.3 Major Minerals

Mineral	RDA [1]	Result of Deficiency	Food Source
Calcium	800–1200 mg	Affects bone and tooth formation, normal clotting of blood, muscle contraction, and relaxation; rickets	Milk, cheese, egg yolk, nuts, whole grains, green leafy vegetables
Chlorine	— [2]	Affects fluid balance maintenance and proper stomach acidity	Abundant in most foods
Magnesium	300–400 mg	Affects protein metabolism, growth, and maintenance processes	Abundant in most foods
Phosphorus	800–1200 mg	Affects acid-base balance in body	Same as calcium
Potassium	— [2]	Affects cellular fluid balance, muscle excitability, metabolism of carbohydrate and protein	Abundant in many foods
Sodium	— [2]	Affects normal fluid balance between inside of cell and its surroundings; affects cell permeability and muscle excitability	Table salt, some foods
Sulphur	— [2]	Affects energy metabolism	Abundant in many foods

[1] U.S. Recommended Daily Allowance for females ages 18 to 35 (first number) and males ages 18 to 35 (second number).
[2] No current recommendation for dietary intake.

Minerals Minerals are divided into two categories: major minerals and trace minerals. The daily dietary need for the major minerals is greater than for the trace minerals. Tables 9.3 and 9.4 list the major and trace minerals, the recommended daily allowance for the 18 to 35-year-old male and female, the results of deficiency, and food sources.

It is fairly easy to obtain the recommended daily allowance if one eats a balanced diet every day. This diet includes the following:

> Milk Foods: Three or more glasses of milk for children, 4 or more glasses for teen-agers, and 2 or more glasses for adults. Servings of ice cream, cheese, cottage cheese, pudding, and creamed soups can be substituted for a glass of milk.

Table 9.4 Trace Minerals

Mineral	RDA [1]	Result of Deficiency	Food Source
Copper	— [2]	Affects iron utilization, bone formation, and brain tissue maintenance	Liver, meat, seafood, nuts, whole grains
Fluorine	1 PPM [3]	Affects teeth and bones	Water
Iodine	100–150 mg	Development of a goiter	Seafood, iodized salt
Iron	18 mg	Affects hemoglobin formation	Liver, meat, egg yolk, whole grains. enriched bread, nuts, green vegetables
Manganese	300–400 mg	Affects protein metabolism, synthesis of fatty acids, and blood sugar oxidation	Cereal, tea, nuts, soybeans
Zinc	15 mg	Liver disease	Liver, seafood

[1] U.S. Recommended Daily Allowance for females ages 18 to 35 (first number) and males ages 18 to 35 (second number).
[2] No current recommendation for dietary intake.
[3] One part per million per gallon of water.

Table 9.5 Nutrients in a Balanced Diet

Food RDA	Calories 2000	Protein 55 g	Fat 66 g	Carbohydrate 275 g
1/2 c. orange juice	60	.5	T	13
1 c. bran flakes	145	4.0	1	40
1 c. 2% milk	145	10.0	5	15
1 slice white enriched toast	70	2.0	1	13
1 t. sugar	13	0	0	4
1 pat butter	35	T [1]	4	T
Coffee, black	0	0	0	0
	468	16.5	11	85
1 c. yogurt	125	8.0	4	13
2 slices white enriched bread	140	4.0	2	26
1 1/4″ thick slice bologna	80	3.0	7	T
1 T. mayonnaise	100	T	11	T
1 8-oz. glass of 2% milk	145	10.0	5	15
1 med. apple	70	T	T	18
	660	25.0	29	72
1/2 chicken breast, fried, 3.3 oz. with bone	155	25.0	5	1
Med. baked potato	90	3.0	T	21
1 T. butter	100	T	12	T
1 c. broccoli stalks cut in 1/2″ pieces	40	5.0	1	7
1 8-oz. glass of 2% milk	145	10.0	5	15
1/2 c. jello	70	2.0	0	17
	600	45.0	23	61
Total	1728	86.5 g	63 g	218 g
Percentage of U.S. Recommended Daily Allowance	86%	157%	95%	79%

[1] T = trace.

Meat Foods: Two or more 4-oz. servings of meats, fish, poultry, eggs, or cheese. Servings of dried beans, peas, and nuts can be substituted for one serving of meat.

Vegetables and Fruits: Four or more servings, including one serving each of dark green or yellow vegetables and citrus fruits.

Food RDA	Calcium .8 g	Iron 18 mg	Vitamin A 5000 IU	Thiamine 1.0 mg	Riboflavin 1.5 mg	Niacin 13 mg	Vitamin C 55 mg
Orange juice	10	.1	135	.08	.01	.4	60
Bran flakes	28	13.5	—	.16	.07	2.7	0
Milk	352	.1	200	.10	.52	.2	2
Sugar	—[1]	.0	0	0	0	0	0
Toast	21	.6	—	.06	.05	.6	—
Butter	2	0	170	0	0	0	0
Coffee	0	0	0	0	0	0	0
	413	14.3	505	.40	.65	3.9	62
Yogurt	294	.1	170	.10	.44	.2	2
Bread	42	1.2	—	.12	.10	1.2	—
Bologna	2	.5	—	.04	.06	.7	0
Mayonnaise	3	.1	40	—	.01	—	0
Milk	352	.1	200	.10	.52	.2	2
Apple	8	.4	50	.04	.02	.1	3
	701	2.4	460	.40	1.15	2.4	7
Chicken	9	1.3	70	.04	.17	11.2	0
Potato	9	.7	—	.10	.04	1.7	20
Butter	3	0	470	0	0	0	0
Broccoli	136	1.2	3880	.14	.31	1.2	40
Milk	352	.1	200	.10	.52	.2	2
Jello	0	0	0	0	0	0	0
	509	3.3	4620	.38	1.04	14.3	162
Total	1623 g	20.0 mg	5585 IU	1.18 mg	2.84 mg	20.6 mg	231 mg
Percentage of U.S. Recommended Daily Allowance	203%	111%	112%	118%	189%	158%	420%

[1] No current recommendation for dietary intake.

Breads and Cereals: Four or more servings of enriched or whole grain products such as bread, macaroni, rice, muffins, cereal.

Tables 9.5 and 9.6 list a daily consumption of foods for two days. These tables compare positive and negative food consumption. It is clear from these tables that a person can

Table 9.6 Nutrients in an Unbalanced Diet

Food RDA	Calories 2000	Protein 55 g	Fat 66 g	Carbohydrate 275 g
1/2 c. orange juice	60	.5	T[1]	13
1 slice white enriched toast	70	2.0	1.0	13
1 t. margarine	33	T	4.0	T
1 t. peanut butter	31	1.3	2.6	1
	194	3.8	7.6	27
3 oz. ground beef patty	245	21.0	17.0	0
1 bun	120	3.0	2.0	21
12 oz. cola	170	0	0	45
1 T. catsup	15	T	T	4
20 potato chips	230	2.0	16.0	20
	780	26.0	35.0	90
1/2 of a 14″-cheese pizza	740	28.0	24.0	108
2 12-oz. beers	300	2.0	0	28
	1040	30.0	24.0	136
1 oz. chocolate covered peanuts	160	5.0	12.0	11
1 cake donut	125	1.0	6.0	16
4 chocolate chip cookies	200	4.0	12.0	24
	485	10.0	30.0	51
Total	2499	69.8 g	96.6 g	304 g
Percentage of U.S. Recommended Daily Allowance	125%	127%	146%	111%

[1] T = trace.

obtain all of the recommended quantities of nutrients while staying within a caloric boundary. Positive eating habits should be established early in life and continued into and throughout later life.

Table 9.5 illustrates a nutritionally sound diet. All quantities of nutrients exceed the recommended allowances except for calories, fats, and carbohydrates. If the body requires more energy than is provided by the caloric intake, the extra 57% of the protein could be used.

Table 9.6 illustrates a nutritionally unsound diet. It shows that none of the food groups provides the recommended daily

Food RDA	Calcium .8 g	Iron 18 mg	Vitamin A 5000 IU	Thiamine 1.0 mg	Riboflavin 1.5 mg	Niacin 13 mg	Vitamin C 55 mg
Orange juice	10	.1	135	.08	.01	.4	60
Bread	21	.6	T[1]	.06	.05	.6	T
Margarine	1	0	156	0	0	0	0
Peanut butter	3	.1	0	T	T	.8	0
	35	.8	291	.14	.06	1.8	60
Beef	9	2.7	30	.07	.18	4.6	0
Bun	30	.8	T	.11	.07	.9	T
Cola	0	0	0	0	0	0	0
Catsup	3	.1	210	.01	.01	.2	2
Potato chips	16	.8	T	.08	.02	2.0	6
	58	4.4	240	.27	.28	7.7	8
Pizza	428	2.8	1160	1.60	.48	2.8	16
Beer	36	T	0	.02	.22	4.8	0
	464	2.8	1160	1.62	.70	7.6	16
Candy	33	.4	T	.10	.05	2.1	T
Donut	13	.4	30	.05	.05	.4	T
Cookies	16	.8	40	.04	.04	.4	T
	62	1.6	70	.19	.14	2.9	T
Total	619 g	9.6 mg	1761 IU	2.22 mg	1.18 mg	20.0 mg	84 mg
Percentage of U.S. Recommended Daily Allowance	77%	53%	35%	222%	79%	154%	153%

[1] T = trace.

allowances of vitamins and minerals. Even though there is only one meat serving in this diet, additional protein is obtained from the cheese on the pizza and the peanuts in the candy. Protein is fairly easy to obtain. Only 77% of the needed calcium is provided because there is a lack of foods from the dairy group. The greatest amount of calcium comes from the cheese on the pizza. The diet provides a little over one-half of the necessary iron. The addition of meat, milk, and vegetables would bring it up to the 18-milligram requirement. Vitamin A is the lowest nutrient, with only 35% of the recommended amount being consumed. Dark green or deep yellow fruits and vegetables would help to increase vitamin A intake. Additional meat and dairy products would bring the riboflavin closer to the 1.5-milligram requirement. This diet also shows an excess in niacin, vitamin C, calories, fats, and carbohydrates. The quantities of niacin and vitamin C pose no health problem because the extra nutrients are discarded by the body. The potential problem lies with the extra fats, carbohydrates, and calories. The extra 499 calories for the day's eating pattern, should it continue, could result in an extra caloric intake of 3493 calories a week, 13,972 calories a month (a 28-day month), and 167,644 calories a year. One pound of fat is the equivalent to 3500 calories. If this individual were to consume the additional 167,644 calories in one year and do nothing to expend this extra energy, the calories would be stored in the body in the form of 48 pounds of fat per year.

Nutritional Status of Americans

Overnutrition rather than undernutrition appears to be a problem with younger age groups. Higher levels of income, greater mobility, and fast-paced lifestyles allow and sometimes encourage younger age groups to purchase commercially prepared and prepackaged foods that have been supplemented with additional nutrients. As pointed out in Chapter 1, surveys show an increase in protein, fat, iron, magnesium, thiamine, riboflavin, niacin, vitamin B_6, and ascorbic acid. Caloric intake has also increased (30, p. 118).

The literature reveals that the diet of many older adults is low in calories or low in one or more of the following nutrients: protein, iron, calcium, magnesium, ascorbic acid, folic acid, riboflavin, and vitamins A and D (7, 22).

Physical and Psychosocial Components of Nutrition

It has been said that we are what we eat. This implies that good nutritional practices create healthy individuals. To a certain extent there is truth in this statement. However, what we eat, how the body utilizes food, the general level of physical and mental health, the availability of money for food, and many other factors influence nutritional practices.

Physical Components of Nutrition Before the body can use the nutrients in foods, digestion must take place. The digestive process begins in the mouth where food is chewed and mixed with saliva. Regardless of age, decayed teeth, missing teeth, poorly fitted dentures, or canker sores can interfere with eating. When oral health is in poor condition, eating foods such as raw fruits and vegetables and some meats is difficult. Some people avoid foods that require much chewing, and thus they eliminate roughage from their diet.

The Esophagus. Once food has been chewed, it is swallowed and travels through the esophagus, which is the tube that connects the mouth and the stomach. The esophagus is about 10 inches in length and contains four specialized layers of tissues. The channel of the esophagus is opened and closed by two strategically placed circular muscles called sphincters, which act like drawstrings. The sphincters normally remain closed except during swallowing.

As age increases, a number of problems can interfere with the consumption of food. Esophageal pain, for example, can be caused by gastric reflux, inflammation of the esophagus, and/or diffused muscular spasms of the sphincters. Sometimes it can result from postural changes such as straining, stooping, lying down, or the ingestion of too much food.

Dysphagia (difficulty in swallowing) is related to a general loss of motility, esophagus and bronchial cancers, stroke, and pseudobulbar palsy. In advanced age a diaphragmatic or hiatal hernia can develop. The hiatus is an opening in the diaphragm through which the esophagus passes from the chest to the abdominal cavity. In the hiatal hernia, a portion of the stomach may protrude into the chest cavity. The symptoms include pain beneath the lower end of the breastbone, difficulty in swallowing, and sometimes bleeding from the lower end of the esophagus or stomach.

The Stomach. After food passes through the esophagus, it enters the stomach. The stomach is J-shaped and mobile, and it contains glands that produce substances that make up gastric juices and produce mucous to protect the lining of the stomach from being digested by its own enzymes. In the digestive process the food that enters the stomach is further broken down before it enters the intestinal tract. Limited nutrient absorption occurs in the stomach. Although physiological changes occur in the stomach as a person ages, researchers still disagree on the degree and rate of these changes. Most agree that hyperacidity and achlorhydria increase with age.

The three most common stomach ailments in later years are peptic ulcer, cancer, and gastritis. Peptic ulcer, although it can develop in later years, often is the extension of an ulcerous condition developed in the middle years. The classic symptoms of weight loss, anemia, and painless vomiting are usually seen. Perforation and great pain may be absent in the older person. One particularly important contributing factor in ulcer development is that the older adult has increased the use of drugs to alleviate other health problems. Some drugs, such as aspirin and cortecosteroids, increase gastric secretions and lower gastric mucosa resistance to other health problems. In most cases, the symptoms can be treated by taking healing medications, eliminating irritating drugs, and cessation of tobacco products. Specific ulcer diets have proved ineffective and therefore are generally not imposed.

Cancer may be suspected if a peptic ulcer has failed to heal within six weeks. As with an ulcer, the symptoms of stomach cancer are often nonspecific. The individual has malaise, has no appetite, loses weight, and is anemic. The classic signs of nausea, indigestion, difficulty in swallowing, bloody vomit, and tarry stools will generally appear at some time.

Gastritis is an inflammation of the gastric mucosa. The symptoms range from mild discomfort to extreme pain. Acute gastritis is usually associated with alcohol, drugs, or bacterial toxins which injure the mucosa. Chronic hypertrophic gastritis is associated with burning, gnawing pains, and indigestion. Chronic atrophic gastritis is associated with reduced acid secretion, atrophy of the mucosa, chronic pancreatitis, and alcoholism. Depending upon the severity of the symptoms, these conditions are controlled through diet, therapy, and medication.

Small Intestine. The small intestine is approximately 20 feet in length and is divided into three sections: the duodenum, the jejunum, and the ileum. The duodenum is the first 12 inches of the small intestine. Its function is more closely related to the function of the stomach and its structures include epithelial villi, various glands, and both circular and smooth muscle fibers. The final stages of digestion take place as the glands produce enzymes which further break down protein, fats, and carbohydrates. The muscles provide a vigorous churning type of peristalsis which completely mixes the food and enzymes.

The last eight inches of the small intestine is divided into two parts called the jejunum and the ileum. This portion of the small intestine comprises many of the same structures as seen in the duodenum. Only slight differences are seen. It is in this section that nutrient absorption takes place through the highly vascular villi. Muscles are stimulated by the nervous system to move the liquid content into the large intestine.

Age-related changes in the small intestine seem to be minimal. Therefore, in the absence of disease, nutrient absorption continues well into old age. The main difficulty associated with the function of the small intestine is in changes in the accessory glands such as the liver, gallbladder, and pancreas. These changes will be discussed later. Researchers do not agree on the changes in the blood vessels (decreased size, permeability, diminished elasticity), the lungs, and delayed peripheral nerve transmission and the effect these changes have on nutrient absorption.

Digestive and absorptive problems are not uncommon in older people. Various conditions that can lead to faulty digestion and malabsorption are listed below (3):

1. Bacterial overgrowth: Invasion of species from *Clostridia, Bacteroides* and *Veillonella* from the large intestine.
2. Cardiovascular abnormalities: Congestive heart failure, constrictive periocarditis, arteriosclerosis intestinal angina.
3. Diseases: Addison's disease, thyroid disease, diabetes, Paget's disease, collagen vascular disease, neoplastic disease, celiac sprue.
4. Drug-Induced: Anticonvulsants, alcohol, diuretics, colchicine, antibiotics, and cathartics.
5. Organ insufficiencies: Amyloidosis, pancreatic insufficiency, decreased bile acid synthesis, gallstones.
6. Radiation: Injury due to exposure.
7. Surgeries: Esophagectomy, gastrectomy, small bowel resection.

Large Intestine. The large intestine receives the liquid residue of digestion. The large intestine is about 5 feet long and is divided into the ascending, transverse, and descending colon.

Structurally, the large intestine contains no villi as seen in the small intestine. The inner epithelial tissue dips and is lined with columnar and mucous-secreting cells. Smooth muscle tissue is also found here. Fluids and food waste travel slowly through the large intestine. Large amounts of fluids are absorbed by the intestine so that a semisolid fecal mass is formed. The feces enter the rectum only when they are about to be evacuated by the body.

It is generally thought that the anatomical changes that interfere with the function of the large intestine include atrophy of the mucosa and connective tissue, abnormalities in cell structure, and arteriosclerosis. The most controversial problem associated with the large intestine is constipation. A great many older people believe that a daily elimination of the bowels is essential for good health. This is not necessarily so. Individual make-up and quantity of food influence whether bowel elimination is necessary. Inactivity, poor diet, misuse of cathartics, and psychological stress increase the occurrence of constipation in most people, but other factors are the cause of constipation in older people. (See Table 9.7).

Accessory Organs. The liver, gallbladder, and pancreas serve important functions in the total digestive process:

1. The functions of the liver are numerous; for example, the liver
   a. Produces bile
   b. Reabsorbs used bile salts for later use
   c. Stores iron
   d. Stores blood plasma, proteins, and other amino acids
   e. Stores carbohydrates
   f. Stores fats
   g. Converts waste products from the blood into a suitable form for use by other organs
   h. Detoxifies oral and respiratory ingested substances
   i. Synthesizes or stores vitamins and proteins needed for blood clotting
   j. Forms blood cells during embryonic development
2. The function of the gallbladder is primarily that of a reservoir for bile.
3. The function of the pancreas in the digestive process is to

Table 9.7 Deviations from Normal Health in the Large Intestine

Cause	Description	Symptoms
Cancer	Large intestine and rectum	Change in bowel habits; loss of appetite; weakness; weight loss; anemia
Diverticulosis	Tiny herniations of the mucous layers through muscles; pocket formations projecting from the bowel collect fecal material and become infected	Abdominal pain; diarrhea or constipation or alternating bouts of each; bleeding
Ischemic Colitis	Arteriosclerosis of mesenteric artery which occludes blood flow to large intestine	Abdominal pain; loose stool with red blood or clots; gassy bowel
Hemorrhoids	Ruptured blood vessels around the anus or within the anal canal; results from constipation, prolonged use of cathartics, straining at the stool	Can be without symptoms or be very painful and bleed

Source: Cary S. Kart, Eileen S. Metress, and James F. Metress, *Aging and Health* (Reading, Mass.: Addison-Wesley Publishing Co., Inc., 1978), pp. 91–97.

produce enzymes for the breakdown of fats, proteins, and carbohydrates. The pancreas also has a function in the endocrine system by providing the bloodstream with insulin which is necessary for carbohydrate regulation and metabolism.

Changes in the accessory structures can have numerous effects on the body's ability to utilize nutrients. The liver, for example, experiences cellular changes that interfere with the production of enzymes and the oxidative capacity of old cells. Protein synthesis is often decreased as a result of these changes.

The most common changes that occur in the gallbladder are changes in the physical composition and quantity of bile and a reduced ability of the gallbladder to empty itself. These changes in the older person often lead to the development of gallstones which block the bile duct. The general symptoms of gallstones are indigestion, nausea, vomiting, fat intolerance, and jaundice, but in many cases the condition is asymptomatic in older adults. Changes in the quality and quantity of bile interfere with the emulsification of fat globules into fatty acids and glycerol in the intestinal tract. Therefore, the body is unable to fully utilize the fats that are consumed in the diet. The function of fats in the body was discussed earlier.

The pancreatic changes may be enzymatic or structurally related. In addition, since the pancreas is controlled by both the endocrine system and the nervous system, changes related to these two systems can affect the efficiency of the pancreatic function. Beginning about age 40 the pancreas produces fewer enzymes, especially the proteolytic enzymes. This can greatly interfere with the breakdown of protein molecules. The structural changes involve not only reduced alveoli cell generation but also obstruction of the pancreatic duct. Both of these conditions can lead to pancreatitis. Pancreatitis may be very mild, with no symptoms or pain, or it may be acute and require hospitalization for the severe pain, disorientation, hallucination, or unconsciousness which can occur.

Psychosocial Components of Nutrition Psychosocial changes or specific diseases are not the only contributors to the development of malnutrition. Another important component of nutrition is the effect of reduced income, loss of mobility, stress, attitude, and loneliness on nutritional practices.

Reduced Income. As age increases the level of income decreases. Men have a higher income than do women and elderly whites have a higher income than do elderly blacks. In 1976 the average income for a married older couple was around $8167 per year. A single man averaged $3692 and a single female averaged $3235 (30, p. 29).

Each year the consumer price index increases. These increases are not as damaging to the fully employed person, but for those on a fixed income they are devastating. The consumer price index between 1960 and 1977 had the greatest increase in medical expenses. The increase for medical expenses was 153.4%, followed by housing 107.9%, food 103.6%, transportation 98.8%, and clothing 98.8% (30, pp. 478–479). Table 9.8 shows all food price increases from as little as 34.9% for eggs to the highest (excluding coffee) of 192.7% for fish.

Many older adults are faced with a difficult task. They must

Table 9.8 Consumer Price Food Index Increases 1960–1977

	1960 Index	1977 Index	Percent Increase
Cereal and bakery	87.1	182.5	109.5
White bread	85.2	162.8	91.0
Meat, poultry, fish	89.1	175.9	97.4
Meat	87.2	171.3	96.4
Poultry	106.9	157.6	47.4
Fish	85.0	248.8	192.7
Dairy products	88.4	173.1	95.8
Milk, fresh, grocery	91.1	161.5	77.2
Fruits and vegetables	88.3	195.1	120.9
Other foods	94.9	224.6	136.6
Eggs	113.2	152.8	34.9
Margarine	88.6	201.8	127.7
Sugar	92.2	187.1	102.9
Coffee	94.0	486.2	417.2
Tea	100.9	173.0	71.4

Source: Ben J. Wattenberg, *1978 The U.S. Fact Book, 98th* ed. Based on statistics from U.S. Bureau of Labor Statistics, *Monthly Labor Review,* pp. 47, 81.

attempt to maintain a well-balanced diet on a reduced income, but they are also forced to reduce their caloric intake while continuing to maintain all other nutrients. This task is not as difficult as it appears. For example, a married couple over the age of 55 with an income of $5000 to $10,000 could spend $26.20 per week on food and maintain a balanced diet. This figure does not include alcoholic beverages, pet food, soap, cigarettes, paper goods, or other nonfood items. These items add another 25 cents of every dollar spent in supermarkets. In addition, these figures would also increase each year as the consumer price index increases (25, pp. 1–3). Table 9.9 suggests the quantity of foods to purchase on a low-cost food plan of $26.20 per week for two people. Other suggestions are offered below (1, pp. 18–21, 26):

Preparing to go to the grocery store

1. Check the newspaper ads and compare grocery items.
2. Avoid smaller markets that provide delivery service because they usually charge higher prices.

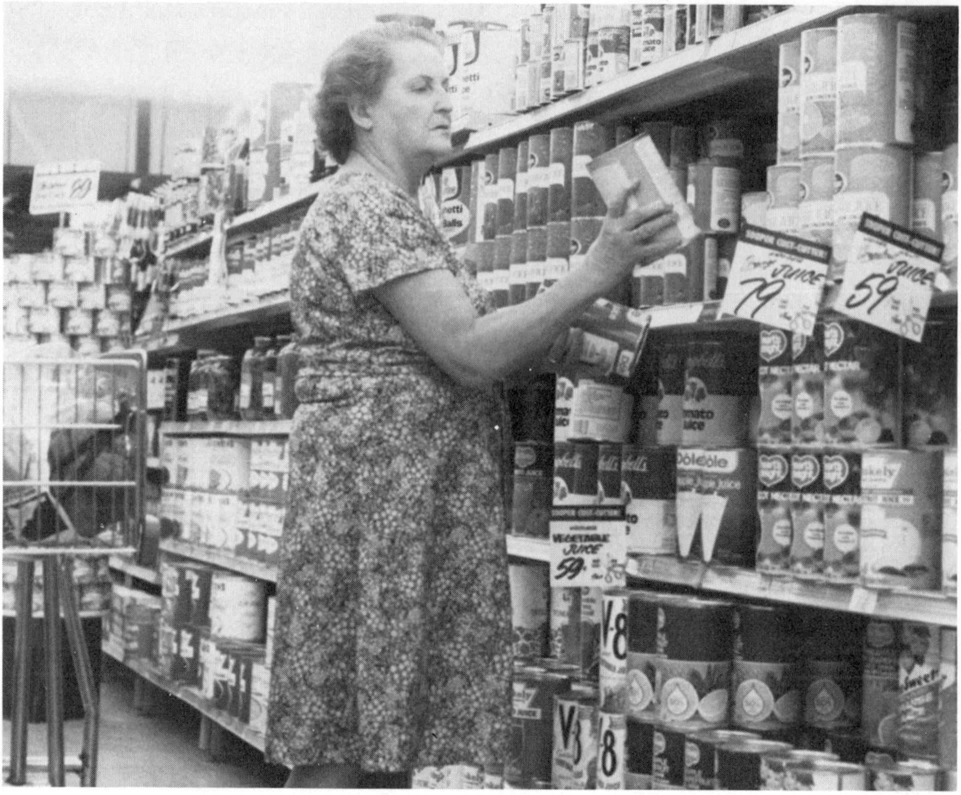

Figure 9.1 A reduced or constant income and ever higher food prices are just two of the problems often facing the older adult.

3. Take advantage of "cents off" coupons, but buy only the items that are really needed.
4. Prepare a list before going to the store and list the price range of items.
5. Use glasses to read labels.

Selecting food

1. Larger loaves of bread are usually less expensive unless the bread will get stale before it can be eaten. Select biscuits and muffins for a change. Always make sure that they are enriched.
2. Cereals that have to be cooked are generally less expensive than ready-to-eat cereals. Cereals in multipacks of individual boxes may cost two or three times as much per ounce as the same cereal in a large box.
3. Manufacturers of canned foods are required by law to list

Table 9.9 Low-Cost Weekly Food plan for a Married Couple Age 55 and Over

	Milk and Cheese	Meat, Fruit, Poultry	Eggs	Dried Beans, Beans, Nuts
Male	2.6 qt.	3.6 lb.	4	.61 lb.
Female	3.0 qt.	2.4 lb.	4	.67 lb.
	Citrus Fruits, Tomatoes	**Dark Green and Deep Yellow Vegetables**	**Potatoes**	**Other Vegetables**
Male	.21 lb.	.61 lb.	1.7 lb.	4.9 lb.
Female	.15 lb.	.62 lb.	1.2 lb.	4.5 lb.
	Cereal	**Flour**	**Bread**	**Other Bakery Products**
Male	1.0 lb.	.62 lb.	1.7 lb.	1.2 lb.
Female	.97 lb.	.58 lb.	1.2 lb.	.86 lb.
	Fats and Oils	**Sugar, Sweets**		
Male	.77 lb.	.90 lb.		
Female	.38 lb.	.64 lb.		

Source: U.S. Department of Agriculture, Agriculture Research, *Family Food Budgeting.* Home and Garden Bulletin No. 94, 1976, p. 5.

ingredients in order of weight. For example, a can of beef stew that lists beef first is a better buy than one that lists water first, carrots second, and beef third.

4. Purchase only the fresh fruits and vegetables that can be eaten as soon as possible. Foods in season are the best buys.
5. Select meat, fish, and poultry that provide the most for the least amount of money. Avoid meat that has excessive bone, gristle, or fat. Use leftover meats in casseroles, salads, sandwiches, soups, and as vegetable flavoring.
6. Select fluid milk for drinking and nonfat dry milk for cooking.
7. Purchase medium-sized eggs by the half dozen.
8. Purchase flour and sugar in small packages.

Loss of Mobility. Increasing age may be accompanied by physiological changes and diseases that restrict activity and mobility. As people become less mobile, they are less likely to go shopping at the supermarket or to dine out.

If special attention is not given to older adults who have limited mobility, it is likely that they will be malnourished. Programs designed to meet these needs will be discussed later.

Men over the age of 65 have more activity restrictions due to poor health than do women of the same age (29). However, most older men are married and unless their wives are restricted, they will continue to plan and prepare meals. Table 9.10 shows the percentage of men and women in two age groups who have activity restrictions for specific health problems.

It is important to note that the specific health conditions that limit activity may not be nearly as restrictive as the mental effort required to adapt to or overcome the inconvenience of the restriction. This does not mean, however, that certain conditions or changes are more phychological than physiological. For example, muscles that have not been used are not strong. The decalcification of bones can result in skeletal instability and broken bones. Osteoporosis can produce kyphosis (humpback) and kyphoscoliosis (lateral spine curvature) which interferes with stability and balance. Changes in the vertebral discs of the spinal column bring about diminished flexibility, misalignment, and back pain. Overall postural changes adversely affect the functioning of other organs (18). In addition, health

Table 9.10 Percentage of Men and Women with Activity Limitations Caused by Selected Chronic Conditions, 1974

Chronic Condition	Male 45–64	65+	Female 45–64	65+
Heart conditions	24.2	25.2	15.6	22.2
Arthritis	12.5	15.6	22.4	29.4
Visual impairments	4.1	8.6	3.8	10.7
Hypertension without heart involvement	5.9	6.0	11.8	10.9
Mental and nervous conditions	5.2	3.0	6.3	3.8

Source: U.S. National Center for Health Statistics, unpublished data.

problems such as hypertension, heart disease, arthritis, vision impairments, and any medications used for these problems can interfere with mobility.

The tasks that healthy people take for granted become complex tasks for those who have restricted activity. Reading a grocery advertisement or a menu, pushing a shopping cart, getting in and out of an automobile, reading labels on grocery items, reaching for an item on a top shelf, carrying a box of groceries, or preparing a meal are all examples of some of the difficulties encountered by those who have restrictions.

Another factor to be considered in mobility loss is the lack of transportation. Some older people are able to operate an automobile, but some have physical limitations that prohibit driving an automobile. In addition, the cost, maintenance, and insurance of owning an automobile may be prohibitive if an individual has a limited income. Public transportation, if it is available, helps with this problem.

Stress Chapter 4 discussed the sources of stress for the aging person (middle age, marriage, widowhood, remarriage, sexual adjustments, employment, retirement, and discrimination and the aging female. These are examples of psychosocial events or stressors. Other stressors can be categorized as physiological stressors (phyical changes, disease, physical activity). Regardless of the source of the stress, each person can respond in several ways. The response can be emotional, behavioral, or physiological. The total stress response is probably a combination of all of the responses.

An emotional response can be expressed in a wide range of feelings from ecstasy to rage. It is usually a subjective response and is based upon perception and past experiences. In comparison, a behavioral response is seen in changes in actions or behavior. The change can be either positive or negative (21).

A physiological response to a stressor is the physical and chemical changes that take place in specific organs and tissues of the body and functional changes in the entire body (19). Food intake and digestion can be affected by stress. An individual can respond behaviorally either by overeating as a means of relieving stress or by not being able to eat. In either case, nutritional status can change if the stressor is not relieved.

A physiological response to stress results in the interaction of the nervous and endocrine systems. According to Selye's stress theory of aging, the exhaustion stage of the general adaption syndrome (GAS) can be likened to old age when adaptive energies are lower than at younger ages (20). Selye found that adrenal function in animals under nonstress conditions remained fairly constant and could maintain life, but under stress conditions the animals were incapable of supporting adaptive reactions (23, p. 548). Whether or not this is true in humans is unknown, but qualitative factors such as the rate of metabolism, including cholesterol metabolism, reduced binding properties of blood protein to hormones, the ratio of free to bound hormones, and the affinity and storage of cortisol by tissues have been determined to result from a stress state (23, p. 550, 4). Consequently, a prolonged stress state and biochemical changes may lead to arteriosclerosis, deficient antibody production, enzyme production, and changes in thyroid, pituitary, and pancreas hormones which in turn affect the function of other body organs. These biochemical changes are precipitated in the older person by such stressors as physical illness, loss of a spouse, injury, changes in financial status, change in residence, marriage, the change in the health of a family member, sex difficulties, or retirement.

Family Attitudes. Nutritional attitudes and practices are established in childhood and seem to be closely tied to family, friends, special occasions, and religious practices. Obese adults establish their eating practices as children and probably were obese children. In the United States where food is plentiful, it it easy to consume large amounts of food. The gradual increase in weight is viewed by many as "something that happens with age." Some adults grew up with the belief that a "fat child is a healthy child." Others believe that it is better to be "pleasingly plump" and happy rather than miserable and constantly dieting.

Nutrition deficiency develops when one or more essential foods are omitted from the diet for any length of time. One's attitude about food can be negatively influenced when a poor emotional climate exists in the home and during meal times. Ignorance of nutritional needs, poor eating habits, and personal dislikes also influence nutritional status.

Prior to older age most people eat to continue life and to maintain some level of health. As people outlive their spouses, friends, and relatives, they also lose their means of social involvement and most of their ". . . landmarks of existence that tell them who they are and where they come from" (24). Therefore, eating and attitudes about eating may take on new meaning. Howell and Loeb (11) divided eating habits into three categories based upon the purposes of eating.

In *category one* is the person who sees eating as a way of remembering. The person uses "food for thought" and gains comfort by reminiscing about the past. The concern is not with the life-giving qualities of the food but with the symbolic meaning of the food.

In *category two* is the person who sees eating as a means of sustaining life. When this person is confronted with physical deterioration, the primary function of food for bodily maintenance becomes increasingly important. In addition, some people see food as a magical solution to restoring youth. Food faddism and hoarding behaviors are commonly seen.

In *category three* is the person who sees food and eating as a way of relating. This person sees the provision, preparation, and consumption of food as activities closely related to basic familial relationships. The woman prepares and serves the food; the man provides and consumes the food. When these classic sex-role identifications are lost through widowhood or divorce, the corresponding identifications with food and eating are weakened.

Eating Alone. It is expensive to purchase and prepare meals for one person because foods are generally packaged in large quantities and it is usually less expensive to buy larger quantities than smaller ones. It is not economical for a single person to purchase large quantities of food unless it can be stored for an extended period of time but many foods cannot be stored for any length of time. In addition, eating alone may encourage an individual to eat foods that require little or no preparation.

Probably more important than having food to maintain physical health is the need for meaningful social involvement. In family situations the preparation and eating of a meal is a social event. Most of the social interaction enhances one's attitude toward eating. The person who lives alone and eats alone misses the social aspects of eating. People who have become accustomed to eating as a social event will find it difficult and unpleasant to plan, prepare, and eat a meal alone. Some older people feel so rejected and lonely that they lose the incentive to eat alone.

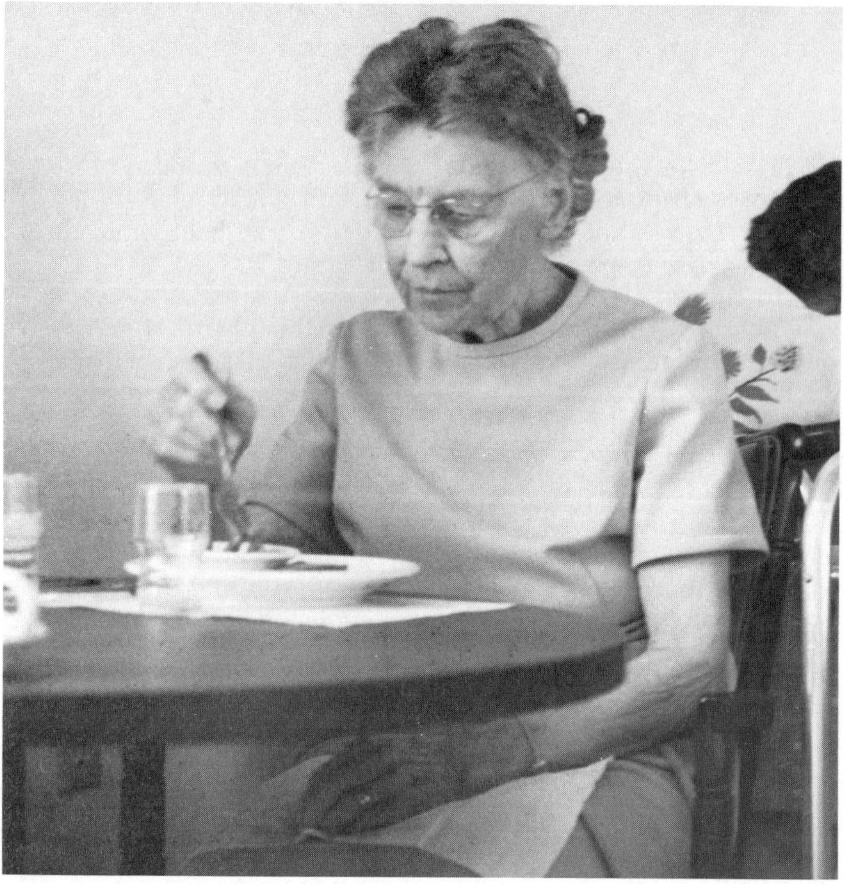

Figure 9.2 A person living and eating alone misses the very important social aspects of eating.

■ Fad Diets

A fad diet is a passing fashion or craze which proposes the consumption of a particular food and claims innumerable benefits. Most fad diets are too expensive for the low incomes of many older people. The only time a fad diet can become a problem is if the diet complicates an existing chronic disease. Many nutritionists feel that food fads may have a beneficial influence on the mental health of some older people because ". . . . they can change one's spirit from embittered defeat to embattled retreat" (12).

The older person may be victimized by a food quack who pretends to have knowledge or training in foods and nutrition that he or she does not have. The contemporary faddists are the old-time medicine men in modern-day clothing. Often they claim to have "miracle" products and say that they have combined the latest scientific findings with reliable methods from the past (1, pp. 15, 28).

A variety of claims (by quacks) have been made about preventing aging, elminating fatigue, and curing disease. For example, it has been claimed that the use of antioxidants, butylated hydroxyanisole (BHA), and butylated hydroxytolunen (BHT) will prevent aging, but these claims have not been substantiated in humans (13). Another claim is that vitamins and minerals will correct fatigue. The food quack often makes appeals such as, "Do you feel tired, lack energy, and have an overall run down feeling?"(17). Vitamins provide no energy and cannot correct fatigue. Others claim that special foods are good for the health, for example, beets make red blood, fish and celery are brain food, cod-liver oil, honey, or vinegar cure arthritis, and blackstrap molasses cures anemia and rheumatism (17). The danger in believing that certain foods will cure diseases is the increased risk of disability or death and most certainly the high expense for delayed medical assistance when a problem does exist.

■ Programs That Enhance Nutritional Status

In 1972 Congress amended the Older Americans Act (Public Law 92–258) and added a new Title VII Nutrition Program for the Elderly. In addition to the nutrition program for providing a balanced meal, the law stipulated that administrators of such programs must provide, as needed:

1. Transportation to and from congregate meal sites
2. Information and referral services
3. Health and welfare counseling services
4. Nutrition education
5. Shopping assistance
6. Recreation activities incidental to the project (5, p. 3)

The benefits of congregate meal programs are numerous. Eating meals with other people provides social interaction and companionship, eliminates the necessity of planning, shopping, and cooking for one, and is usually more economical. Nevertheless, a small number of older people will not participate in a congregate meal program. Some older people fear leaving the confines and security of their homes. They fear physical harm, especially if they live in a dangerous neighborhood. Occasionally, cultural factors or religious beliefs may prevent them from participating in a program sponsored by a race or religious sect other than their own. Some consider the congregate meal program a "welfare" program and will not participate because they oppose welfare programs. Even though the law requires that transportation services be provided to and from the meal site, transportation is not always available because drivers, program directors, and participants cannot agree on a schedule. Long rides to and from the meal sites are exhausting. Special physical handicaps often present problems because not all vehicles are equipped to accommodate all kinds of handicaps. As a result, some people choose not to participate in the congregate meal program.

Nutrition education may be obtained through organized programs such as the program developed by Rutgers University (17), a slide series called "Rules to Shop By" (5, p. 12), the revival of victory gardens (5, p. 15), or the many available books, pamphlets, and articles especially printed for the older consumer (see Table 9.11).

Table 9.11 Selected References on Food and Nutrition in the Senior Years

---

Cooking for One: In the Senior Years by M. Washbon, An Extension publication of the New York State College of Human Ecology, Cornell University, Ithaca, N.Y., 11 pages, September, 1971.

Cooking for One or Two: In Leisure Years by M. S. Mindman, Clemson University Cooperative Extension Service, Clemson, S.C., H.E. Circular 243, 12 pages, October, 1970.

Cooking for Two by D. W. Davis and B. K. McGeary, Program Aid No. 1043, Food and Nutrition Service, U.S. Dept. of Agriculture, available from Superintendent of Documents, U.S. Government Printing Office, Washington, D.C. 20402, 89 pages, November, 1973, $1.10.

Eat and Keep Healthy After 60, published by Home Economics Service, Community Service Society, 105 East 22nd Street, New York, N.Y. 10010, 8 pages, $.10.

Food: Flavor, Facts and Fun for Folks After Fifty by H. E. Spence,

Table 9.11 *(continued)*

H. McLachlan, published under the auspices of the Durham Golden Age Society, 810 Proctor Street, Durham, N.C., 9 pages.

The Single Burner Chef Cookbook by Deborah L. Craig, published by the New Hampshire Network, Box 2, Durham, N.H. 03824, 39 pages, 1973.

Food Guide for Older Folks by M. A. Walker and M. M. Hill, U.S. Dept. of Agriculture, Home and Garden Bulletin, No. 17, available from the Superintendent of Documents, U.S. Government Printing Office, Washington, D.C. 20402, 19 pp., revised February, 1972, $.20.

Food Hints for Mature People: More Years to Life—More Life to Years by C. G. King and G. Britt, Public Affairs Pamphlet No. 336, published by Public Affairs Committee, 2 E. 38th Street, New York, N.Y., 28 pages, 1962, $.25.

Food to Keep Fit as the Years Go By, published by Department of Health, The City of New York, 125 Worth Street, New York, N.Y. 10013, 4 pages.

To Your Health—In Your Second Fifty Years, published by the National Dairy Council, 111 N. Canal Street, Chicago, Ill. 60606, 7 pages, 1974.

To Your Health—In Your Second Fifty Years (adapted from the National Dairy Council booklet), Dairy Council of Metropolitan New York, 60 East 42nd Street, New York, N.Y. 10017, 4 pages, 1974.

Your Retirement Food Guide by Florence Grodd, published by the American Association of Retired Persons and National Retired Teachers Association, 215 Long Beach Blvd., Long Beach, Calif. 90801, 31 pages, 1971.

How to Add Life to Your Years, published by the Evaporated Milk Association, 910 Seventeenth Street, N.W. Washington, D.C. 20006, 6-page foldout, 1970.

Eats in My Room, published by the Department of Social and Health Services, Health Services Division, P.O. Box 1788, Olympia, Wash. 98504, 6 page foldout, 1972.

Grand Food for Grandparents—Or Those Who Could Be, published by the Tennessee Commission of Aging, Capitol Tower Apartment, 510 Gay Street, Nashville, Tenn. 37219, 17 pages, revised ed., 1973.

Nutrition for Older Adults, a series of seven 4-page booklets available with the following subtitles: Eat Well to Feel Well, Food and Diet Aids, Resources in Your Community, Preparing Food Safely, Eating Out Tips, Goodbuys Hello Dollars and Plan Ahead and Safe, developed and published by Project INSTEP, P.O. Box 1175, Tallahassee, Fla. 32302, 1974.

After the Kids Have Gone (Special Nutritional Needs for the Later Years), published by General Mills Nutrition Service, 9200 Wayzata Blvd., Minneapolis, Minn. 55440, 8 pages, 1974.

Mas Salud en la Edad Avanzada (Better Health for the Older Citizen), published in Spanish by the Nutrition Program Nursing Home Nutritionist, Nursing Home

Table 9.11 (*continued*)

Division, Dept. of Health, San Juan, Puerto Rico, 10 pages, 1973.

Good Eating Keeps You Swinging Even After Fifty, published by the Carnation Co., Home Service Department, Dept. G. E., Los Angeles, Calif. 90036, 11 pages, 1970.

Lower Cost Meals That Please: In Our Senior Years, published by the National Dairy Council, 111 N. Canal St., Chicago, Ill. 60606, 11 pages, 1971.

Many Happy Returns: To The Forties, the Fifties, the Sixties and Over, published by the National Dairy Council, 111 N. Canal St., Chicago, Ill. 60606, 13 pages, 1967.

Meal Planning for the Golden Years, published by General Mills, Inc., Nutrition Service, Dept. 5, 9200 Wayzata Blvd. Minneapolis, Minn. 55440, 16 pages, 1966.

Meals for One, published by Home Economics Service, Community Service Society, 105 East 22nd Street, New York, N.Y. 10010, 8 pages, 1965, $.10.

Nutrition and the Adult: Suggestions That May Make You Feel Better, available from the New England Gerontology Center, 15 Garrison Avenue, Durham, N.H. 03824, 4 pages, 1974.

Forget Birthdays . . . Enjoy Good Eating, published by The American Dietetic Association, 430 N. Michigan Avenue, Chicago, Ill. 60611, 6 pages, revised September, 1961.

What to Eat During Your Second Fifty Years, published by the N.H. Nutrition Committee, c/o Public Health Nutrition Services, 61 S. Spring Street, Concord, N.H. 03301, 6 pages, 1975.

For Older People . . . Eating Right for Less, Consumers Union Guide to Food and Nutrition, Orangeburg, N.Y. 10962, $2.00.

Additional services to improve and/or maintain the diet of older Americans are listed below:

1. Garden plots donated for use by older adults (5, p. 17; 7, p. 15)
2. Training programs for supermarket employees which provide information on the older person as a shopper (5, p. 24)
3. Transportation provided by supermarkets (5, p. 30)
4. Co-op food buying (15, pp. 16–18; 14, pp. 3–5)
5. Ethnic nutrition food services (15, pp. 6–8)
6. Hotel coffee shops used for meal sites (6, pp. 10–11)

7. Candlelight dining at congregate meal sites (8, p. 11)
8. Home-delivered meals (2, 10, 16)

Summary

The nutritional needs are the same for all ages with the exception of calorie requirements. Older adults require fewer calories. Each age group experiences some degree of nutritional deficiency. The nutritional status of the older adult is influenced by both physical and psychosocial factors. Physical factors include such things as physical change, disease, and disorders. Psychosocial factors include a lack of finances, loss of mobility, stress, attitudes toward eating, and eating alone. Fad diets, although not a significant problem in the older age groups, can influence the nutritional practices of some people. Many programs are available to improve the nutritional status and health of the older adult.

References

1. American Association of Retired Persons and National Retired Teachers Association. *Your Retirement Food Guide,* 1970.
2. Anon. " 'Meals-on-Wheels' Avert Hospitalization." *Journal of The American Medical Association* 222 (1972):531–32.
3. Balachi, J. A., and Dobbins, W. V. "Maldigestion and Malabsorption: Making up for Lost Nutrients." *Geriatrics.* 29 (1974):157–66.
4. Berliner, D. L., Keller, N., and Dougherty, T. F. "Mediated and Direct Effects of ACTH and Corticosteroids in Stress." In *Physiology and Pathology of Adaptation Mechanisms,* edited by E. Bajusz. Elmsford, N. Y.: Pergamon Press, 1969.
5. Carlin, Joseph, ed. *Nutrition Education for the Older American,* p. 3. New England Gerontology Center, n.d.
6. ——. "Coffee Shop Fertile Ground for Dakota Meal Site." *Aging* 274 (1977):10–11.

7. ——. "Do It Yourself: Texas Gardeners Grow Bumper Crop." *Aging* 274 (1977):15.

8. Freedman, Martha H. "Candlelight and Vintage Years." *Aging* 274 (1977):9.

9. Guthrie, H., Black, K., and Madden, J. P. "Nutritional Practices of Elderly Citizens in Rural Pennsylvania." *The Gerontologist* 12 (1972):33.

10. Henry, C. E. "Feeding Elderly People in Their Homes." *Journal of the American Dietetics Association* 35 (1959): 149–51.

11. Howell, S., and Loeb, M. B. "Adult Stress and Diet." *The Gerontologist* 9 (1969):40–49.

12. Kart, Cary S., Metress, Eileen S., and Metress, James F. *Aging and Health,* p. 114. Reading, Mass.: Addison-Wesley 1978.

13. Mayer, Jean. "Aging and Nutrition." *Geriatrics* 34 (1979): 57–59.

14. ——. "Nutrition California Co-Op Cuts Bills in Half." *Aging* 274 (1977):3–5.

15. ——. "Nutrition—Kosher Meals a Specialty at New York Luncheon Club." *Aging* 274 (1977):6–8.

16. Pelcovits, J., and Wolgamot, I. H. "Nutritional Programs for the Elderly: Selecting a Meal Delivery System." *Journal of Home Economics* 66 (1974):43–45.

17. Rutgers The State University of New Jersey. "Modern Medicine Man." *Nutrition for the Elderly, Mini-Lesson Kit.* P.O. Box 231, New Brunswick, N. J. 08903, n.d.

18. Saxon, Sue V., and Etten, Mary Jean. *Physical Change and Aging,* pp. 28–30. New York: Tiresias Press, 1978.

19. Selye, Hans. *The Stress of Life.* New York: McGraw-Hill, 1956.

20. Selye, H., and Prioreschi, P. "Stress Theory of Aging." In *Aging—Some Social and Biological Aspects,* edited by N. W. Shock. Washington, D.C.: American Association for the Advancement of Science, 1960.

21. Tanner, Ogden, ed. *Stress.* New York: Time-Life Books, 1976.

22. Ten-State Nutrition Survey 1968–1970. Washington, D.C.: Center for Disease Control, 1972.

23. Timiras, P. S. *Developmental Physiology and Aging.* New York: Macmillan, 1972.

24. Troll, Lillian E. "Eating and Aging." *Journal of the American Dietetics Association* 59 (1971):5–9.

25. U.S. Department of Agriculture, Agriculture Research Service. *Family Food Budgeting for Good Meals and Good Nutrition.* Home and Garden Bulletin No. 94, 1976.

26. U.S. Department of Agriculture, Agriculture Research Service. *Food Guide for Older Folks.* Home and Garden Bulletin No. 7, 1974, pp. 7–8.

27. U.S. Government Printing Office. *Dietary Goals for the United States,* 2nd ed. December, 1977.

28. U.S. Department of Health, Education and Welfare, *FDA Consumer Memo—Quackery.* DHEW Publication No. (FDA) 74–1017. March, 1974.

29. U.S. National Center for Health Statistics, unpublished data.

30. Wattenberg, Ben. J. *The U.S. Factbook,* 98th ed. New York: Grosset & Dunlap, 1978.

31. Young, V. R., Perera, W. D., Winterer, J. C., and Scrimshaw, N. S. In *Nutrition and Aging,* edited by M. Winick, pp. 77–118. New York: John Wiley, 1976.

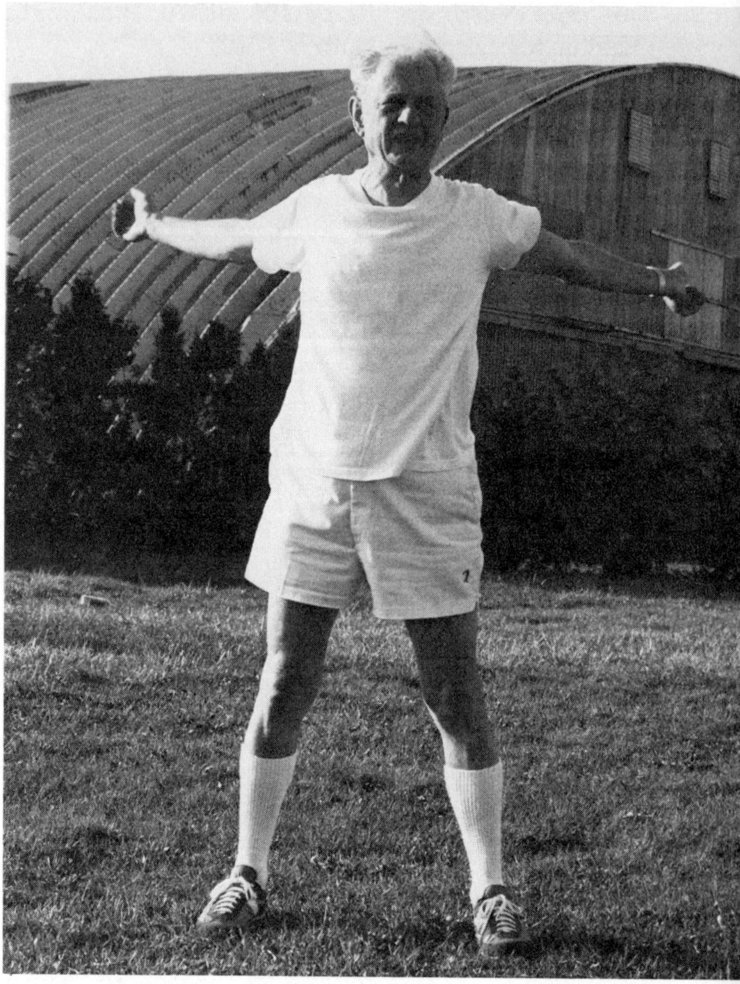

■ Chapter 10

Physical Fitness

Major Concepts

1. Total physical fitness includes strength, flexibility, muscular endurance, and cardiorespiratory endurance.
2. Levels of physical fitness vary in different age groups.
3. Certain health problems may limit the amount and type of exercise in which a person can participate.
4. There are many organized exercise and fitness programs for older adults.

■ Components of Physical Fitness

Physical fitness is defined as ". . . the capability of the heart, blood vessels, lungs, and muscles to function at optimal efficiency" (14, p. 9). Physical fitness is divided into four components: strength, muscular endurance, flexibility, and cardiorespiratory endurance. These four components will be discussed below in relation to the physiological changes that occur as older adults participate in exercise programs.

Strength The capacity of a muscle to exert a single maximum contraction against a resistance is known as strength. The average male reaches his peak muscular strength at age 17 and a female generally reaches her maximum strength at the onset of puberty (6, p. 9). The person who engages in the appropriate type and amount of exercise will experience an increased muscle mass. Large muscle masses will continue to exist throughout most of a person's life if the person continues to exercise.

Regardless of age, inactivity results in decreased muscle mass. Nonfunctional changes with age (decreased hormone production, decreased deposits of collagen and elastic fibers in muscles) also tend to reduce the power of muscles. Decreased muscular strength was demonstrated in a study in which manual cranking ability and arm strength were measured in men between the ages of 20 and 89. For men ages 20 to 69, the strength scores were the same. For men in their seventies, the scores declined 20 points and they declined 45 points for men in their eighties. Cranking ability, maximum power output, declined progressively after age 39 (30).

Muscular Endurance The ability of a muscle to contract, either through a prolonged static contraction or through repeated exertion, is called muscular endurance. Increasing age reduces the possibilities of a person's achieving a performance level equal to that achieved in younger years. There are, however, cases of older people being capable of high physical and motor performances. For example, distance runner Clarence DeMar and runner Larry Lewis both set records (14, p. 10).

Scientific studies have concluded that physical work capacity, work load limit, and general muscular endurance increase in both men and women of all ages who participate in an appropriate training program. Again, the degree and rate of improvement in increased muscular endurance are higher in younger subjects (1, 3, 11, 12, 32).

Flexibility The ability to move the joints in a wide range of motion is called flexibility. The combination of general aging and inactivity cause joint tissue to thicken and lose elasticity. Regular exercise that includes a wide range of movements offsets these changes. In addition, exercise and joint mobility may also delay or reduce the chances of developing arthritis (8, p. 13).

Cardiorespiratory Endurance The capacity of the heart, lungs, and blood vessels to adjust to the requirements of large muscle group contractions for long periods of time is called cardiorespiratory endurance. This component of fitness is probably the most important of the four components.

Up until age 25 there is little change in resting heart rate. After the age of 25 the normal heart beat decreases 6 beats per minute for every 5 years (5). Normal blood pressure is 120/72 for men and slightly lower for women. Both systolic and diastolic pressures increase over the span of adult life by 10 to 15 milligrams mercury. Cardiac output, the amount of blood pumped by the heart per minute, is about equal for all ages (16).

Somewhere between 20% and 25% of the lung function is lost with increasing age. Changes include decreases in:

1. Vital capacity
2. Maximal oxygen intake
3. Forced expiratory volume
4. Maximal ventilation
5. Residual volume
6. Employing of the lungs
7. Elasticity of the lungs
8. Flexibility of the thorax (6, p. 9)

For years researchers wondered whether or not a vigorous training program could delay or reverse the changes which are considered normal for the heart and lungs of an inactive person. The evidence over the last 20 years substantiates that it can prevent some of the changes. Kasch and Wallace (18) studied 16 middle-aged men for 10 years. The men participated in a

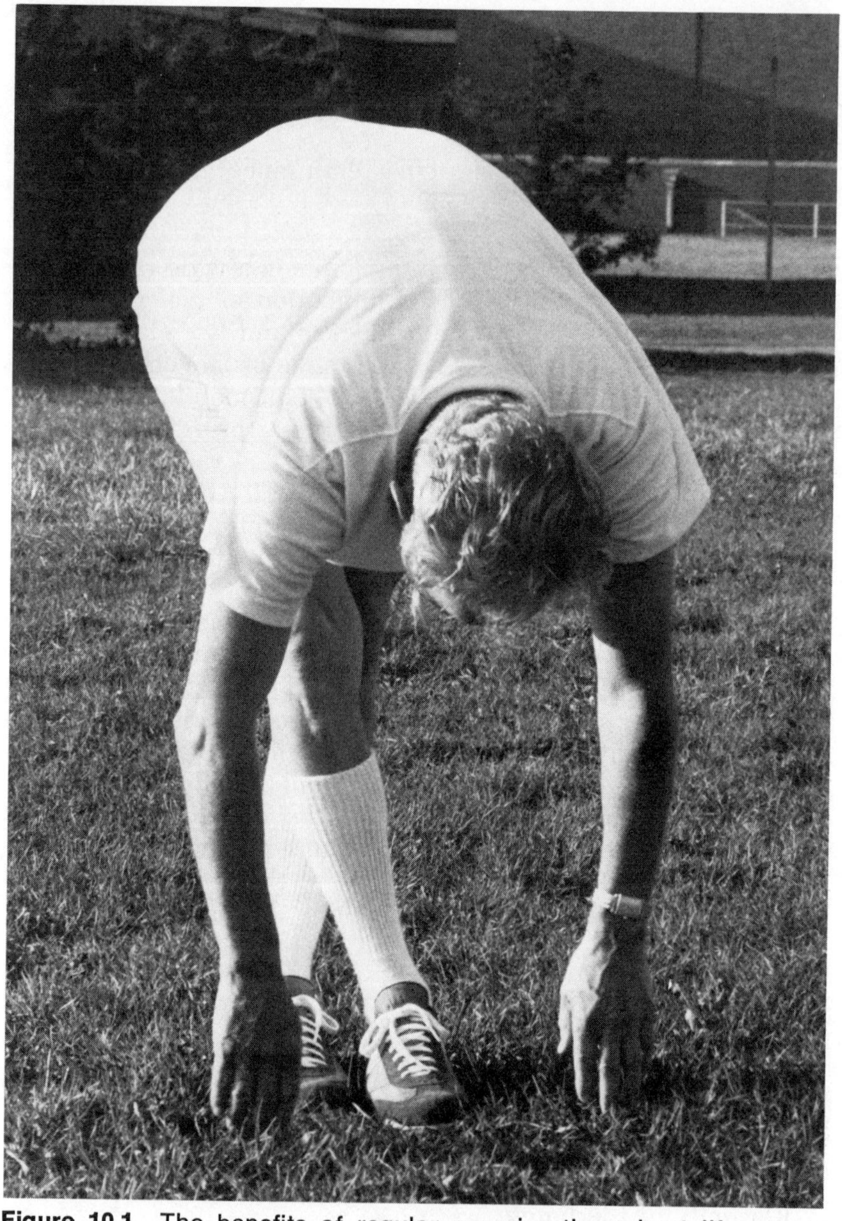

Figure 10.1 The benefits of regular exercise throughout life can be enormous.

regular exercise program of jogging or swimming. The subjects maintained a constant body weight, resting heart rate, blood pressure, and maximum oxygen intake. Pulmonary ventilation improved (18).

Studies by de Vries (12), Barry et al. (3), Adams and de Vries (1), and Cureton (10) concluded that regular training of older adults improved oxygen intake capacity, cardiovascular and respiratory tests, resting heart rate, physical work capacity, oxygen transport systems, and pulmonary ventilation..

Other long-term benefits of fitness have been documented over the years and include the following:

1. Reduced risk factors associated with coronary heart disease through increased respiratory endurance, reduced triglyceride levels, reduced blood cholesterol, increased red blood cells and blood volume, improved myocardial vascularization, and collateral circulation development (6, p. 4).
2. Reduced body fat and increased lean body mass (21).
3. Reduced risk of developing hyperkinetic diseases such as diabetes, ulcers, low back pain, and emotional difficulties. Hyperkinetic diseases are any physical or mental derangements induced by inactivity (19, 20).
4. Psychosocial problems are reduced. People who exercise regularly appear to have reduced tension, improved general learning potential for a given intelligence level, and positive self-concepts and are more confident, more self-sufficient, and more controlled (6, p. 3; 11; 33, p. 11; 34).
5. Positive changes occur in human growth hormone (HGH) and cortisol levels. HGH regulates anabolism (food changes into living tissue) and cortisol regulates catabolism (tissue changes into food). Generally, training effects increase levels of HGH, especially in older and unfit individuals. Cortisol levels increase only under stressful exhaustive exercise (29).

The literature does not indicate that regular exercise and high levels of physical fitness will stop the aging process, but many of the degenerative diseases that are associated with chronological age can be delayed or averted. This is especially true when exercise programs are combined with good eating habits, regular and adequate sleep, rest and relaxation, and avoidance of tobacco, alcohol, and indiscriminate use of drugs.

Exercise and Fitness Levels

The benefits of exercise and fitness in terms of quality and perhaps quantity of life are explicit. However, in order for a person to benefit in both quality and quantity of life, positive

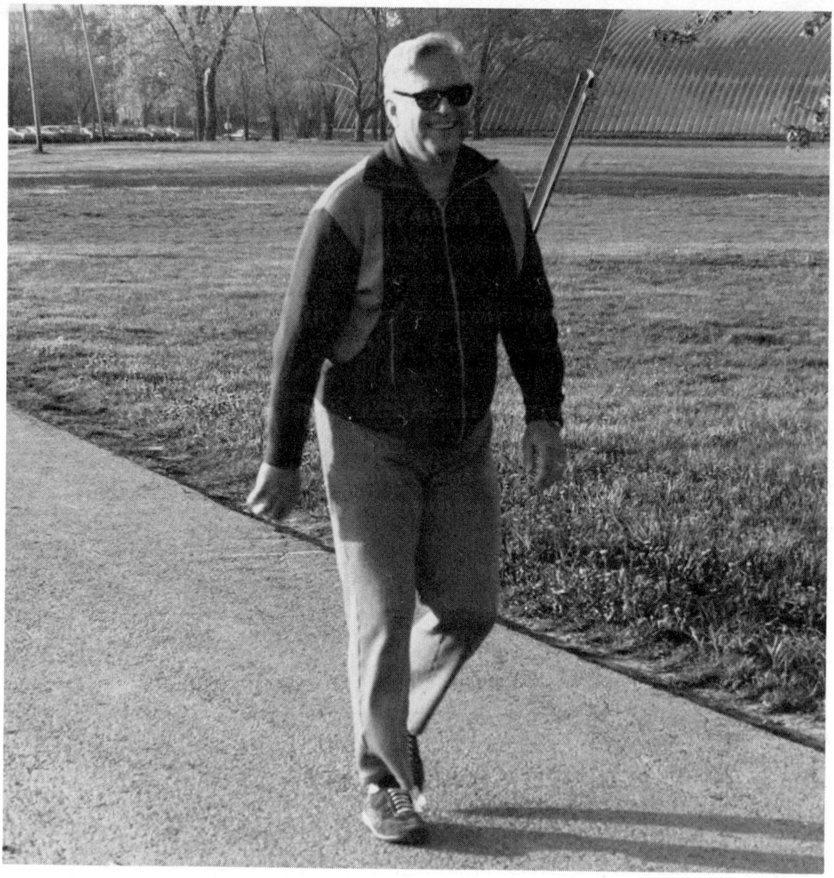

Figure 10.2 Don't overlook the many benefits of walking as a regular exercise.

attitudes toward and practices of exercise should be established as young as possible.

In the past 10 years the level of physical fitness in American youth has decreased. The Research Council of the American Alliance for Health, Physical Education and Recreation conducted the AAHPER Youth Fitness Test in 1958, 1965, and 1975. Between 1958 and 1965 the test scores of both males and females improved dramatically. Test scores for 1965 and 1975 were almost identical (7). Reiff and Hunsicker (26) speculate that this stabilization of test scores and a general lack of improvement can be attributed to three factors. (1) Schools, for economic reasons, cut back or dropped physical education. (2) During the Kennedy Administration national physical fitness was a priority. This interest has slowly declined. (3) Views and programming on fitness have changed as the physical education program emphasizes "lifetime sports."

It appears from the minimal information that has been collected that as age increases the level of physical activity decreases. In 1972 the Opinion Research Corporation conducted a National Adult Fitness Survey for the President's Council on Physical Fitness. The survey involved 2,000 men and women. Of those aged 60 and over, only 39% reported getting any systematic exercise. The favorite form of exercise for men (46%) and women (33%) was walking. Only small percentages participated in calisthenics (6%), swimming (4%), bicycling (3%), or jogging (1%) (6, p. 1). Tables 10.1 and 10.2 list the percentages of men and women in different age groups who participated in 1975 in specific types of exercise.

Two factors contribute to inactivity in later years: lack of knowledge about exercise and negative attitudes toward exercise Elderly individuals did not have the opportunity to learn about exercise and fitness in their school years because few schools provided physical education classes. If people do not know that exercise is important or if they fear exercise, they will not participate in it. Conrad (8, p. 11) described the attitudes of older people toward exercise as follows:

1. Some believe that as they get older the need for exercise diminishes.

Table 10.1 Percentage of Men and Women Ages 20 to 44 Engaged in Physical Exercise, 1975

	Percentage of Population	
Type of Exercise	Men [1]	Women [2]
Bicycling	14.9	17.2
Calisthenics	17.5	17.1
Jogging	10.6	4.1
Weight lifting	10.1	1.1
Swimming	18.8	15.0
Walking	31.4	36.0

Source: U.S. National Center for Health Statistics, unpublished data.

[1] Total population: 34,268.
[2] Total population: 36,816.

Table 10.2 Percentage of Men and Women Ages 45 to 65+ Engaged in Physical Exercise, 1975

Type of Exercise	Men 45–64 [1]	Men 65+ [2]	Women 45–64 [3]	Women 65+ [4]
Bicycling	6.7	4.3	6.4	1.8
Calisthenics	10.1	5.9	11.4	6.3
Jogging	3.8	2.1	1.6	—
Weight lifting	2.6	— [5]	—	—
Swimming	8.1	4.1	7.8	1.9
Walking	31.4	39.4	34.2	33.0

(Percentage of Population)

Source: U.S. National Center for Health Statistics, unpublished data.

[1] Total population: 20,567.
[2] Total population: 8830.
[3] Total population: 22,579.
[4] Total population: 112,595.
[5] Base less than minimum required for reliability.

2. Some believe that after middle age the risks involved in vigorous exercise are very high.
3. Some overrate the benefits of sporadic and/or light exercise.
4. Some underestimate their capacities and abilities.

Many programs have been designed and implemented in an attempt to improve the level of fitness and change negative attitudes toward exercise. These programs will be discussed later in this chapter.

■ Physical Limitations

Older people who have been inactive for years can participate in exercise programs. They cannot expect to perform at levels once performed when they were young, but their performance can improve. Carefully planned programs of exercise can help improve problems such as heart conditions, arthritis, obesity, and diabetes.

Heart Conditions Once cardiovascular disease is diagnosed, many people automatically assume a restricted lifestyle. They fear that physical activity will stimulate a heart attack. Under carefully designed and supervised exercise programs, individuals who have a heart condition can greatly improve the condition.

In a study by deVries (12, p. 325) seven men with various cardiovascular problems participated in a training program of calisthenics, stretching exercises, and walking. Maximum heart rate was kept at 120 beats per minute. They exercised for six weeks, and upon retesting, were found to have improvements in oxygen pulse and minute ventilation, vital capacity, decreased body fat, physical work capacity, and both systolic and diastolic blood pressure.

The improvement in a heart condition, as a result of appropriate exercise, was seen in the case of Sidney Meadows. Meadows had practiced weightlifting for several years. When he was tested, he was found to be very strong, but there were marked deficits in cardiovascular tests. These deficits included shortness of breath when running, depressed brachial pulse wave after running in place for one minute, and extremely high heart beat and blood pressure. Further examination by a cardiologist revealed that Meadows had had a heart attack about four years earlier. After being tested, Meadows substituted aerobic exercise for weightlifting. On his 65th birthday, three years after the heart condition was detected, he had eliminated all of the orginal cardiovascular weaknesses and was able to run 10 miles in 1 hour and 17 minutes (9).

Arthritis Exercise for the rheumatoid arthritic patient includes quiet exercises that include a full range of motion. Strenuous or athletic activity is not usually recommended. A correct balance of exercise and rest helps to correct and prevent deformities (2, p. 12).

The amount and type of exerise the osteoarthritic patient can perform depends upon the joints that are involved and upon the severity of the case. As in rheumatoid arthritis, the treatment, in part, includes individually tailored exercises (2, p. 16).

In arthritis, exercise can help to improve the condition.

Pritikin et al., while studying the effects of exercise and controlled diet on peripheral vascular disease, found that the participants in the experimental group who had arthritis improved in both the peripheral vascular disease and the arthritis (25).

Obesity Excessive fat on the body is called obesity. According to Getchell (14, p. 240), a body fat value of 10% to 12% in men and from 18% to 20% in women is ideal. Any time a person exceeds 25% (men) or 30% (women) of body fat, he or she is considered obese.

Obese people put a strain on their hearts, joints, and other parts of the body. They also run the risk of developing diseases like arthritis, diabetes, or heart disease.

The obese person has probably been inactive for years. The inactivity, coupled with the extra fat and weight, makes it difficult for the person to engage in a vigorous or strenuous exercise program. In the absence of any serious disease, the obese person can begin mild-stretching, flexibility, and muscular strengthening exercises along with walking or perhaps bicycling. Walking a 17-minute mile on a grassy surface expends 3.8 calories per minute. Bicycling a 6.4-minute mile expends 6.7 calories per minute (14, p. 246). These figures are for a person weighing 154 pounds but not overweight. The obese person would expend an even greater amount of energy engaging in these activities. As the fat decreases, the intensity and duration of the exercise should be increased.

Diabetes Unless the diabetic has a secondary complication from the disease that completely removes the possibility of physical activity, the diabetic should engage in regular exercise.

Recent findings by Dr. David Costill, Director of the Human Performance Laboratory, Ball State University, Muncie, Indiana, indicate that regular vigorous exercise lowers blood glucose. Dr. Costill and his associates observed that diabetics who exercised for 30 or more minutes a day saw a 30% to 40% reduction in insulin needs (14, p. 263). Exercise promotes insulin production, promotes better utilization of glucose by the body, and helps to maintain a lean body mass. According to Briggs and Calloway, diabetes is much less likely to develop in people who are physically active and who maintain a normal body weight (4).

Components of a Physical Fitness Program

Whether a person has high-level wellness or is infirmed, the beginning of any exercise program should be planned carefully. Any physical fitness program contains three components: intensity, duration, and frequency of exercise. There are some differences in these components between young and older adults.

Intensity of Exercise In order to improve cardiorespiratory function, exercise levels must be increased to above the resting heart rate. A person should seek an intensity level somewhere between resting heart rate and maximal heart rate.

The maximal heart rate of young adults is between 180 and 200 beats per minute. Most authorities believe that a workout of 75% of the heart rate maximum is sufficient to produce cardiorespiratory fitness (14, p. 94).

Morehouse and Goss (22) and Clarke (5) proposed that the maximal heart rate in people over the age of 60 be based on a figure which subtracts age from a maximal heart rate of 220 beats per minute. Among sedentary people the maximal heart rate declines with age. The Morehouse–Goss formula for the intensity level of exercise identifies five categories ranging from 50% heart rate maximum to 100% heart rate maximum. At each level of heart rate maximum the training heart rate varies with age. For instance, a workout at 70% heart rate maximum at age 60 would result in training heart rate of 112 beats per minute. As age increases, the training heart rate decreases (6, p. 21).

Duration of Exercise The recommended duration of exercise for all age groups is 30 minutes a day. Beginners should not attempt a 30-minute workout at 75% heart rate maximum but should gradually work up in time (14, p. 98; 22).

Frequency of Exercise Exercising three to four times a week seems to be sufficient for all age groups to produce beneficial results. In young adults this requires a work load of 75% maximum heart rate for 30 minutes a day 3 or 4 days a week. In older adults the duration and frequency are the same as for young people, but the intensity may vary (15, 31). The greater the frequency of training, the greater the improvements. That is, the training effect will be greater if a person exercises five times a week compared to three times a week.

Programs That Enhance Physical Fitness

There were few physical fitness programs for older adults prior to the development of the "Join the Active People Over 60" program. The National Association for Human Development (NAHD), through a grant funded by the Administration on Aging under Titles III and VII of the Older Americans Act, worked in cooperation with the President's Council on Physical Fitness (PCPF) to develop model programs of health information and fitness activities for older Americans. The goals of the program are to educate, inform, motivate, and enlist support and participation of older persons in physical activities for the purpose of health enhancement.

Pilot workshops were implemented in Ohio, Delaware, Maryland, and Texas. The workshops were designed to educate community leaders about the importance of physical activity for older adults and about the causes of cardiovascular and other diseases associated with aging. In addition, regimens of exercises for people over age 60 were demonstrated. Discussions were held on ways to recruit community resources to implement the program. The statewide workshops generated not only regional and local workshops but also nationwide interest in the program.

Three booklets have been published which include series of exercises and activities for basic, moderate, and advanced levels of fitness. Each program includes exercises for the development of flexibility, strength, and endurance (23, 33).

Many programs and activities have been conducted across the country in an attempt to enhance fitness levels in older people. In California the "Life Begins at Sixty Super Marathon" is an annual event. In 1972 seven men ages 60 to 72 ran in relays from Hollywood, California, to Las Vegas, Nevada (290 miles) in 44 hours and 6 minutes (28).

The Cohoes Community Center in Waterford, New York, began a program called "Drownproofing—Hydro-Exercise Program." Participants ranged in age from 62 to 80. Before entering the program, each participant was given a physical examination that included a check on blood pressure and heart and lung function. The results of the examination were given to the participant and the instructor so that both would know the participant's degree of endurance and strength. Local physicians recommended the program for therapeutic reasons to their arthritic patients and to their patients whose muscle tone was poor.

Each session began with exercises and education. Classes in learning to swim were offered and "drownproofing" classes were offered to those who feared the water (17).

In West Virginia a program called "Preventicare" was established for older adults. It consisted of low-level mobility exercises to improve circulation, respiration, and digestion, to strengthen and tone the muscles, and to improve motion in all joints. The major emphasis was on peripheral circulation and only cardiorespiratory exercises that kept the heart rate below 120 beats per minute were used. The program was developed primarily for people over the age of 60. All participants were required to obtain physician approval (13).

"Let Me Light Your Bunsen Burner" is a program developed in College Park, Maryland. The program includes a variety of beginning physical activities. The objectives of the program are:

1. To enhance mobility, flexibility, agility, strength, eye-hand/eye-foot coordination, tactile awareness, depth perception, and endurance.
2. To enhance body image and self-concept.
3. To develop an awareness of latent and suppressed capabilities (27).

In September, 1978, the second annual Senior Olympics was held in Springfield, Illinois. Almost 300 seniors participated in the 10-mile bike ride, archery, bowling, 200-yard free-style swim, 50-yard dash, 3-mile run, and standing broad jump. In December, 1978, members of the Dancers of the Third Age from the Roosevelt Hotel for Senior Citizens in Washington, D.C., performed at a lunch given by the National Council on Aging (24).

Physical activity and fitness are important qualities of health which everyone should possess. Younger people should develop the habit of engaging in regular exercise. Not only will exercise delay premature physiological aging, but it will also delay the onset of many diseases associated with inactivity.

Older adults also need to be involved in regular exercise because it can correct some of the health problems and physiological changes of aging and it helps to eliminate the risk

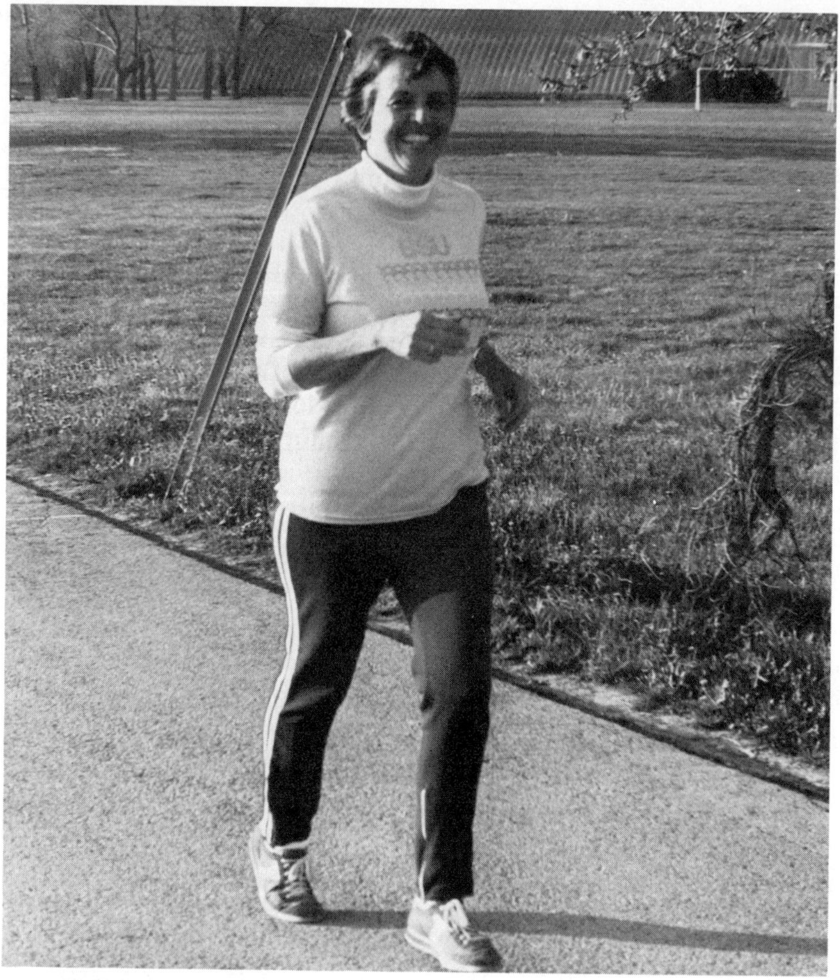

Figure 10.3 Maintaining your physical fitness can be enjoyable, as well as good for your health.

of acquiring health problems associated with inactivity. High levels of wellness enhance independence. The person who feels good mentally and physically and who has mobility will also be independent.

■ Summary

Physical fitness involves strength, flexibility, muscular endurance, and cardiorespiratory endurance. Although the older adult cannot regain the level of performance achieved at a younger age, he or she can participate in a fitness program and show marked improvement in all levels of fitness. Fitness levels in young people have not improved over the past years. Although no comprehensive testing has been done with large numbers of older adults, a small number are increasing their level of fitness. Heart conditions, arthritis, obesity, and diabetes may limit the type and amount of physical activity for some people, but in many cases, exercise will help these conditions. Over the past years many programs across the country have been developed in an attempt to enhance the fitness of older adults.

■ References

1. Adams, Gene M., and DeVries, Herbert A. "Physiological Effects of an Exercise Training Regimen Upon Women, Aged 52 to 79." *Journal of Gerontology* 28 (1973):50.
2. Arthritis Foundation. *Arthritis The Basic Facts.* Atlanta, Ga.: Arthritis Foundation, 1976.
3. Barry, Alan J., Daly, J. W., Pruett, E. D. "The Effects of Physical Conditioning on Older Individuals, I. Work Capacity, Respiratory Function and Work Electrocardiogram." *Journal of Gerontology* 21 (1966):182.
4. Briggs, George W., and Calloway, Doris H. *Bogert's Nutrition and Physical Fitness,* 10th ed., p. 567. Philadelphia: Saunders, 1979.
5. Clarke, David H. *Exercise Physiology.* Englewood Cliffs, N.J.: Prentice-Hall, 1975.
6. Clarke, H. Harrison, ed. "Exercise and Aging." *Physical Fitness Research Digest.* Washington, D. C.: President's Council on Physical Fitness and Sports, 1977.
7. Clarke, H. H. *Physical Fitness Research Digest,* p. 2. Washington, D.C.: President's Council on Physical Fitness and Sports, 1976.
8. Conrad, C. Carson. "When You're Young at Heart." *Aging* (April, 1976):13.
9. Cureton, Thomas K. "A Case Study of Sydney Meadows." *Journal of Association for Physical and Mental Rehabilitation* 19 (1965):36.
10. ——. "A Physical Fitness Case Study of Joie Ray." *Journal*

of Association for Physical and Mental Rehabilitation 17 (1963):14.

11. ———. "Improvement of Psychological States by Means of Exercise Fitness Programs." *Journal of Association for Physical and Mental Rehabilitation* 17 (1963):14.
12. deVries, Herbert A. "Physiological Effects of an Exercise Training Regimen Upon Men Aged 52–88." *Journal of Gerontology* 25 (1970):325.
13. Frankel, Lawrence J., and Richard, Betty B. *Be Alive as Long as You Live Mobility Exercises for the Older Person.* Charleston, W.Va.: Preventicare Publications, 1976.
14. Getchell, Bud. *Physical Fitness a Way of Life,* 2nd ed. New York: John Wiley, 1979.
15. Gettman, Larry A., Melesis, Chris, and Pollock, Michael. "Physiological Responses of Adult Men to Different Durations and Frequencies of Training." *Abstracts: Research Papers 1976 AAHPER Convention.* Washington, D.C.: American Alliance of Health, Physical Education and Recreation, 1976.
16. Granoth, A., Jansson, B., and Strandell, T. "Circulation in Healthy Old Men, Studied by Right Heart Catheterization at Rest and During Exercise in Supine and Sitting Position." In *Physical Activity and Aging,* edited by D. Brunner and E. Jokl, p. 48. Baltimore: University Park Press, 1970.
17. Gullie, Robert A. "New York Elderly Swim Their Way to Fitness." *Aging* (July–Aug., 1976) 10–12.
18. Kasch, Fred W., and Wallace, Janet P. "Physiological Variables During 10 Years of Endurance Training." *Medicine and Science in Sports* 8 (1976):5.
19. Kraus, Hans. *Backache, Stress and Tension: Their Cause, Prevention and Treatment.* New York: Simon & Schuster, 1965.
20. Kraus, Hans, and Wilhelm, Raab. *Hypokinetic Disease.* Springfield, Ill: Charles C Thomas, 1961.
21. Mayer, Jean. *Overweight: Causes, Cost, and Control.* Englewood Cliffs, N.J.: Prentice-Hall, 1968.

22. Morehouse, Lawrence, E., and Gross, Leonard. *Total Fitness.* New York: Simon & Schuster, 1975.

23. National Association for Human Development. *Join the Active People Over 60.* Washington, D.C.: Administration on Aging, 1976.

24. ———. "Older Americans Make Their Mark." *AAHPER News Kit on Programs for the Aging.* Washington, D.C.: American Alliance of Health, Physical Education and Recreation, 1979.

25. Pritikin, Nathan, and Associates. "Diet and Exercise as a Total Therapeutic Regimen for the Rehabilitation of Patients with Severe Peripheral Vascular Disease." In *Physical Fitness Research Digest,* edited by H. Harrison Clarke, p. 4. Washington, D.C.: The President's Council on Physical Fitness and Sports, 1977.

26. Reiff, Guy G., and Hunsicker, Paul A. "Youth Fitness: 1975." *AAHPER Update* (June, 1976):3.

27. Santoro, Linda Campanelli. "Let Me Light Your Bunsen Burner." Presented at the Second Workshop on Aging at the AAHPER Convention, New Orleans, La., March, 1979.

28. ———. "Seven 60+ Men Run 290-Mile Marathon, Los Angeles–Las Vegas." *Aging* (Jan.–Feb., 1976):22.

29. Shephard, Roy J., and Sidney, K. H. "Effects of Physical Exercise on Plasma Growth Hormone and Cortisol Levels in Human Subjects." In *Exercise and Sports Science Review,* Vol. 3, edited by Jack H. Wilmore and Jack F. Keogh, pp. 1–30. New York: Academic Press, 1975.

30. Shock, N. W., and Norris, A. H. "Neuromuscular Coordination as a Factor in Age Changes in Muscular Exercise." In *Physical Activity and Aging,* edited by D. Brunner and E. Jokl, p. 92. Baltimore: University Park Press, 1970.

31. Tooshi, Ali. "Effects of Three Different Durations of Endurance Training on Serum Cholesterol, Body Composition and Other Fitness Measures." Doctoral Dissertation, University of Illinois, 1970.

32. Vittorio, Gary R. "The Rate of Development and the Effects of Double Work Periods on Endurance in Varying Age

Groups." Master's Thesis, Pennsylvania State University, 1961.

33. ———. "Workshops Spark Fitness Programs." *Aging* 258 (1976):14.

34. Young, R., and Ismail, A. H. "Personality Differences of Adult Men Before and After a Physical Fitness Program." *Research Quarterly* 47 (1976):513.

Index

Page numbers in italic indicate illustrative material.